Diabetic Foot Reconstruction

Joon Pio Hong • Hyunsuk Suh
Editors

Diabetic Foot Reconstruction

A Practical Guide

Springer

Editors
Joon Pio Hong
Department of Plastic Surgery
Asan Medical Center, University of Ulsan
Seoul, Korea (Republic of)

Hyunsuk Suh
Department of Plastic Surgery
Asan Medical Center, University of Ulsan
Seoul, Korea (Republic of)

ISBN 978-981-16-9815-6 ISBN 978-981-16-9816-3 (eBook)
https://doi.org/10.1007/978-981-16-9816-3

This Springer imprint is published by the registered company Springer Nature Singapore Pte Ltd.
The registered company address is: 152 Beach Road, #21-01/04 Gateway East, Singapore 189721, Singapore

Foreword

This important book by Joo Pio Hong (JP) and his colleague Hyunsuk Peter Suh focuses on one of, if not the, most difficult areas of reconstructive surgery—the ulcerated diabetic foot. Some at some stage will have witnessed the disaster where surgery on the gangrenous toe of a diabetic has resulted in a series of proximal amputations that end below or above the knee. The culprit—undiagnosed vascular disease. The authors have set out to avoid this scenario by selecting experts for each chapter whose wisdom contributes to provide a combined approach. This encompasses not only important "tips" from the surgeon based on experience, but an overview of the entire pathogenesis of the diabetic ulceration, preliminary investigations, infection control, debridement and, in some cases, procedures to improve limb circulation.

A healthy foot should be sensate, well vascularized, mobile, and free of deformity. Diabetes undermines these ideals. With a high incidence of arteriosclerosis, especially involving the crural arteries near the knee, this often leads insidiously to altered sensation in the cutaneous nerves and deformity. The latter due to atrophy of small foot muscles, over action of long toe extensors and shortening of the tendo Achilles. With abnormal gait, pressure points, skin vascular compromise, and numbness that may have been undetected by the patient, the stage is set for ulceration and infection.

The old adage "to be forewarned is to be fore armed" is a must for the surgeon so that he or she will "do no harm." JP and his co-authors have presented a text that provides us with goals that emphasize the need for a combined approach that focuses on:

(i) A clear understanding of the disease process.
(ii) The need for a compliant and informed patient to minimize recurrence after surgery.
(iii) Meticulous history and examination.
(iv) Investigation, especially CT angiography to locate the site and extent of vascular disease.
(v) Preliminary procedures including debridement and infection control, intra vascular stenting and vascular bypass surgery, and finally
(vi) An experienced surgeon, especially if microsurgery and free flap transfer are contemplated.

JP, one of the new young "stars on the horizon" with his team have, based on considerable experience, provided the reader with much insight into the problem of the ulcerated diabetic foot. They focus on the careful selection of vessels for anastomosis both pre and intra operative for "the flap to match the patch" and the postoperative care. It is notable that one of the favorites is the groin flap that JP has modified from our original "Free Flap" in 1973 to provide a much thinner refined procedure. Nevertheless, notwithstanding the need, it still demands not only super microsurgery but a surgeon with similar skills to tackle very small vessels.

With the incidence of diabetes increasing rapidly, this book is timely. JP Hong and his co-authors provide us with a very important guideline overview, not only of the surgery but of the entire management of the diabetic patient with important insight into the pathogenesis of their ulcerated foot. This text is a must, not only for the one contemplating reconstructive surgery for this challenging problem, but for the management of the patient before and after surgery.

G. Ian Taylor
University of Melbourne, Melbourne, Australia
g.taylor@unimelb.edu.au

Foreword

To say I am amazed that the number of plastic surgery or other subspecialty trainees who upon completion of their requisite training program continue to advance within the realm of reconstructive microsurgery including microvascular tissue transfer is such an abysmal group would be an understatement. Actually, it is quite understandable, now that I reflect back on my own long pathway. Once upon a time I drained a lot of *blood, sweat, and tears* so to speak. Long hours, roadblocks at every turn, constant interruption of the basic essentials of life, like "sleep," and every expert outsider was a disbeliever. Free flaps just didn't work. Add to that often truly these were "free" "free-flaps, [1]" which made the business side of a private practice a constant nightmare.

My biased purview of the world today makes me wonder then if this fork in the road were taken, why of all the choices would a rationale individual decide to concentrate on reconstruction of the lower extremity? The "head & neck" always has great inflow, "breast" reconstruction at least in the good ol' U.S.A. has legally mandatory insurance coverage, while the "upper extremity" gets thanks for restoration of the activities of daily living. The lower extremity is NOT the golden child, so frightening to so many. Maybe so because the dysvascular patient increases the risk of microanastomotic thrombosis [and the inconvenience of not so-infrequent take-backs], with a larger than their share of co-morbidities as witnessed when sometimes the flap lives . . . & the bearer does not; or in general in this anatomical region, wounds just don't heal as well nor quickly enough, requiring a disproportionate amount of hand wrenching during post-operative management.

All that said, there can be nothing but respect for all our colleagues from Asan Medical Center as they have not only taken on the challenge of the lower extremity, but they have mastered it. Lo and behold, they then went a step some may say further downward—how to reconstruct the diabetic foot at risk? Most of us like myself have always shied away from what actually is quite a frequent problem today around the world that cannot be escaped. If we are real doctors, not just mere cosmetologists, we need to note that the 5-year survival rate after diabetic limb salvage is significantly better than that for those undergoing some form of amputation. This indeed is a life-saving endeavor which deserves to be so recognized, maybe even someday by those more interested in the so-called health economics?

How to properly go about ensuring a diabetic foot salvage will predetermine the outcome. The editors are quite humble in stressing in each section of this pragmatically oriented book that a multidisciplinary approach is totally essential. More often than not, it is the medical aspects that are more important for success than just the minute input of us as surgeons. The overall systemic condition of the patient must be understood and maximized, vasculopathy overcome, and infection so common eradicated. Before the soft tissue reconstruction begins, debridement and wound bed preparation must be meticulous following our basic principles of anatomy including the angiosome. An orthoplastic approach always will minimize the risk of failure now and later recurrence. Finally, as in this "Table of Contents," comes the surgeons' role. There we must realize that if the relative simplicity of a local flap is not possible, in spite of our predestined fears of futility for our efforts, a free flap should be selected as the success rate is no different than that expected of the usual lower extremity population.

For those of you whom I have not yet met, I am just one of the few aliens in this small world of ours who has been lucky enough to have had the privilege of visiting not just the remarkable edifices of most of these authors, but also to have witnessed their approach to patient care in their office, in their clinics, and in their operating rooms. This encompassed not just observing the actions of the doctors, but the nurses in the operating room and on the floors, the orderlies, and all the rest of their staff without whom their doors could not remain open. And remember, one does not always have to be a *supermicrosurgeon* to achieve successes such as shown in this timely book. But Dr. Suh and Dr. Hong are just that.

Geoffrey G. Hallock, M.D.
Sacred Heart Campus, St. Luke's Hospital
Allentown, Pennsylvania, USA

Reference

1. Hallock GG. Are "Free Flaps" "Free" Flaps. J Reconstr Microsurg. https://doi.org/10.1055/s-0041-1732429.

Preface

Despite the enormous evolution in reconstruction for traumatized, congenitally deformed, cancer related, and other miscellaneous defects, reconstruction for diabetic foot still remains ignored, overlooked, and even neglected. This is most likely due to the complexity that diabetic foot has, requiring knowledge not only in reconstruction but in various other fields of medicine. The goal of this book is to give you an overview of the essential knowledge that is needed to perform diabetic foot reconstruction. Why is blood sugar control important? why is vascular status important? or how do we make reconstruction reliable? These are some of the questions that we had to learn the hard way through trials and errors. This is the biggest reason we decided to write this book to answer the basic questions in regards to reconstructing diabetic foot. We hope that this book will guide you to make the practical decisions for reconstruction.

In most countries, about 8 to 15% will be diabetic and 10% of these patients will have some problems with their foot. Despite the high incidence of diabetic foot, only a small number of patients will ever undergo reconstruction. As reconstructive surgeons, we have the capability to reconstruct and salvage the limb. Along the journey of diabetic foot reconstruction, it is always a great pleasure to share the same passion with other colleagues. However, there is only a handful of reconstructive surgeons. I was very fortunate to have great partners like Hyunsuk Peter Suh, my coauthor of the book, and Changsik John Pak making this journey exciting and able to share pain along the way. Great many surgeons like Drs Chris Attinger, Paul Kim, Larry Laverey, Raja Sabapathy, Rica Tanaka, Scott Levin, Geoffrey Hallok, and others give us new knowledge and motivations to go on. We do hope that many other colleagues will join us in this journey and this book be a practical guide in their journey.

On behalf of the contributors of this book, we hope this will be the first step in the many other steps toward the evaluation for treating diabetic foot. Thank you.

Seoul, Republic of Korea

Joon Pio Hong
Hyunsuk Peter Suh

Acknowledgements

First of all, I would like to thank my co-author and friend, Dr Hyunsuk Peter Suh. Every step of the way in the making of this book, never was there a dull moment. Working with my partner was a huge treat and sharing the hope that this book will bring more reconstructive surgeons to be confident in providing reconstruction for diabetic foot cases.

Along my journey of plastic surgery, I was privileged to have many wonderful mentors and there are few mentors that have really had a profound impact and shaped me the way I am today. My life as a reconstructive surgeon all started with Professor Yoon Kyu Chung back at Wonju, Korea. He showed and opened my eyes to reconstruction. He taught me that there is always something to learn from a good as well as a bad experience. I still consult with him on various cases today and feel grateful that I have a "reconstruction family home" to go to when I am facing a challenge. Dr David Chang from the University of Chicago has shown me the importance of sharing. Not only sharing knowledge with your peers but to serve in places of need. His guidance has made me realize what my calling is. To be part of peoples' path and help them grow. When I started the professorship at Asan Medical Center, Professor Kyung Suk Koh guided me and taught me what being a true professor means. How to serve the patients and attend to their needs. Most of all how to face a challenge on push on. Dr Geoffrey Hallock has been more than just a teacher but a true friend. To share your passion and knowledge is a gift in life. Jason Yoon, the former Chairman to Daewoong Pharmaceutical and my confidant, has led me to understand the world of business. He taught me how to use constraint and to be consciously aware of decisions you make in your life. Finally my father, Soon-Young Hong, who passed away few years ago. He has always taught me to follow the right path even though it meant taking the long road. I miss him dearly as I walk along this road of life today.

I am grateful that I have a wonderful team led by my friends and partners Dr Hyunsuk Peter Suh and Changsik John Pak. Working with them, plastic surgery colleagues, anesthesiologists, fellows, residents, nurses, and other specialists is an unbelievable experience at Asan Medical Center. It is always a pleasure coming to work and in engaging with this group of professionals in aiming to provide better solutions to help our patients. All the past fellows and residents, to be part of your path is a privilege.

Finally, I want to thank God, family, and friends. Without God's never ending grace, mercy, and provision I would not have had this wonderful life to serve others. Without my family's support and love, I would not be where

I am today. Never ending communications with friends is always a huge pleasure.

Thank you.

—Joon Pio (Jp) Hong, MD, Ph.D., MMM

I clearly remember the day that I was stood quietly gazing upon a surgical field as an intern. When the artery was connected to the latissimus dorsi muscle on the leg, the muscle became alive. It was the first free flap I've ever seen. When the red, brown, and loppy muscle became pinkish, lively, and sprightly, I was so stunned into silence that I could hear my heartbeat. It was a spectacular scene made by Professor Hong, making me a microsurgeon. I am so grateful to Professor Hong from that moment until today for teaching and encouraging me to follow the way he showed us. He always was a good teacher, a great mentor, and a best friend.

I want to thank the authors. They are the pioneers and experts in diabetic patient care. They taught me to do better practice and showed me their steadfast endeavor to salvage the diabetic limb.

Finally, I want to thank my family. I would not have become the person I am today without my family's support. I will forever owe my achievement to my dedicated, caring, and thoughtful wife.

Thank you.

—Hyunsuk Peter Suh M.D., Ph.D.

Contents

1 Understanding Diabetes for Reconstruction

Jiwoo Lee and Woo Je Lee

1.1 Why Understanding Diabetes from the Medical Perspective Matters for Reconstruction

The prevalence of diabetes mellitus (DM) is growing at epidemic proportions worldwide [1]. Globally, approximately 463 million adults (20–79 years) are living with diabetes, and by 2045, this is expected to increase to 700 million [1].

Diabetic foot complications are one of the major complications of diabetes that lead to a significant number of hospitalizations, medical expenses, disabilities, and deaths [2]. Diabetic foot problems can occur as a result of ischemic or neuropathic ulcers, traumatic wounds, skin cracks or fissures, or other infections in the skin of the foot or nail beds (paronychia) [3]. The initiating problem, usually a minor trauma that causes cutaneous ulceration, can often be identified.

Diabetic foot complications are estimated to affect 40–60 million people with diabetes worldwide [1]. In patients with diabetes, the lifetime incidence of diabetic foot ulcers may be as high as 34% [4]. The risk of death at 5 years for a patient with diabetic foot ulcers is 2.5 times higher than that of a patient with diabetes who does not have foot ulcers [5]. More than 50% of cases of diabetic ulcers are infected, and approximately 20% of moderate or severe diabetic foot infections result in amputation [6]. Mortality after amputation related to diabetic foot problems exceeds 70% after 5 years [7].

Several risk factors such as neuropathy, vascular disease, and foot deformities can predict ulcers and amputation. Early recognition and management of risk factors are important for decreasing diabetic foot problems [4].

Neuropathy is a disease that affects the nerves, leading to impaired sensation, movement, and other health aspects depending on the nerve affected. Diabetic neuropathy is the most common complication of diabetes, with a lifetime prevalence rate of 60% [8]. Neuropathy is the most crucial risk factor underlying the development of foot ulcers. Peripheral neuropathy manifests as sensory, motor, and autonomic neuropathy [9]. Sensory neuropathy is a more frequent complaint than motor neuropathy. Sensory neuropathy presents as "glove and stocking" in the feet as hyperesthesia, hypoesthesia, or anesthesia. Motor neuropathy manifests as weakness of the foot or clawing of the toes [10]. Autonomic neuropathy presents as tachycardia when stable, orthostatic hypotension, gastric paralysis, overactive bladder, erectile dysfunction, and hypoglycemic unawareness [11, 12]. Neuropathic disturbances

J. Lee · W. J. Lee (✉)
Department of Internal Medicine, Asan Medical Center, University of Ulsan College of Medicine, Seoul, Republic of Korea

J. P. Hong, H. Suh (eds.), *Diabetic Foot Reconstruction*,
https://doi.org/10.1007/978-981-16-9816-3_1

in sensory, motor, and autonomic functions result in loss of skin integrity [13].

In patients with diabetes, loss of sensation in a joint may lead to a chronic, progressive, and destructive foot deformity. Charcot arthropathy is the typical deformity. It is related to tabes dorsalis and is characterized by the slow degeneration of the neural tracts, primarily in the dorsal root ganglia of the spinal cord. The pathogenesis of this condition remains unclear, but it is likely to be multifactorial, such as a combination of mechanical and vascular factors and diabetic neuropathy [14].

Peripheral arterial disease (PAD) is an atherosclerotic occlusive disease of the lower extremity. Diabetes is a significant risk factor for PAD [15]. PAD can appear in up to 50% of patients with diabetic foot ulcers and is a risk factor for poor recovery and amputation [16]. In addition, the presence of PAD is notably related to reduced survival in the patients with diabetic foot ulcers, which are responsible for 70% mortality due to diabetes [17]. Patients with diabetes have a higher incidence of atherosclerotic occlusion of the large and medium-sized arteries, e.g., aortoiliac or femoropopliteal arteries, which causes ischemia. With digital artery disease, improper arterial blood supply and, thus, peripheral ischemia worsen foot ulcers and cause poor wound healing [6, 15]. Less arterial perfusion also causes infection, chronic impaired wound healing, and amputation [15].

The strategy for managing diabetic foot is prevention. For this, the most fundamental strategy is to control diabetes itself by optimizing glycemic control [8]. For type 1 and type 2 diabetes, glycemic control can reduce complications, as demonstrated in landmark trials (The Diabetes Control and Complications Trial (DCCT) [18] and UK Prospective Diabetes Study (UKPDS) [19]). The DCCT demonstrated that intensive glucose control was associated with improved long-term outcomes [20]. Follow-up for more than 10 years after active treatment in the DCCT showed there were less microvascular complications in the group that received intensive treatment [21]. The UKPDS demonstrated that intensive glycemic control significantly reduced microvascular complications in patients with type 2 diabetes [19]. Long-term follow-up of the UKPDS groups showed lasting effects of early glycemic control on microvascular complications [22].

The major factor that leads to the development of a diabetic ulcer is neuropathy. Glycemic control could contribute to reducing the incidence of neuropathy, but it can not completely prevent it, as shown in the UKPDS [19, 22]. Patients with decreased sensation in the feet due to neuropathy can benefit from several strategies to develop an overall plan for preventive management. Early recognition of new lesions in a patient with a diabetic foot ulcer is critically important for reducing the risk of complications. Diabetic foot ulcers are often accompanied with infection and PAD, resulting in complex wound problems [6, 16]. Thus, moderate or severe ulcers lead to amputation [6], which reduces the quality of life and increases mortality [7]. Reconstruction has been developed and used for the treatment of diabetic foot ulcers and reduction of the number of amputations [23]. Despite the comprehensive strategy for prevention, ulceration of the foot may occur. In this situation, surgical reconstruction of the skin may be necessary for treatment. Skin reconstruction, such as skin grafts or local flaps, can be used for discrete areas that do not heal easily [24]. The greatest advantage of reconstruction is to provide the opportunity for bipedal ambulation by salvaging the limb. However, assessment of vascularity should be made before reconstruction to evaluate the likelihood of healing [25]. If the vascularity to the foot is poor, then reconstruction may fail.

1.2 Medical Diabetes

1.2.1 Definition

Diabetes mellitus is a chronic metabolic disorder of glucose homeostasis leading to hyperglycemia. It is caused by an absolute deficiency of insulin (type 1 DM) or by a relative deficiency of insulin combined with a decrease in insulin sensitivity, known as insulin resistance (type 2 DM). Insulin, a peptide hormone, is produced by the pancreatic β-islet cells and plays a crucial role in regulating blood glucose levels. Insulin allows cells to absorb glucose for use as fuel or storage and suppresses glucose formation by the liver. It also stimulates protein synthesis and inhibits the breakdown of fat.

Type 1 DM is autoimmune process that destroys pancreatic β-islet cells and is triggered by unknown precipitating events such as a viral illness in a susceptible host. It usually leads to absolute insulin deficiency. It is not a lifestyle-related disease and tends to occur in children and younger adults.

Type 2 DM is caused by progressive loss of appropriate β-cell insulin secretion and insulin resistance. It tends to occur in patients with a strong family history and those with environmental factors such as sedentary lifestyles or obesity. Therefore, type 2 DM generally occurs in older and overweight adults, and nowadays, it is also common in obese children and adolescents. Worldwide, 463 million people, or 9.3% of adults, have diabetes, and this number in growing exponentially. By 2045, 700 million people or 10.9% of adults are expected to have diabetes [1]. Half of those with diabetes (50.1%) do not know that they have diabetes [1].

Many asymptomatic people have "prediabetes," either impaired fasting glycemia (IFG) or impaired glucose tolerance (IGT). Prediabetes means that glucose levels do not meet the criteria for diabetes but are higher than normal [18]. IFG is defined as fasting plasma glucose (FPG) levels between 100 and 125 mg/dL, and IGT is defined as a 2-h plasma glucose during 75 g oral glucose tolerance test (OGTT) levels between 140 and 199 mg/dL [26]. Prediabetes is a risk factor for diabetes, cardiovascular disease, obesity, dyslipidemia, and hypertension [26]. The global incidence of IGT is estimated to be 7.5% (374 million) in 2019 and is expected to increase to 8.6% (548 million) by 2045 [1].

1.2.2 Diagnosis

Hyperglycemia is measured through laboratory findings of elevated plasma glucose levels, either fasting, random, or OGTT (Table 1.1). Diagnosis is made based on the results of two abnormal tests from the same sample or in two separate test samples. In the presence of typical symptoms, only one elevated plasma glucose result is required.

Clinical symptoms of hyperglycemia are polyuria, nocturia, dehydration, weight loss, tiredness, and blurred vision. In Type 1 DM, these symptoms may be acute at onset, and the patient may become ill with diabetic ketoacidosis. However, type 2 DM shows a more insidious onset, and symptoms usually go unnoticed for many years.

1.3 Complications of Diabetes Mellitus

Diabetes mellitus is a major cause of morbidity and mortality and is sixth-leading cause of death in the USA. It is also a major underlying cause of coronary heart disease and cerebrovascular disease. In many studies, the mortality rate of indi-

Table 1.1 Diagnosis of diabetes mellitus

FPG ≥ 126 mg/dL[a]
OR
2-h PG ≥ 200 mg/dL during OGTT[b]
OR
A1C ≥ 6.5%
OR
Random plasma glucose ≥200 mg/dL (in a patient with classic symptoms of hyperglycemia or a hyperglycemic crisis)

FPG fasting plasma glucose, *OGTT* oral glucose tolerance test, *2-h PG* 2-h plasma glucose

[a]Fasting is defined as no caloric intake for at least 8 h

[b]The test should be performed using a glucose load containing the equivalent of 75 g anhydrous glucose dissolved in water

viduals with DM is two times higher than that of individuals without diabetes.

1.3.1 Acute Complications of Diabetes Mellitus

DM leads to infection, caused by either bacteria and fungi, and may result in hyperglycemic crises such as diabetic ketoacidosis and hyperglycemic hyperosmolar syndrome. Treatment of diabetes with oral agents or injections may cause complications such as hypoglycemia (Table 1.2).

1.3.2 Chronic Complications of Diabetes Mellitus

Diabetes affects both small vessels (microvascular complications) and large vessels (macrovascular complications). Microvascular complications include diabetic retinopathy, diabetic nephropathy, and diabetic neuropathy (Table 1.3). Macrovascular complications include coronary heart disease, cerebrovascular disease, and PAD (Table 1.4).

Among the many complications of diabetes, neuropathy and PAD are most likely to affect the incidence of diabetic foot and reconstruction outcomes. Diabetic neuropathies are a heterogeneous group of disorders with diverse clinical manifestations. Diabetic neuropathy is the most common complication in diabetes, with a lifetime prevalence rate of 60% [8]. Up to 50% of cases of diabetic peripheral neuropathy may be symptomatic. The most common manifestations of neuropathy are diabetic peripheral neuropathies such as distal symmetric sensorimotor polyneuropathy and autonomic neuropathy [27]. Distal symmetric sensorimotor polyneuropathy is the most common type of diabetic neuropathy and is often considered synonymous with the term diabetic neuropathy. It is characterized by a progressive loss of distal sensation correlating with the loss of sensory axons, followed by motor weakness and motor axonal loss. Classic "stocking-glove" sensory loss is typical in this disorder [8]. Diabetic autonomic neuropathy is a common complication of diabetes. It is diagnosed by exclusion and may be unnoticed because of multiorgan involvement and its insidious onset. However, it can lead to severe dysfunction of a single organ, such as postural hypotension, gastroparesis, and genitourinary disturbance [28].

Table 1.2 Acute complications of diabetes mellitus

Diabetic ketoacidosis	Hyperglycemic crisis with a high anion gap due to acidic substances called ketones
Hyperglycemic hyperosmolar syndrome	Hyperglycemic crisis with increased serum osmolarity
Hypoglycemia	Overdose of diabetes medication relative to food intake

Table 1.3 Microvascular vascular complications of diabetes mellitus

Disease	Clinical and laboratory features
Diabetic retinopathy	
Non-proliferative	Microaneurysms, exudates, macular edema
Proliferative	Vulnerable new vessels, vitreous hemorrhage, retinal detachment
Diabetic nephropathy	Microalbuminuria: Urine Alb/Cr ≥ 30 and <300 mg/g or 24 h urine albumin ≥30 and <300 mg/day
	Macroalbuminuria: Urine protein/Cr ≥ 0.3 mg/g or 24 h urine protein ≥ 0.3 g/day
	End-stage chronic kidney disease
Diabetic neuropathy	Motor: Abnormal posture or feet deformities, e.g., clawed toes
	Sensory: Reduction in vibration, monofilament, touch sensation, and proprioception
	Autonomic: Postural hypotension, gastroparesis, diarrhea, neurogenic bladder, impotence, dry feet

Table 1.4 Macrovascular vascular complications of diabetes mellitus

Disease	Clinical and laboratory features
Coronary heart disease	Angina pectoris, myocardial infarction (MI), heart failure
Cerebrovascular disease	Stroke, hemorrhage
Peripheral arterial disease	Intermittent claudication, rest pain, ulcer, gangrene

PAD, defined as atherosclerosis in the arteries of the lower extremities, is also a strong risk factor for diabetic foot problems [29]. Moreover, PAD causes significant long-term disability in patients with diabetes [30]. PAD affects approximately one-third of those with comorbid DM [30]. The prevalence of PAD may be underestimated in patients with diabetes owing to the asymptomatic nature of less severe PAD and the often concomitant diabetic neuropathy [30]. The clinical manifestations of PAD, which include claudication, rest pain, ulceration, and gangrene, are predominantly caused by progressive luminal stenosis or occlusion.

1.4 Treatment of Diabetes Mellitus

Both Type 1 and Type 2 DM require lifestyle modifications, i.e., regular exercise for a duration of 150 min/week [31], and regular, calorie-regulated meals with less simple sugars, and more complex carbohydrates, fiber, and low glycemic index foods [32]. Diabetes patients should stop smoking cigarettes and consume a moderate amount of alcohol to reduce cardiovascular risks.

1.4.1 Type 1 Diabetes Mellitus

Type 1 DM patients require insulin to live. An intensive insulin regimen, multiple daily injections (MDI), or an insulin pump are preferred for better glycemic control and fewer microvascular complications [18]. Traditionally, short-acting soluble insulin, such as Humulin R, is administered with intermediate-acting NPH insulin, such as Humulin N. Nowadays, insulin analogs are available, which are more convenient to use with fewer hypoglycemic episodes. For example, rapid-acting insulin analogs such as Insulin Lispro, Glulisine, Aspart, or faster Aspart can be injected immediately before and after eating each meal. Longer acting insulin analogs such as Glargine, Detemir, or Degludec can help provide peakless basal insulin, leading to fewer hypoglycemic episodes (Table 1.5).

Table 1.5 Type of insulin

Insulin	Compound
Rapid-acting	Lispro
	Glulisine
	Aspart
	Inhaled insulin
Short-acting	Human regular
Intermediate-acting	Human NPH
Concentrated human regular insulin	U-500 human regular insulin
Long-acting	Glargine
	Detemir
	Degludec
Premixed insulin products	NPH/regular 70/30
	NPH/Lispro 50/50
	NPH/Lispro 75/25
	NPH/Aspart 70/30

1.4.2 Type 2 Diabetes Mellitus

Various oral hypoglycemic agents are available with different mechanisms of action and effects (Table 1.6). Metformin has been initially recommended for diabetes patients for many years. Sulfonylureas have also been regularly used for many years. Thiazolidinediones (or glitazones) have been shown to improve insulin sensitivity. More recently, incretin mimetics, dipeptidyl peptidase-4 inhibitors (DPP-4 inhibitors), and glucagon-like peptide-1 receptor agonists (GLP-1 RAs), which act by increasing the active level of the hormone glucagon-like peptide-1 (GLP-1) secreted by the small intestine, are available in the form of tablets and injections, respectively. SGLT2 inhibitors inhibit renal glucose reabsorption. However, after acquiring type 2 diabetes for 10 years, many patients need insulin therapy. Initially, once-daily long-acting insulin added to oral agents may control the diabetes, but eventually, patients may need more frequent insulin injections.

Table 1.6 Type of oral hypoglycemic agents

Class	Name
Biguanide	Metformin
Sulfonylureas (2nd generation)	Glyburide, Glibornuride, Gliclazide, Glipizide, Gliquidone, Glisoxepide, Glyclopyramide, Glimepiride
Meglitinides (glinides)	Repaglinide, Nateglinide, Mitiglinide
Glucosidase inhibitors	Acarbose, Miglitol, Voglibose
Thiazolidinediones	Pioglitazone, Rosiglitazone, Lobeglitazone
DPP-4 inhibitors	Sitagliptin, Saxagliptin, Linagliptin, Alogliptin, Vildagliptin, Gemigliptin, Teneligliptin, Anagliptin, Evogliptin, Trelagliptin, Omarigliptin, Gosogliptin
GLP-1 receptor agonists	Exenatide, Extended-release exenatide, Liraglutide, Albiglutide, Dulaglutide, Lixisenatide, Semaglutide
SGLT2 inhibitors	Canagliflozin, Dapagliflozin, Empagliflozin, Ertugliflozin, Ipragliflozin, Luseogliflozin, Remogliflozin etabonate, Tofogliflozin

1.5 Management of Diabetes Complications

1.5.1 Glycemic Control

The UKPDS [19] and Kumamoto Study [33] demonstrated that intensive glycemic control significantly reduced rates of microvascular complications in patients with short-duration type 2 diabetes. Long-term follow-up of the UKPDS showed enduring effects of early glycemic control on most microvascular complications [22]. Thus, achieving A1C targets of 7% has been observed to decrease microvascular complications of type 1 and type 2 diabetes when instituted early in the course of disease [34]. Therefore, treatment for diabetes aims at tight control of glucose levels, and therefore, frequent monitoring of these parameters is essential (Table 1.7).

Among hospitalized patients, careful management of diabetes has benefits. A HbA1c test on all hospitalized patients with diabetes or hyperglycemia (blood glucose >140 mg/day) is recommended. Insulin therapy should be initiated for persistent hyperglycemia (≥180 mg/dL). Once insulin therapy is initiated, a target glucose range of 140–180 mg/dL is recommended for the majority of critically and noncritically ill patients [35, 36]. When caring for hospitalized patients with diabetes, consult with a specialized diabetes or glucose management team.

Table 1.7 Glycemic recommendations for adults with diabetes

A1C	7.0%
Preprandial capillary plasma glucose	80–130 mg/dL[a]
Peak postprandial capillary plasma glucose	180 mg/dL[a]

[a]More or less stringent glycemic goals may be appropriate for individual patients. Goals should be individualized based on the duration of diabetes, age/life expectancy, comorbidities, known CVD or advanced microvascular complications, hypoglycemia unawareness, and individual patient considerations

1.5.2 Management of Peripheral Neuropathy and PAD

Symptomatic diabetic neuropathy is generally not reversible, and management aims to slow further progression and prevent complications such as diabetic foot ulcers. Optimal glycemic control has an important role in slowing the progression of neuropathy [28]. In patients with neuropathy, foot care is essential to help reduce the risk of complications. In addition, symptomatic therapies for neuropathic pain are important for management. Pain medications are not useful for nonpainful symptoms of neuropathy, such as numbness. Pharmacotherapy options for painful diabetic neuropathy include several antidepressants (e.g., duloxetine, venlafaxine, amitriptyline, and other tricyclic drugs) and gabapentinoid antiepileptic drugs (pregabalin, gabapentin) [37]. Among these, pregabalin, duloxetine, and gabapentin are recommended as initial pharmacologic treatments for neuropathic pain in diabetes [8].

The management of patients with diabetes and PAD is focused on relieving symptoms and lowering the risk of cardiovascular disease progression and complications. Smoking cessation, lipid-lowering therapy, antihypertensive therapy, glycemic control, diet, and exercise are recommended to reduce the risk of future cardiovascular events, including limb-related events [38, 39]. Long-term antithrombotic therapy using aspirin (75–100 mg/day) or clopidogrel (75 mg/day) is recommended for all diabetes patients with PAD to reduce the risk of overall cardiovascular events and death [40, 41]. Unless there is a clear indication, dual antiplatelet therapy is not routinely recommended for patients with DM and PAD [42]. Patients with DM and chronic limb-threatening ischemia may require revascularization procedures.

1.6 Significance of Multidisciplinary Care

Care for patients with diabetic foot problems is complicated from asymptomatic to critically ischemic limb, which needs amputation. This complexity of diabetic foot is due to a series of comorbidities, including diabetes, vascular disease, and neuropathy that exceed the boundaries of usual medical or surgical care. Of these comorbidities, the treatment must begin with strict glycemic control and nutritional support while managing the wound and infection [43]. With managing these systemic factors, peripheral vascular diseases have to be reviewed, and play a crucial role to improve circulation for further reconstruction.

Patients with diabetic foot problems have poor glycemic control and thus need the comprehensive treatment from an endocrinologist. An infectious disease specialist is also required because patients with diabetic foot problems often have severe infections. Moreover, because many patients have peripheral vascular disease with poor blood supply, an experienced cardiologist and a vascular surgeon are also needed to improve the limb salvage rate. Orthopedic and plastic surgeons perform debridement of the wound or remove the infected soft tissue and bone. Plastic and reconstructive surgery helps the restoration of the form and function of the foot. Specialized wound podiatrists and nurses also play crucial roles in managing diabetic foot problems. To effectively manage these complicated aspects in patients with diabetic foot problems, multidisciplinary team approach would be helpful.

A multidisciplinary diabetic foot team has been working at Asan Medical Center (AMC) since 2015. This team is mainly composed of endocrinologists, plastic surgeons, orthopedic surgeons, cardiologists (specialized for peripheral artery intervention), and specialized nurses. In AMC, if patients with diabetic foot problem need hospitalization, whatever specialist evaluated the patients, they were admitted to endocrinology department. Patients with diabetic foot problem often have various medical problems such as poor glycemic control, chronic kidney disease, or cardiovascular disease. Therefore, after the patients were hospitalized to endocrinology department, conservative treatments including glycemic control, antibiotics use, and fluid & electrolyte imbalance correction were performed. Depending on the patient's condition, plastic surgeon, orthopedic surgeon, and cardiologist conducted debridement, amputation, and angioplasty, respectively. The multidisciplinary diabetic foot team in AMC had a conference once a week to discuss and decide the patients' treatment directions.

Moreover, when patients with diabetic foot problem who need emergent surgical treatment came to emergency room, plastic or orthopedic surgeons perform emergency debridement within 24 h, which contribute to stabilization of the patients' condition. After hospitalization, the patient is continuously treated with team approach as described above.

This kind of multidisciplinary team approach is important to limit the spread of acute infection and lead to limb salvage. This team approach provides efficiency because time is not wasted for waiting specific department's consultations. The team approach provides the link between the departments to work closely together when making challenging medical and surgical decisions.

The comorbidities of diabetic foot result in poor ulcer healing and eventually increase the risk of major amputation [44]. A multidisciplinary team approach for individuals with foot ulcers and high-risk feet is important to optimally deal with these comorbidities to reduce major amputations [8]. Several systemic reviews evaluated the impact of multidisciplinary team care on diabetic foot disease outcomes [32, 45, 46]. In these studies, multidisciplinary teams were related to significant decreases in major (above-ankle) amputations for patients with diabetic foot problems. Multidisciplinary team care is an effective strategy for the highest risk patients, especially those with severe ulcers requiring hospitalization and underlying peripheral vascular disease. This is consistent with expert opinion guidelines suggesting a comprehensive approach to care [47].

Therefore, it is important to form a multidisciplinary team comprising an endocrinologist, an infectious disease specialist, a cardiologist, an orthopedic surgeon, a plastic surgeon, a vascular surgeon, a podiatrist, specialized nurses, and other allied health professionals to handle various problems in patients with diabetes. Multidisciplinary teams, composed of physicians who are able to control glycemic levels, manage peripheral vascular disease, properly care for infections, and provide localized wound management, were related to a decreased risk of major amputation for patients with severe diabetic foot disease.

References

1. Saeedi P, Petersohn I, Salpea P, Malanda B, Karuranga S, Unwin N, et al. Global and regional diabetes prevalence estimates for 2019 and projections for 2030 and 2045: results from the International Diabetes Federation Diabetes Atlas, 9(th) edition. Diabetes Res Clin Pract. 2019;157:107843.
2. Frykberg RG, Zgonis T, Armstrong DG, Driver VR, Giurini JM, Kravitz SR, et al. Diabetic foot disorders. A clinical practice guideline (2006 revision). J Foot Ankle Surg. 2006;45(5 Suppl):S1–66.
3. Jeffcoate WJ, Harding KG. Diabetic foot ulcers. Lancet. 2003;361(9368):1545–51.
4. Armstrong DG, Boulton AJM, Bus SA. Diabetic foot ulcers and their recurrence. N Engl J Med. 2017;376(24):2367–75.
5. Walsh JW, Hoffstad OJ, Sullivan MO, Margolis DJ. Association of diabetic foot ulcer and death in a population-based cohort from the United Kingdom. Diabet Med. 2016;33(11):1493–8.
6. Lipsky BA, Berendt AR, Cornia PB, Pile JC, Peters EJ, Armstrong DG, et al. 2012 Infectious Diseases Society of America clinical practice guideline for the diagnosis and treatment of diabetic foot infections. Clin Infect Dis. 2012;54(12):e132–73.
7. Lavery LA, Hunt NA, Ndip A, Lavery DC, Van Houtum W, Boulton AJ. Impact of chronic kidney disease on survival after amputation in individuals with diabetes. Diabetes Care. 2010;33(11):2365–9.
8. American Diabetes Association. 11. Microvascular complications and foot care: standards of medical care in diabetes-2020. Diabetes Care. 2020;43(Suppl 1):S135–s51.
9. Boulton AJ, Gries FA, Jervell JA. Guidelines for the diagnosis and outpatient management of diabetic peripheral neuropathy. Diabet Med. 1998;15(6):508–14.
10. Boulton AJ, Vinik AI, Arezzo JC, Bril V, Feldman EL, Freeman R, et al. Diabetic neuropathies: a statement by the American Diabetes Association. Diabetes Care. 2005;28(4):956–62.
11. Vinik AI, Ziegler D. Diabetic cardiovascular autonomic neuropathy. Circulation. 2007;115(3):387–97.
12. Vinik AI, Maser RE, Mitchell BD, Freeman R. Diabetic autonomic neuropathy. Diabetes Care. 2003;26(5):1553–79.
13. Tentolouris N, Voulgari C, Liatis S, Kokkinos A, Eleftheriadou I, Makrilakis K, et al. Moisture status of the skin of the feet assessed by the visual test neuropad correlates with foot ulceration in diabetes. Diabetes Care. 2010;33(5):1112–4.
14. Jeffcoate WJ, Game F, Cavanagh PR. The role of proinflammatory cytokines in the cause of neuropathic osteoarthropathy (acute Charcot foot) in diabetes. Lancet. 2005;366(9502):2058–61.
15. American Diabetes Association. Peripheral arterial disease in people with diabetes. Diabetes Care. 2003;26(12):3333–41.
16. Moulik PK, Mtonga R, Gill GV. Amputation and mortality in new-onset diabetic foot ulcers stratified by etiology. Diabetes Care. 2003;26(2):491–4.
17. Boyko EJ, Ahroni JH, Smith DG, Davignon D. Increased mortality associated with diabetic foot ulcer. Diabet Med. 1996;13(11):967–72.
18. Nathan DM, Genuth S, Lachin J, Cleary P, Crofford O, Davis M, et al. The effect of intensive treatment of diabetes on the development and progression of long-term complications in insulin-dependent diabetes mellitus. N Engl J Med. 1993;329(14):977–86.
19. Intensive blood-glucose control with sulphonylureas or insulin compared with conventional treatment and risk of complications in patients with type 2 diabetes (UKPDS 33). UK Prospective Diabetes Study (UKPDS). Group Lancet. 1998;352(9131):837–53.
20. Cleary PA, Orchard TJ, Genuth S, Wong ND, Detrano R, Backlund JY, et al. The effect of intensive glycemic treatment on coronary artery calcification in type 1 diabetic participants of the Diabetes Control and Complications Trial/Epidemiology of Diabetes Interventions and Complications (DCCT/EDIC) Study. Diabetes. 2006;55(12):3556–65.

21. Nathan DM, Cleary PA, Backlund JY, Genuth SM, Lachin JM, Orchard TJ, et al. Intensive diabetes treatment and cardiovascular disease in patients with type 1 diabetes. N Engl J Med. 2005;353(25):2643–53.
22. Holman RR, Paul SK, Bethel MA, Matthews DR, Neil HA. 10-year follow-up of intensive glucose control in type 2 diabetes. N Engl J Med. 2008;359(15):1577–89.
23. Edmonds M, Bates M, Doxford M, Gough A, Foster A. New treatments in ulcer healing and wound infection. Diabetes Metab Res Rev. 2000;16(Suppl 1):S51–4.
24. Santema TB, Poyck PP, Ubbink DT. Skin grafting and tissue replacement for treating foot ulcers in people with diabetes. Cochrane Database Syst Rev. 2016;2(2):Cd011255.
25. Joret MO, Osman K, Dean A, Cao C, van der Werf B, Bhamidipaty V. Multidisciplinary clinics reduce treatment costs and improve patient outcomes in diabetic foot disease. J Vasc Surg. 2019;70(3):806–14.
26. American Diabetes Association. 2. Classification and diagnosis of diabetes standards of medical care in diabetes-2020. Diabetes Care. 2020;43(Suppl 1):S14–s31.
27. Booth J, Young MJ. Differences in the performance of commercially available 10-g monofilaments. Diabetes Care. 2000;23(7):984–8.
28. Pop-Busui R, Boulton AJ, Feldman EL, Bril V, Freeman R, Malik RA, et al. Diabetic neuropathy: a position statement by the American Diabetes Association. Diabetes Care. 2017;40(1):136–54.
29. Hingorani A, LaMuraglia GM, Henke P, Meissner MH, Loretz L, Zinszer KM, et al. The management of diabetic foot: a clinical practice guideline by the Society for Vascular Surgery in collaboration with the American Podiatric Medical Association and the Society for Vascular Medicine. J Vasc Surg. 2016;63(2 Suppl):3s–21s.
30. Marso SP, Hiatt WR. Peripheral arterial disease in patients with diabetes. J Am Coll Cardiol. 2006;47(5):921–9.
31. Umpierre D, Ribeiro PA, Kramer CK, Leitão CB, Zucatti AT, Azevedo MJ, et al. Physical activity advice only or structured exercise training and association with HbA1c levels in type 2 diabetes: a systematic review and meta-analysis. JAMA. 2011;305(17):1790–9.
32. Musuuza J, Sutherland BL, Kurter S, Balasubramanian P, Bartels CM, Brennan MB. A systematic review of multidisciplinary teams to reduce major amputations for patients with diabetic foot ulcers. J Vasc Surg. 2020;71(4):1433–46.e3.
33. Ohkubo Y, Kishikawa H, Araki E, Miyata T, Isami S, Motoyoshi S, et al. Intensive insulin therapy prevents the progression of diabetic microvascular complications in Japanese patients with non-insulin-dependent diabetes mellitus: a randomized prospective 6-year study. Diabetes Res Clin Pract. 1995;28(2):103–17.
34. Lind M, Pivodic A, Svensson AM, Ólafsdóttir AF, Wedel H, Ludvigsson J. HbA(1c) level as a risk factor for retinopathy and nephropathy in children and adults with type 1 diabetes: Swedish population based cohort study. BMJ. 2019;366:l4894.
35. American Diabetes Association. 15. Diabetes care in the hospital: standards of medical care in diabetes-2020. Diabetes Care. 2020;43(Suppl 1):S193–s202.
36. van den Berghe G, Wouters P, Weekers F, Verwaest C, Bruyninckx F, Schetz M, et al. Intensive insulin therapy in critically ill patients. N Engl J Med. 2001;345(19):1359–67.
37. Griebeler ML, Morey-Vargas OL, Brito JP, Tsapas A, Wang Z, Carranza Leon BG, et al. Pharmacologic interventions for painful diabetic neuropathy: an umbrella systematic review and comparative effectiveness network meta-analysis. Ann Intern Med. 2014;161(9):639–49.
38. Gerhard-Herman MD, Gornik HL, Barrett C, Barshes NR, Corriere MA, Drachman DE, et al. 2016 AHA/ACC guideline on the management of patients with lower extremity peripheral artery disease: a report of the American College of Cardiology/American Heart Association Task Force on Clinical Practice Guidelines. J Am Coll Cardiol. 2017;69(11):e71–e126.
39. Newman JD, Schwartzbard AZ, Weintraub HS, Goldberg IJ, Berger JS. Primary prevention of cardiovascular disease in diabetes mellitus. J Am Coll Cardiol. 2017;70(7):883–93.
40. CAPRIE Steering Committee. A randomised, blinded, trial of clopidogrel versus aspirin in patients at risk of ischaemic events (CAPRIE). Lancet. 1996;348(9038):1329–39.
41. Bhatt DL, Marso SP, Hirsch AT, Ringleb PA, Hacke W, Topol EJ. Amplified benefit of clopidogrel versus aspirin in patients with diabetes mellitus. Am J Cardiol. 2002;90(6):625–8.
42. Berger JS, Krantz MJ, Kittelson JM, Hiatt WR. Aspirin for the prevention of cardiovascular events in patients with peripheral artery disease: a meta-analysis of randomized trials. JAMA. 2009;301(18):1909–19.
43. Suh HS, Oh TS, Hong JP. Innovations in diabetic foot reconstruction using supermicrosurgery. Diabetes Metab Res Rev. 2016;32(Suppl 1):275–80.
44. Brennan MB, Hess TM, Bartle B, Cooper JM, Kang J, Huang ES, et al. Diabetic foot ulcer severity predicts mortality among veterans with type 2 diabetes. J Diabetes Complicat. 2017;31(3):556–61.
45. Khan N, Sapsed S. Diabetes foot complication: assessing primary and secondary outcomes of multidisciplinary team versus standard care (a systematic review). Int J Diabetes Dev Countries. 2017;37(2):129–36.
46. Buggy A, Moore Z. The impact of the multidisciplinary team in the management of individuals with diabetic foot ulcers: a systematic review. J Wound Care. 2017;26(6):324–39.
47. Wennberg L, Widgren S, Axelsson R, Gerok-Andersson K, Åkerlund B. Multidisciplinary diabetic foot care in Sweden—a national survey. Diabetes Res Clin Pract. 2019;149:126–31.

Vasculopathy in Diabetic Foot

2

Chang Hoon Lee and Seung-Whan Lee

Key Points

- Vasculopathy is one of pathophysiologic triads including neuropathy and infection in diabetic foot.
- Diabetic foot is a clinical presentation of peripheral arterial disease (PAD) among macrovasculopathy complications.
- Management of PAD is important to reconstruction, wound healing, and preventing recurrence of diabetic foot.
- Endovascular procedure is an emerging therapeutic option for patients with diabetic foot with obstructive PAD.

2.1 Introduction

Diabetic vasculopathies are microvascular and macrovascular complications which are caused by endothelial dysfunction, systemic inflammation, thrombogenic condition, and vascular tone alteration [1]. Among macrovascular diabetic vasculopathies, peripheral artery disease (PAD) is the third leading cause of atherosclerotic cardiovascular (CV) morbidity, following coronary artery disease (CAD) and stroke [2]. Diabetic foot is the most common and financially heavy clinical presentations of PAD, and includes lower extremity infection, ulcer formation, and/or deep tissue damage, caused by a combination of neuropathy and varying degrees of vascular disease [3, 4]. Notably, diabetic foot ulcer (DFU) is the most frequently recognized complication. The lifetime incidence of DFU has been estimated to be 15–25% among patients with diabetes mellitus (DM) [5]. Furthermore, the natural history of a DFU is grave. DFUs are associated with the increased risk of death by 2.5 times [6]. More than half of DFUs become infected [7], of which approximately 20% leads to some level of amputation [8]. The recurrence rate of DFU has been estimated roughly 40% within 1 year after ulcer healing, almost 60% within 3 years, and 65% within 5 years [5]. Because of the high risk of mortality, infection, amputation, and a heavy economic burden to society, the prevention and management of DFU is one of the most important topics in the current approach to diabetic foot [9, 10].

Recent guidelines from the International Working Group on the Diabetic Foot (IWGDF) are established with the participation of a multi-

C. H. Lee
Department of Cardiology, Veterans Health Service Medical Center, Seoul, South Korea
e-mail: chlee@bohun.or.kr

S.-W. Lee (✉)
Department of Cardiology, Asan Medical Center, University of Ulsan College of Medicine, Seoul, South Korea
e-mail: seungwlee@amc.seoul.kr

J. P. Hong, H. Suh (eds.), *Diabetic Foot Reconstruction*,
https://doi.org/10.1007/978-981-16-9816-3_2

disciplinary working group of independent experts [10–12]. Among the specialist areas such as endocrinology, vascular surgery, orthopedics, and cardiology, plastic surgery for soft tissue reconstruction plays as a goalkeeper in the management of unhealed ulcer to avoid amputation [13]. Due to the variety in treatment modalities, treatment intensity, and patient adherence, it is likely that there are differences in the effectiveness of standard care as well. Therefore, although multidisciplinary approach (pressure offloading, debridement tissue, infection control, wound dressing, control of blood glucose, and revascularization of PAD) is the current standard therapy, skin grafts and substitutes are the last resort of nonhealing DFU [4, 12]. In particular, previous studies of skin graft and substitutes have been conducted on the premise of nonischemic and noninfected DFU [13–17]. As a prerequisite for a successful reconstructive surgery, the infection should be resolved, and abundant blood flow must be provided to the surgical site and the donor. In addition, blood flow should be maintained for as long as necessary for the skin graft and replacement to survive after reconstructive surgery (Fig. 2.1). Therefore, the treatment of PDA plays an important role in reconstruction of DFU, in addition to its own effect of wound healing and reducing DM foot amputation [18, 19]. In this chapter, we review the diagnosis and management of PAD associated with diabetic foot based on recently reported articles.

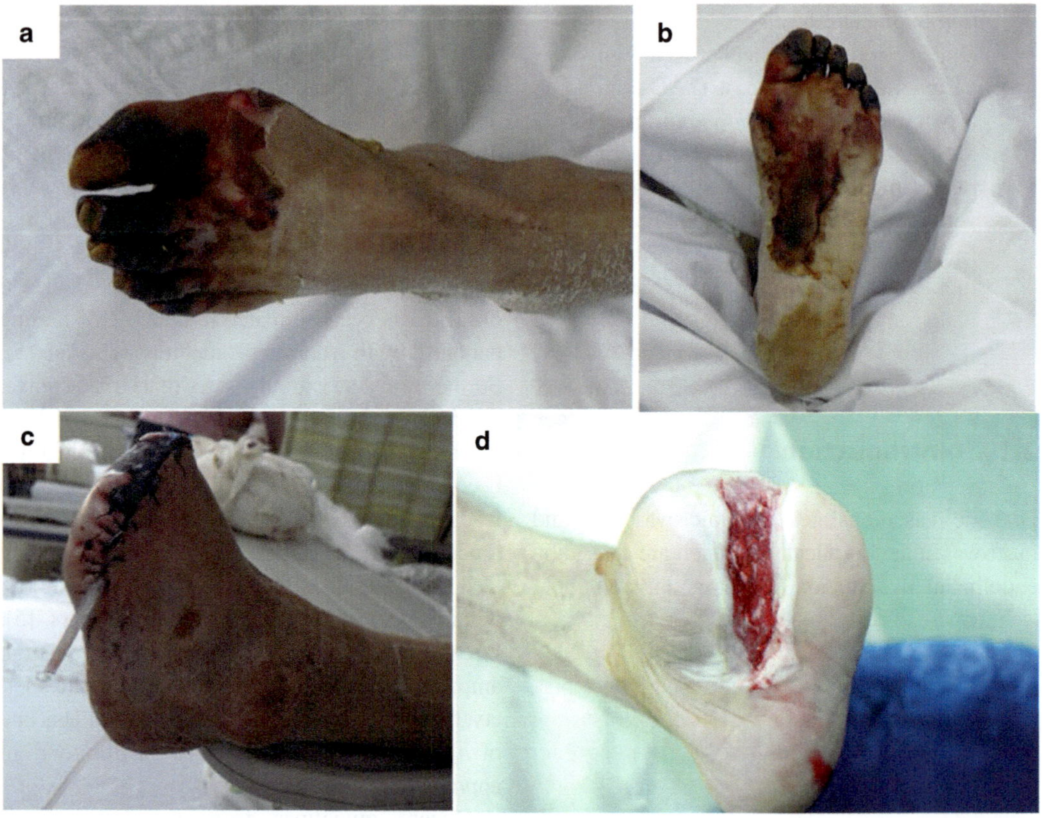

Fig. 2.1 Unhealed wound after amputation of all toes. The figures of (**a**) and (**b**) depict the clinical appearance of an ischemic wound on the forefoot, especially at the toes and plantar aspect of metatarsal-phalangeal joints. The figure of (**c**) depicts an ischemic wound following amputation of all digits at the metatarsal-phalangeal joint level. As a result of failing revascularization, a wound base remains without evidence of healing such as granulation tissue or epithelial ingrowth (**d**)

2.2 Pathophysiology of Peripheral Artery Disease in Diabetic Foot

The pathophysiology of PAD in DM is similar to that in nondiabetic patients, but is amplified by hyperglycemia, dyslipidemia, and insulin resistance which are characteristics of DM. These metabolic abnormalities enhance vascular inflammation, endothelial dysfunction, vasoconstriction, and platelet activation in the pathophysiology of PAD in DM [20].

2.2.1 Hyperglycemia

Endothelial cell dysfunction is the main features of diabetic vasculopathy favoring a pro-inflammatory/thrombotic state which ultimately leads to atherothrombosis [21]. Macro- and microvascular diabetic complications are mainly due to persistent exposure to hyperglycemia including with other risk factors such as arterial hypertension and dyslipidemia [20]. The initial step of endothelial dysfunction due to hyperglycemia is the imbalance between nitric oxide (NO) bioavailability and reactive oxygen species (ROS) [21]. In healthy blood vessels, endothelial cells synthesize nitric oxide (NO), which is a potent vasodilator that inhibits platelet activation and vascular smooth muscle cell migration [22]. While the protein kinase C (PKC) of endothelial cells is activated due to hyperglycemia, ROS is overproduced, and NO availability is rapidly reduced [23]. With a lack of NO, the activation of PKC promotes the production of endothelin-1 (ET-1) which is involved in vasoconstriction and platelet aggregation [24]. Accumulation of superoxide anion also triggers upregulation of pro-inflammatory genes monocyte chemoattractant protein-1 (MCP-1), vascular cell adhesion molecule-1 (VCAM-1), and intracellular cell adhesion molecule-1 (ICAM-1) via activation of nuclear factor kappa-light-chain-enhancer of activated B cell (NF-kB) signaling [21, 25]. These events lead to vascular inflammation as well as proliferation of smooth muscle cell, accelerating the atherosclerotic process. Endothelial dysfunction in DM also derives from increased synthesis of thromboxane A2 (TXA2) via upregulation of cyclooxygenase (COX-2) following activation of PKC [26]. Furthermore, ROS increases the synthesis of glucose metabolite methylglyoxal leading to activation of advanced glycation end product/receptor for AGE (AGE/RAGE) signaling and the pro-oxidant hexosamine and polyol pathway flux [27].

2.2.2 Insulin Resistance and Dyslipidemia

The persistent exposure of hyperglycemia results in insulin resistance in patients with DM. In particular, in terms of adipose tissue as an active source of inflammatory mediators and free fatty acids (FFA), obesity plays an important role in this phenomenon [28]. Free fatty acids bind Toll-like receptor (TLR) and activate NF-kB triggering tissue inflammation due to upregulation of inflammatory genes IL-6 and TNF-α [21]. In addition, TLR activation by FFA induces phosphorylation of insulin receptor substrate-1 (IRS-1) by c-Jun amino-terminal kinase (JNK) and PKC, altering the ability to activate downstream target phosphatidylinositol 3-kinase (PI3K) and Akt [21]. These molecular phenomena lead to downregulation of the glucose transporter type 4 (GLUT-4) and thereby insulin resistance [29]. Consequently, downregulation of PI3K/Akt induced by insulin resistance leads to eNOS inhibition and decreased NO production in endothelial cell [30]. In addition, intracellular oxidation of stored FFAs produces ROS, which leads to vascular inflammation, AGE synthesis, reduced PGI2 synthetase activity, and PKC activation [30].

Dyslipidemia such as high triglycerides, low HDL cholesterol, increased remnant lipoproteins, elevated apolipoproteins B, as well as small and dense LDL could highly affect the atherogenic effects of insulin resistance [31]. Atherogenic dyslipidemia is a reliable predictor of CV risk, and its pharmacological modulation reduces vascular events in subjects with type 2 diabetes and metabolic syndrome [32].

In platelets, lack of insulin impairs the IRS-1/PI3K pathway resulting in Ca^{2+} accumulation and increased platelet aggregation [21]. In addition, insulin resistance enhances atherothrombosis through increased cellular synthesis of PAI-1 and fibrinogen and reduced production of tissue plasminogen activator [21]. Therefore, platelets from DM patients show faster response and increased aggregation compared with those from healthy subjects [33].

2.2.3 Thrombosis and Coagulation

Due to deregulation of coagulation factors and platelet activation, diabetic patients have an increased risk of coronary events and CV mortality when compared to nondiabetic patients [34, 35]. The pathogenesis of this prothrombotic condition is associated with insulin resistance and hyperglycemia [21]. Insulin resistance increases plasminogen activator inhibitor-1 (PAI-1) and fibrinogen and decreases tissue plasminogen activator (t-PA) levels [36]. Hyperinsulinemia-induced increase of tissue factor (TF) levels activates thrombin-converting fibrinogen to fibrin [37]. Fibrin organization is further enhanced due to high PAI-1 and reduced t-PA levels. These events are reinforced by hyperglycemia [37]. In addition, low-grade inflammation induces TF expression in the vascular endothelium of diabetics, which contributes to atherothrombosis [37].

2.3 Diagnosis of Peripheral Artery Disease

2.3.1 Physiologic and Non-invasive Testing

As per the IWGDF guidelines, all patients with diabetes (even those without foot ulcers) have their peripheral arteries examined at least annually through a medical history and pedal pulse palpation [38]. When patients with symptoms and high risk or history of PAD are present, assessment review should be increased to at least once every 1–3 months, or even more often. During review of history and physical examination for PAD, physicians should pay attention to absence of hair growth, onychodystrohpy, thinning skin, and temperature gradient [4]. For patients with an appropriate history and physical examination, the diagnosis of PAD is established with the measurement of the ankle-brachial index (ABI) [39]. In addition to ABI, non-invasive tests such as the toe-brachial index (TBI) and transcutaneous oxygen pressure ($TcPO_2$) can improve the diagnostic accuracy of lower limb ischemia [4].

ABI is currently the first choice for evaluating PAD, which is characterized by its simplicity, affordability, reproducibility, and high specificity [40]. In patients with a history or physical examination suggestive of PAD, the ABI has good validity with sensitivities ranging from 68 to 84% and specificities from 84 to 99% [40]. Patients with ABI ≤ 0.9 are diagnosed with PAD (normal reference value of the ABI is 0.9–1.4) [39]. Values >1.4 indicate incompressible arteries secondary to vascular calcification, which is more common among individuals with DM and advanced chronic kidney disease (CKD). Values with ABI 0.5–0.9 indicate vascular stenosis; those with ABI 0.3–0.5 indicate severe stenosis; and those with ABI < 0.3 indicate the possibility of gangrene. Although those with ABI 0.91–0.99 are acceptable, they may possibly have PAD and increased CV risks including stroke and CAD [41].

TBI is recently preferred for evaluating PAD because the digital arteries are less likely to be calcified. Although the reference values remain controversial, values with TBI > 0.7 are generally considered normal; those <0.7 suggest arterial occlusion and may indicate symptoms of intermittent claudication; those <0.2 may be associated with resting pain; and a toe pressure <55 mmHg suggests poor wound healing [42]. In a case-control study to compare TBI with ABI in DM with PAD, TBI was not superior to the ABI to determine lower limb perfusion except in cases where the ABI is >1.3, in which the TBI performs significantly better [43].

$TcPO_2$ is a measurement of skin perfusion that is also unaffected by calcification of the medial arteries. In a study to evaluate the values of $TcPO_2$ measurement in diabetic patients compared with nondiabetic patients, $TcPO_2$ value was significantly lower in diabetic patients than nondiabetic patients (50.02 ± 8.92 vs. 56.04 ± 8.8 mmHg, $p < 0.001$). And $TcPO_2$ was significantly associated with diabetic patients (correlation coefficient = 0.258, $p = 0.004$) [44]. The sensitivity and specificity of $TcPO_2$ are better than those of ABI (sensitivity 0.86; 95% confidence interval [CI], 0.68–0.95 vs. 0.52; 95% CI, 0.42–0.63 and specificity 0.72; 95% CI, 0.61–0.81 vs. 0.48; 95% CI, 0.36–0.61) [45]. The efficacy of PTA to significantly improve TcPO2 after procedure was highly predictive of limb salvage even though in cases of recanalization failure by angiographic outcome criteria [46].

Currently, there are no clear cutoff values indicating normal lower limb vessels. Generally, the possibility of PAD is lower when the ABI is 0.9–1.3, the TBI is >0.7, and a triphasic waveform is seen on Doppler ultrasound. Indicators such as skin perfusion pressure ≥ 40 mmHg, TBI ≥ 30 mmHg, or TcPO2 ≥ 25 mmHg suggest an increase in healing rate of at least 25% in DFU with PAD [4].

2.3.2 Advanced Imaging Test

Because of no single test that has proven to be optimal, if physiologic testing suggests an abnormality, the patient may require advanced imaging test such as ultrasound, computed tomography angiography (CTA), magnetic resonance angiography (MRA), or digital subtraction angiography (DSA) of the lower extremities for revascularization strategy.

Ultrasound is an imaging method that is used to evaluate the location and extent of vascular disease, arterial hemodynamics, and lesion morphology [47]. Each mode such as Type B, continuous-wave, pulsed-wave Doppler, and two-dimensional ultrasound provides specific information. In particular, duplex ultrasound scanning (DUS; B mode + Doppler flow detection) is very useful in identifying proximal arterial disease. A prospective, blinded, comparative study for DUS and DSA showed that DUS had 88% sensitivity, 79% specificity, and 95% accuracy [48]. In general, the ratio of the peak systolic velocity (PSV) within stenotic lesion is compared with the PSV in the vessel just proximal to it to estimate the degree of stenosis. For the lower extremity arteries, a PSV ratio of <2.0 indicates <50% arterial stenosis, and a ratio of ≥2.0 indicates ≥50% arterial stenosis [49].

CTA can provide the number, length, lumen diameter, and morphology of arterial lesions in the lower limbs, the severity of calcification, and the status of the distal runoff vessels, allowing accurate preoperative planning in terms of surgical path, balloon selection, and long-term patency expected after intervention [49]. In addition, chronic total occlusion can be clearly displayed through evaluating adequately collateral vessels. Therefore, CTA is often obtained first in the absence of contraindications to intravenous contrast. Previous meta-analysis has reported that CTA appeared slightly inferior to contrast-enhanced MRA with sensitivities of 89–99% and specificities of 83–97% [50], but recent study using dual-energy CTA has shown improvement of the sensitivity and specificity of PAD diagnosis in DM, reaching 100% and 93.1% after multi-level reconstruction and 99% and 91.8% after maximum intensity projection, respectively [51]. Furthermore, in a comparison study for the preoperative evaluation of PAD, there were no differences between CTA and DSA about the endovascular and surgery ratio (1.8 vs. 1.4, $p = 0.305$), reintervention rates (21 vs. 16%, $p = 0.517$), and major amputation (9 vs. 11%, $p = 1.0$) [52].

The meta-analysis found that contrast-enhanced MRA has excellent accuracy, with sensitivities ranging from 92 to 99.5% and specificities from 64 to 99% for the evaluation of lower extremity arterial stenosis >50% [50]. However, the accuracy of MRA for DM with infrapopliteal arterial stenosis is unclear. A systemic review that included only three studies (83 patients) found that the sensitivity of MRA on infrapopliteal arteries was 86% (95% CI, 0.86–0.91) and the specificity was 93% (95% CI, 0.90–0.95) [53]. This analysis based on low patient numbers suggests that MRA for infrapopliteal arteries in DM risks adoption of incorrect revascularization strategies. Hence, contrast-enhanced MRA may be more suitable for screening than diagnosis for detection of infrapopliteal arterial stenosis in diabetic patients. Recently, to avoid the side effect of contrast and obtain high-quality images, many nonenhanced MRA methods such as quiescent-interval single-shot MRA are increasingly used to evaluate the severity of PAD and have shown good results [54].

Because of obtaining the highest spatial resolution and image quality after injection of a contrast agent through femoral artery puncture, DSA is considered the gold standard for arterial vascular imaging [49]. In a comparative study with CTA, DSA had an advantage over CTA in determining the severity of lower limb ischemia and vascular density, especially in distal segment lesion with Trans-Atlantic Inter-Society Consensus (TASC) grade C or D classification (DSA vs. CTA, 25 vs. 0%, $p = 0.001$), as well as scarcity of runoff vessels (DSA vs. CTA, 72 vs. 26%, $p = 0.001$) [52]. In addition, DSA has the benefit of image magnification and allows endovascular treatment to be performed simultaneously. However, DSA has potential side effects related to arterial puncture, higher doses of radiation, contrast-induced nephropathy, and allergic reaction.

2.4 Management of Peripheral Artery Disease in Diabetic Foot

Recent practical recommendations for the management of patients with DM and PAD focus primarily on the modification of risk factors for CV disease including hypertension (<140/90 mmHg), hyperglycemia (Hemoglobin A1c < 7%), dyslipidemia, and antithrombotic therapy (e.g., aspirin 100 mg) [4, 12, 40, 55, 56]. Together with these general medical therapy, local wound care, management of infection, and mechanical offloading should be combined in patients with DFU. Optimal medical therapy and wound care could achieve a greater than 40–50% surface area reduction or reduction of depth by 4 weeks [57]. Thus, vascular imaging and revascularization in patients with DFU should be considered when the ulcer does not improve within 6 weeks despite appropriate management or unhealed ulcer with either an ankle pressure < 50 mmHg or ABI < 0.5 [12]. In addition, urgent vascular imaging and revascularization should be performed in patients with DFU where the toe pressure is <30 mmHg or the TcPO2 < 25 mmHg [12].

The aim of revascularization in patients with DFUs and PAD is to restore direct blood flow to at least one of the foot arteries [58], preferably an artery within the ulcer and to achieve a minimum skin perfusion pressure ≥ 40 mmHg, a toe pressure ≥ 30 mmHg, or a TcPO2 ≥ 25 mmHg [12]. Bypass grafting and endovascular treatment can be used for revascularization, but there is inadequate evidence to establish which revascularization technique is superior [59]. Therefore, therapeutic option should be made in a multidisciplinary team on a number of individual factors, such as lesion characteristics of PAD, availability of autogenous vein, patient's comorbidities, and physician's skill [60]. Herein, we discuss mainly interventional techniques for revascularization of PAD.

2.4.1 Endovascular Revascularization

Endovascular revascularization of the lower extremity arteries begins by obtaining vascular access, most commonly through a contralateral common femoral artery retrograde approach or an ipsilateral common femoral artery antegrade approach [61, 62]. However, various access sites such as brachial, popliteal, and pedal arteries may be used according to lesion complexity. After placement of the sheath, a baseline arteriogram is performed to identify the extent and severity of the target lesions, status of the runoff vessels, and collateral vessels as well as to define the baseline status of distal circulation prior to intervention [61]. As classifying the anatomic complexity of occlusive disease, the original TASC classification helped to decide therapeutic option between endovascular and surgical revascularization. However, with the advancement of the endovascular technique, the length of femoropopliteal lesions for which endovascular intervention is recommended has increased over the years and TASC II has been recently used for interpreting the complexity of the lesions rather than helping in choice of therapeutic option [60, 63, 64].

2.4.2 Plain Balloon Angioplasty (Fig. 2.2)

Plain balloon angioplasty (PBA) was established as the standard of care for endovascular procedures. While PBA is temporarily able to restore blood flow, there are limitations such as abrupt vessel closure, dissection, and restenosis. Therefore, PBA has been recently used for simple lesions in femoropopliteal arteries. However, PBA continues to be the method all other technologies are compared against in recent trials. Unlike femoropopliteal lesions, PBA in infrapopliteal lesions has been the mainstay of endovascular treatment. The In.PACT DEEP trial that randomized 358 patients with infrapopliteal lesions to DCB or PBA did not show significant different clinically driven TLR (DCB vs. PBA 9.2 vs. 13.1%, $p = 0.291$) and late lumen loss (LLL) (DCB vs. PBA 0.61 ± 0.78 vs. 0.62 ± 0.78, $p = 0.950$) between two treatment arms [65]. In two randomized multicenter studies comparing bare metal stents (BMS) with PBA in patients with infrapopliteal stenosis, BMS has also not shown to improve patency over PBA [66, 67]. Based on these data, PBA is the most common intervention in the infrapopliteal arteries, and typically long balloons (up to 21 cm in length) with prolonged inflation times (at least 3 min) are used to minimize the recoil or dissections and the need for stents at this location.

2.4.3 Drug-Coated Balloon

Drug-coated balloons (DCBs) designed to decrease intimal hyperplasia are effective in reducing restenosis rate in femoropopliteal lesions. Recent many studies have investigated different DCBs against PTA with encouraging results including primary patency and clinically driven TLR [61]. Therefore, DCBs can be used as alternative to PBA for the medium to long length lesions in femoropopliteal arteries. In the IN. PACT SFA trial, paclitaxel-coated balloon angioplasty improved primary patency compared to PBA (69.5 vs. 45.1%, $p < 0.001$) and freedom from clinically driven TLR at 3 years (84.5 vs. 68.9%, $p = 0.002$) [68]. Furthermore, in the LEVANT II trial comparing DCB with PBA, DCB showed a significant difference in patients-centric metrics such as quality of life (QOL) and walking impairment questionnaire (WIQ) [69]. While DCBs have advantages to avoid the complications associated with stents such as fracture, in-stent restenosis (ISR), and stent thrombosis, heavy calcified lesions can limit the efficacy of DCBs by impeding the release of drugs [70]. To overcome calcified lesions before treating with DCB, debulking the plaque by directional atherectomy (DA) could improve procedural success rate (DA + DCB vs. DCB, 89.6 vs. 64.2%, $p = 0.004$) and decrease flow-limiting dissection (DA + DCB vs. DCB, 2 vs. 19%, $p = 0.01$) [71].

2.4.4 Stent (Fig. 2.3)

Stents have been designed to maintain lumen patency by preventing recoil and tacking down intimal flaps. The type of stent according to deploying method and shape is balloon expandable or self-expanding and bare or covered. Nitinol bare metal, self-expanding stents are the most frequently used stents in the femoropopliteal lesions because of good radial force and easy distensibility [61]. For lesions >10 cm in length (TASC II B/C), primary stent placement can be considered. The FAST trial, a randomized comparative study of BMS vs. PBA, evaluated the lesion <10 cm but did not show a benefit in stenting short SFA lesions over PBS (TLR of BMS vs. PBA 14.9 vs. 18.3%, $p = 0.595$) [72]. However, the ABSOLUTE trial, comparing BMS to PBA in lesions >10 cm, reported significantly lower restenosis rate (37 vs. 63%, $p < 0.001$) [73]. Notably, for patients with long-segment

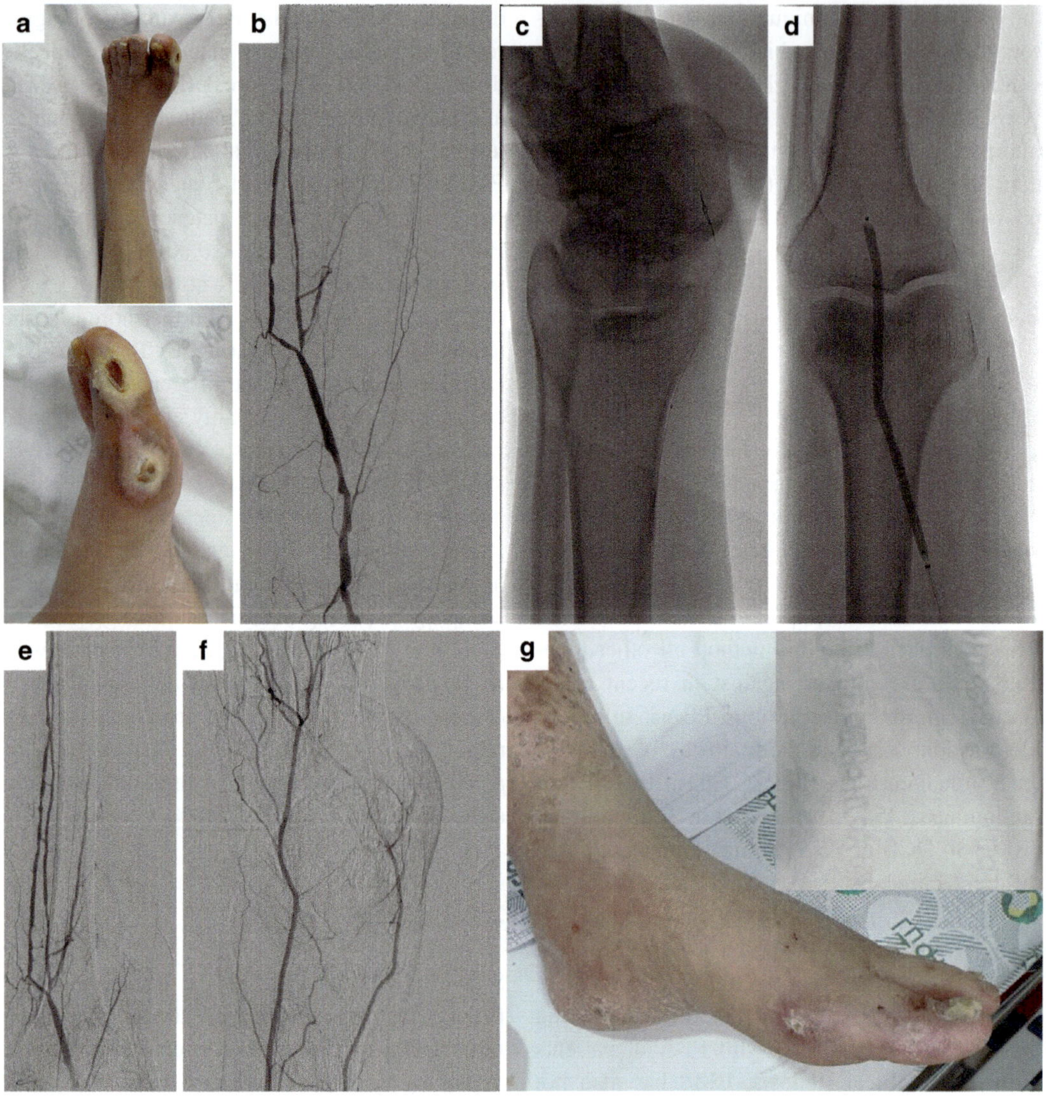

Fig. 2.2 A 72-year-old man presented with severe claudication and was not responding to medical management. He presented with bullae and ulcer in medial aspect of left foot (**a**). The digital subtraction angiography (DSA) demonstrates moderate stenosis of popliteal artery and severe tibial vessel disease with diffuse long stenosis of anterior tibial artery and chronic total occlusion of posterior tibial artery (**b**). Each of the lesions of tibial vessel was crossed using 014 wire, and subsequently each was treated with plain balloon angioplasty (**c**). The stenotic lesion of popliteal artery was treated with drug-eluting balloon angioplasty (**d**). Final DSA demonstrated inline revascularization of each vessel to the foot (**e** and **f**). At 3 months after treatment, his left foot ulcer has been healed and became a remission state (**g**)

occlusions (>15 cm, TASC II C/D), nitinol stents have been frequently used. In the STELLA registry which included patients with a mean lesion length of 26 cm, primary patency at 30 months was 62% [74]. Polytetrafluoroethylene (PTFE) covered stent seems to be an option for long segment lesions in femoropopliteal arteries. In VIASTAR trial comparing heparin-bonded covered stent to BMS, covered stent showed improved 12-month patency rate in long femoropopliteal lesions (covered stent vs. BMS 71.3 vs. 36.8%, $p = 0.01$) [75]. However, when covered

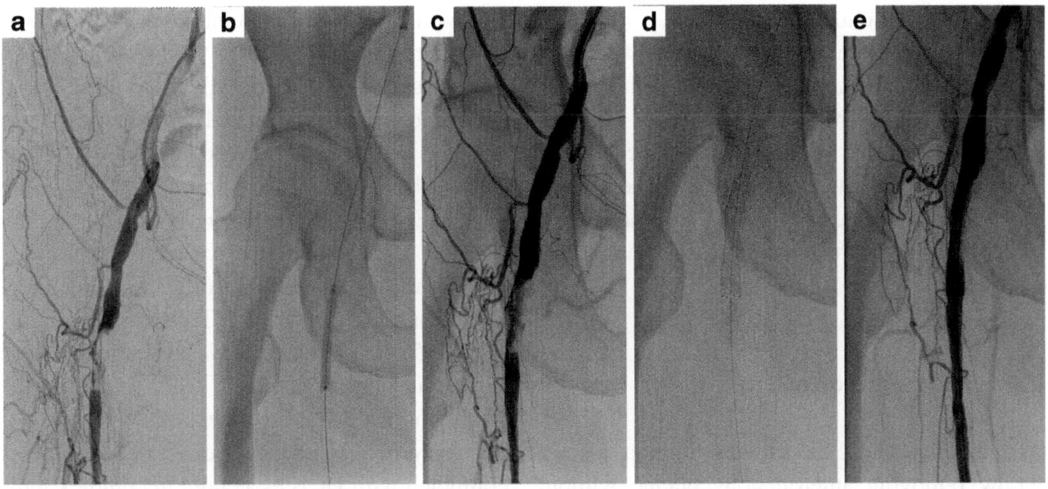

Fig. 2.3 A 69-year-old man complained of severe claudication in the right leg. His right ankle-brachial index (ABI) was 0.57, indicating vascular stenosis. The digital subtraction angiography (DSA) showed severe stenosis of proximal superficial femoral artery (SFA) with calcification and collaterals (**a**). After balloon angioplasty and directional atherectomy with TurboHawk™ system, the lesion of SFA still remained moderate stenosis (**b** and **c**). By using a stent (**d**), the complex stenosis of proximal SFA was revascularized (**e**)

stents fail, stent thrombosis and acute limb ischemia are often the presenting features and frequently lead to limb threatening possibly due to loss of collaterals [61].

2.4.5 Drug-Eluting Stent

Drug-eluting stents (DES) have been used in the femoropopliteal lesions and also selectively used at the infrapopliteal lesions when PBA has failed. In the Zilver PTX randomized trial to evaluate DES for femoropopliteal lesions, long-term results comparing DES (primary and provisional) with standard care (defined as PTA with provisional BMS) have been reported [76]. Overall DES group, compared to standard care, showed significant difference in clinical benefit (freedom from persistent or worsening symptoms of ischemia; 79.8 vs. 59.3%, $p < 0.01$), patency (66.4 vs. 43.4%, $p < 0.01$), and freedom from reintervention (target lesion revascularization, 83.1 vs. 67.6%, $p < 0.01$) at 5 years [76]. In the REAL PTX trial for comparing DES with DCB in femoropopliteal lesions, rates of primary patency were 79 and 80% for DES and DCB at 12 months ($p = 0.96$) and decreased to 54 and 38% through 36 months ($p = 0.17$) [77]. Therefore, after the predilatation, DES is considered when dissection or residual stenosis occurs, and in patients with heavy calcified lesions or high risk of embolization. Generally, DCB is preferred in patients without dissection or residual stenosis after the predilatation.

In the ACHILLES trial of DES application in infrapopliteal lesions, 200 patients were randomized to DES or PBA. Treatment with DES was associated with higher 1-year patency (75.0 vs. 57.1%, $p = 0.025$) as well as lower angiographic restenosis rates (22.4 vs. 41.9%, $p = 0.019$) compared to PBA [78]. To compare DES with BMS, DESTINY trial randomized 140 patients with infrapopliteal lesion to DES or BMS [79]. Primary patency at 12 months was significantly higher with the use of DES than BMS (85 vs. 54%, $p = 0.0001$). The use of the DES significantly reduced the need for repeat intervention (DES vs. BMS, 9 vs. 34%, $p = 0.001$) [79]. DES have also been compared to DCB for treatment in long infrapopliteal lesions [80]. In the IDEAS trial, DES are related to significantly lower residual immediate post-procedure stenosis (9.6 ± 2.2% vs. 24.8 ± 3.5%, $p < 0.0001$) and have shown significantly reduced vessel restenosis at 6 months (28 vs. 57.9%, $p = 0.0457$) [80]. Based on these data, DES can be used safely in infrapopliteal lesions and are associated with superior patency rates compared to PBA or BMS. However, the treated lesions in recent trials were mostly short lesions (<3 cm), whereas the most commonly treated lesions in practice are more complex with longer stenosis and occlusions [62].

2.4.6 Atherectomy (Fig. 2.4)

Atherectomy device can increase luminal diameter by removing atheromatous plaque without leaving foreign body such as a stent in the vessel. A variety of debulking atherectomy devices have been introduced: directional, rotational, orbital, and laser atherectomy. In a study for comparing DA with PBA in infrainguinal vessels, there was no difference in TLR (16.7 vs. 11.1%) between two groups [81]. The COMPLIANCE 360 trial evaluated orbital vs. PTA and did not report a significant difference in freedom from TLR at 12 months (81.2 vs. 78.3%, $p = 0.99$) [82]. In the EXCITE-ISR trial comparing laser atherectomy (LA) to PTA in patients with femoropopliteal ISR, there was a significant difference in TLR at 6 months (LA + PTA vs. PTA, 73.5 vs. 51.8%, $p < 0.005$) [83]. Atherectomy can be used in short to medium-length calcified lesions with device protection for distal embolization. With promising early results, recent use of atherectomy is combined with DCB especially in complex femoropopliteal lesions [71]. However, the risk of complications such as dissection, perforation, and distal embolization remains concerns along with the long-term durability.

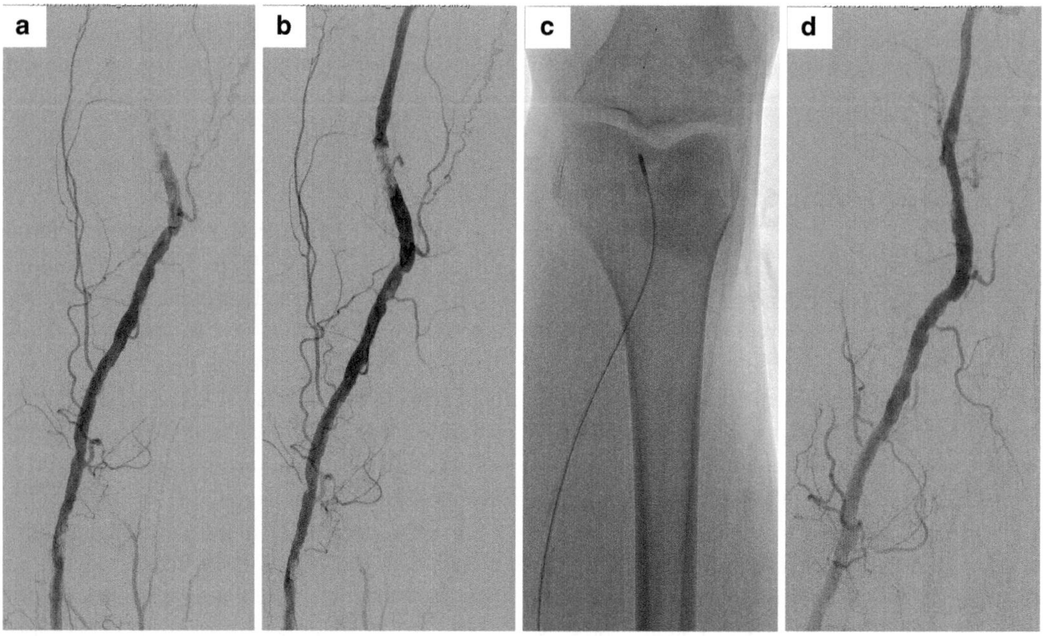

Fig. 2.4 A 79-year-old man complained of severe claudication in the right leg. His right ankle-brachial index (ABI) was 0.35, indicating severe stenosis. The digital subtraction angiography (DSA) showed moderate stenosis of distal superficial femoral artery (SFA) and chronic total occlusion (CTO) with huge calcification and abundant collaterals at popliteal artery (Zone P2) (**a**). In the figure (**b**), selective angiography reveals filling defects in the popliteal artery following balloon angioplasty due to the huge calcification. Since stent implantation was not recommended in the zone P2 of popliteal artery, remaining calcified lesion was treated with atherectomy using Jetstream™ and drug-eluting balloon (**c**). After directional atherectomy with antirestenotic therapy (DAART), completion arteriography demonstrated effective restoration of flow in the distal SFA and popliteal artery (**d**)

Disclosure Statement The authors have nothing to disclose.

References

1. Mota RI, Morgan SE, Bahnson EM. Diabetic vasculopathy: macro and microvascular injury. Curr Pathobiol Rep. 2020;8(1):1–14.
2. Fowkes FG, et al. Comparison of global estimates of prevalence and risk factors for peripheral artery disease in 2000 and 2010: a systematic review and analysis. Lancet. 2013;382(9901):1329–40.
3. Parker CN, et al. Differences between national and international guidelines for the management of diabetic foot disease. Diabetes Metab Res Rev. 2019;35(2):e3101.
4. Wang A, et al. Guidelines on multidisciplinary approaches for the prevention and management of diabetic foot disease (2020 edition). Burns Trauma. 2020;8:tkaa017.
5. Armstrong DG, Boulton AJM, Bus SA. Diabetic foot ulcers and their recurrence. N Engl J Med. 2017;376(24):2367–75.
6. Walsh JW, et al. Association of diabetic foot ulcer and death in a population-based cohort from the United Kingdom. Diabet Med. 2016;33(11):1493–8.
7. Prompers L, et al. High prevalence of ischaemia, infection and serious comorbidity in patients with diabetic foot disease in Europe. Baseline results from the Eurodiale study. Diabetologia. 2007;50(1): 18–25.
8. Lavery LA, et al. Diabetic foot syndrome: evaluating the prevalence and incidence of foot pathology in Mexican Americans and non-Hispanic whites from a diabetes disease management cohort. Diabetes Care. 2003;26(5):1435–8.
9. Bakker K, et al. The 2015 IWGDF guidance documents on prevention and management of foot problems in diabetes: development of an evidence-based global consensus. Diabetes Metab Res Rev. 2016;32(Suppl 1):2–6.
10. Bus SA, et al. Guidelines on the prevention of foot ulcers in persons with diabetes (IWGDF 2019 update). Diabetes Metab Res Rev. 2020;36(Suppl 1):e3269.
11. Game FL, et al. IWGDF guidance on use of interventions to enhance the healing of chronic ulcers of the foot in diabetes. Diabetes Metab Res Rev. 2016;32(Suppl 1):75–83.
12. Hinchliffe RJ, et al. IWGDF guidance on the diagnosis, prognosis and management of peripheral artery disease in patients with foot ulcers in diabetes. Diabetes Metab Res Rev. 2016;32(Suppl 1):37–44.
13. Santema TB, Poyck PP, Ubbink DT. Skin grafting and tissue replacement for treating foot ulcers in people with diabetes. Cochrane Database Syst Rev. 2016;2(2):Cd011255.
14. Rose JF, et al. Split-thickness skin grafting the high-risk diabetic foot. J Vasc Surg. 2014;59(6):1657–63.
15. Veves A, et al. Graftskin, a human skin equivalent, is effective in the management of noninfected neuropathic diabetic foot ulcers: a prospective randomized multicenter clinical trial. Diabetes Care. 2001;24(2):290–5.
16. Caravaggi C, et al. HYAFF 11-based autologous dermal and epidermal grafts in the treatment of non-infected diabetic plantar and dorsal foot ulcers: a prospective, multicenter, controlled, randomized clinical trial. Diabetes Care. 2003;26(10):2853–9.
17. Marston WA, et al. The efficacy and safety of Dermagraft in improving the healing of chronic diabetic foot ulcers: results of a prospective randomized trial. Diabetes Care. 2003;26(6):1701–5.
18. Khanolkar MP, Bain SC, Stephens JW. The diabetic foot. QJM. 2008;101(9):685–95.
19. Faglia E, et al. Long-term prognosis of diabetic patients with critical limb ischemia: a population-based cohort study. Diabetes Care. 2009;32(5):822–7.
20. Creager MA, et al. Diabetes and vascular disease: pathophysiology, clinical consequences, and medical therapy: part I. Circulation. 2003;108(12):1527–32.
21. Paneni F, et al. Diabetes and vascular disease: pathophysiology, clinical consequences, and medical therapy: part I. Eur Heart J. 2013;34(31):2436–43.
22. Marso SP, Hiatt WR. Peripheral arterial disease in patients with diabetes. J Am Coll Cardiol. 2006;47(5):921–9.
23. Nishikawa T, et al. Normalizing mitochondrial superoxide production blocks three pathways of hyperglycaemic damage. Nature. 2000;404(6779):787–90.
24. Geraldes P, King GL. Activation of protein kinase C isoforms and its impact on diabetic complications. Circ Res. 2010;106(8):1319–31.
25. Kouroedov A, et al. Selective inhibition of protein kinase Cbeta2 prevents acute effects of high glucose on vascular cell adhesion molecule-1 expression in human endothelial cells. Circulation. 2004;110(1):91–6.
26. Cosentino F, et al. High glucose causes upregulation of cyclooxygenase-2 and alters prostanoid profile in human endothelial cells: role of protein kinase C and reactive oxygen species. Circulation. 2003;107(7):1017–23.
27. Yan SF, Ramasamy R, Schmidt AM. The RAGE axis: a fundamental mechanism signaling danger to the vulnerable vasculature. Circ Res. 2010;106(5):842–53.
28. Bhatia LS, et al. Non-alcoholic fatty liver disease: a new and important cardiovascular risk factor? Eur Heart J. 2012;33(10):1190–200.
29. Kim JA, et al. Reciprocal relationships between insulin resistance and endothelial dysfunction: molecular and pathophysiological mechanisms. Circulation. 2006;113(15):1888–904.
30. Du X, et al. Insulin resistance reduces arterial prostacyclin synthase and eNOS activities by increas-

ing endothelial fatty acid oxidation. J Clin Invest. 2006;116(4):1071–80.
31. Zhang H, Dellsperger KC, Zhang C. The link between metabolic abnormalities and endothelial dysfunction in type 2 diabetes: an update. Basic Res Cardiol. 2012;107(1):237.
32. Lee M, et al. Efficacy of fibrates for cardiovascular risk reduction in persons with atherogenic dyslipidemia: a meta-analysis. Atherosclerosis. 2011;217(2):492–8.
33. Ferreira IA, et al. Platelet inhibition by insulin is absent in type 2 diabetes mellitus. Arterioscler Thromb Vasc Biol. 2006;26(2):417–22.
34. Haffner SM, et al. Mortality from coronary heart disease in subjects with type 2 diabetes and in nondiabetic subjects with and without prior myocardial infarction. N Engl J Med. 1998;339(4):229–34.
35. Vazzana N, et al. Diabetes mellitus and thrombosis. Thromb Res. 2012;129(3):371–7.
36. Lemkes BA, et al. Hyperglycemia: a prothrombotic factor? J Thromb Haemost. 2010;8(8):1663–9.
37. Boden G, Rao AK. Effects of hyperglycemia and hyperinsulinemia on the tissue factor pathway of blood coagulation. Curr Diab Rep. 2007;7(3):223–7.
38. Hingorani A, et al. The management of diabetic foot: a clinical practice guideline by the Society for Vascular Surgery in collaboration with the American Podiatric Medical Association and the Society for Vascular Medicine. J Vasc Surg. 2016;63(2 Suppl):3s–21s.
39. Aboyans V, et al. Measurement and interpretation of the ankle-brachial index: a scientific statement from the American Heart Association. Circulation. 2012;126(24):2890–909.
40. Gerhard-Herman MD, et al. 2016 AHA/ACC guideline on the management of patients with lower extremity peripheral artery disease: a report of the American College of Cardiology/American Heart Association Task Force on Clinical Practice Guidelines. Circulation. 2017;135(12):e726–79.
41. Del Conde I, Benenati JF. Noninvasive testing in peripheral arterial disease. Interv Cardiol Clin. 2014;3(4):469–78.
42. Andersen CA. Noninvasive assessment of lower extremity hemodynamics in individuals with diabetes mellitus. J Vasc Surg. 2010;52(3 Suppl):76s–80s.
43. Brooks B, et al. TBI or not TBI: that is the question. Is it better to measure toe pressure than ankle pressure in diabetic patients? Diabet Med. 2001;18(7):528–32.
44. de Meijer VE, et al. Reference value of transcutaneous oxygen measurement in diabetic patients compared with nondiabetic patients. J Vasc Surg. 2008;48(2):382–8.
45. Wang Z, et al. A systematic review and meta-analysis of tests to predict wound healing in diabetic foot. J Vasc Surg. 2016;63(2 Suppl):29S–36S.e1–2.
46. Redlich U, et al. Superiority of transcutaneous oxygen tension measurements in predicting limb salvage after below-the-knee angioplasty: a prospective trial in diabetic patients with critical limb ischemia. Cardiovasc Intervent Radiol. 2011;34(2):271–9.
47. Olin JW, et al. Atherosclerotic vascular disease conference: writing group IV: imaging. Circulation. 2004;109(21):2626–33.
48. Eiberg JP, et al. Duplex ultrasound scanning of peripheral arterial disease of the lower limb. Eur J Vasc Endovasc Surg. 2010;40(4):507–12.
49. Ota H, et al. Quantitative vascular measurements in arterial occlusive disease. Radiographics. 2005;25(5):1141–58.
50. Collins R, et al. A systematic review of duplex ultrasound, magnetic resonance angiography and computed tomography angiography for the diagnosis and assessment of symptomatic, lower limb peripheral arterial disease. Health Technol Assess. 2007;11(20):iii–iv, xi–xiii, 1–184.
51. Schabel C, et al. Diagnostic accuracy of dual energy CT angiography in patients with diabetes mellitus. Radiologe. 2015;55(4):314–22.
52. Dias-Neto M, Marques C, Sampaio S. Digital subtraction angiography or computed tomography angiography in the preoperative evaluation of lower limb peripheral artery disease—a comparative analysis. Rev Port Cir Cardiotorac Vasc. 2017;24(3–4):174.
53. Healy DA, et al. Contrast-enhanced magnetic resonance angiography in diabetic patients with infragenicular peripheral arterial disease: systematic review. Int J Surg. 2013;11(3):228–32.
54. Varga-Szemes A, et al. Accuracy of noncontrast quiescent-interval single-shot lower extremity MR angiography versus CT angiography for diagnosis of peripheral artery disease: comparison with digital subtraction angiography. JACC Cardiovasc Imaging. 2017;10(10 Pt A):1116–24.
55. Everett E, Mathioudakis N. Update on management of diabetic foot ulcers. Ann N Y Acad Sci. 2018;1411(1):153–65.
56. Beckman JA, et al. Diabetes and vascular disease: pathophysiology, clinical consequences, and medical therapy: part II. Eur Heart J. 2013;34(31):2444–52.
57. Sheehan P, et al. Percent change in wound area of diabetic foot ulcers over a 4-week period is a robust predictor of complete healing in a 12-week prospective trial. Plast Reconstr Surg. 2006;117(7 Suppl):239s–44s.
58. Iida O, et al. Impact of angiosome-oriented revascularization on clinical outcomes in critical limb ischemia patients without concurrent wound infection and diabetes. J Endovasc Ther. 2014;21(5):607–15.
59. Adam DJ, et al. Bypass versus angioplasty in severe ischaemia of the leg (BASIL): multicentre, randomised controlled trial. Lancet. 2005;366(9501):1925–34.
60. Aboyans V, et al. 2017 ESC guidelines on the diagnosis and treatment of peripheral arterial diseases, in collaboration with the European Society for Vascular Surgery (ESVS): document covering atherosclerotic disease of extracranial carotid and vertebral, mesenteric, renal, upper and lower extremity arteries Endorsed by: the European Stroke Organization (ESO) The Task Force for the Diagnosis and

Treatment of Peripheral Arterial Diseases of the European Society of Cardiology (ESC) and of the European Society for Vascular Surgery (ESVS). Eur Heart J. 2018;39(9):763–816.
61. Kansal A, et al. Endovascular treatment of femoropopliteal lesions. Clin Cardiol. 2019;42(1):175–83.
62. Armstrong EJ, Bishu K, Waldo SW. Endovascular treatment of infrapopliteal peripheral artery disease. Curr Cardiol Rep. 2016;18(4):34.
63. Setacci C, et al. Chapter IV: treatment of critical limb ischaemia. Eur J Vasc Endovasc Surg. 2011;42(Suppl 2):S43–59.
64. Jaff MR, et al. An update on methods for revascularization and expansion of the TASC lesion classification to include below-the-knee arteries: a supplement to the Inter-Society Consensus for the Management of Peripheral Arterial Disease (TASC II). J Endovasc Ther. 2015;22(5):663–77.
65. Zeller T, et al. Drug-eluting balloon versus standard balloon angioplasty for infrapopliteal arterial revascularization in critical limb ischemia: 12-month results from the IN.PACT DEEP randomized trial. J Am Coll Cardiol. 2014;64(15):1568–76.
66. Brodmann M, et al. Percutaneous transluminal angioplasty versus primary stenting in infrapopliteal arteries in critical limb ischemia. Vasa. 2011;40(6):482–90.
67. Schulte KL, et al. Primary self-EXPANDing nitinol stenting vs balloon angioplasty with optional bailout stenting for the treatment of Infrapopliteal artery disease in patients with severe intermittent claudication or critical limb ischemia (EXPAND study). J Endovasc Ther. 2015;22(5):690–7.
68. Schneider PA, et al. Treatment effect of drug-coated balloons is durable to 3 years in the femoropopliteal arteries: long-term results of the IN.PACT SFA randomized trial. Circ Cardiovasc Interv. 2018;11(1):e005891.
69. Rosenfield K, et al. Trial of a paclitaxel-coated balloon for femoropopliteal artery disease. N Engl J Med. 2015;373(2):145–53.
70. Fanelli F, et al. Calcium burden assessment and impact on drug-eluting balloons in peripheral arterial disease. Cardiovasc Intervent Radiol. 2014;37(4):898–907.
71. Zeller T, et al. Directional atherectomy followed by a paclitaxel-coated balloon to inhibit restenosis and maintain vessel patency: twelve-month results of the DEFINITIVE AR study. Circ Cardiovasc Interv. 2017;10(9):e004848.
72. Krankenberg H, et al. Nitinol stent implantation versus percutaneous transluminal angioplasty in superficial femoral artery lesions up to 10 cm in length: the femoral artery stenting trial (FAST). Circulation. 2007;116(3):285–92.
73. Schillinger M, et al. Sustained benefit at 2 years of primary femoropopliteal stenting compared with balloon angioplasty with optional stenting. Circulation. 2007;115(21):2745–9.
74. Davaine JM, et al. Primary stenting of TASC C and D femoropopliteal lesions: results of the STELLA register at 30 months. Ann Vasc Surg. 2014;28(7):1686–96.
75. Lammer J, et al. Heparin-bonded covered stents versus bare-metal stents for complex femoropopliteal artery lesions: the randomized VIASTAR trial (Viabahn endoprosthesis with PROPATEN bioactive surface [VIA] versus bare nitinol stent in the treatment of long lesions in superficial femoral artery occlusive disease). J Am Coll Cardiol. 2013;62(15):1320–7.
76. Dake MD, et al. Durable clinical effectiveness with paclitaxel-eluting stents in the femoropopliteal artery: 5-year results of the Zilver PTX randomized trial. Circulation. 2016;133(15):1472–83. discussion 1483
77. Bausback Y, et al. Drug-eluting stent versus drug-coated balloon revascularization in patients with femoropopliteal arterial disease. J Am Coll Cardiol. 2019;73(6):667–79.
78. Scheinert D, et al. A prospective randomized multicenter comparison of balloon angioplasty and infrapopliteal stenting with the sirolimus-eluting stent in patients with ischemic peripheral arterial disease: 1-year results from the ACHILLES trial. J Am Coll Cardiol. 2012;60(22):2290–5.
79. Bosiers M, et al. Randomized comparison of everolimus-eluting versus bare-metal stents in patients with critical limb ischemia and infrapopliteal arterial occlusive disease. J Vasc Surg. 2012;55(2):390–8.
80. Siablis D, et al. Paclitaxel-coated balloon angioplasty versus drug-eluting stenting for the treatment of infrapopliteal long-segment arterial occlusive disease: the IDEAS randomized controlled trial. JACC Cardiovasc Interv. 2014;7(9):1048–56.
81. Shammas NW, et al. Percutaneous lower-extremity arterial interventions with primary balloon angioplasty versus Silverhawk atherectomy and adjunctive balloon angioplasty: randomized trial. J Vasc Interv Radiol. 2011;22(9):1223–8.
82. Dattilo R, Himmelstein SI, Cuff RF. The COMPLIANCE 360° trial: a randomized, prospective, multicenter, pilot study comparing acute and long-term results of orbital atherectomy to balloon angioplasty for calcified femoropopliteal disease. J Invasive Cardiol. 2014;26(8):355–60.
83. Dippel EJ, et al. Randomized controlled study of excimer laser atherectomy for treatment of femoropopliteal in-stent restenosis: initial results from the EXCITE ISR trial (EXCImer Laser Randomized Controlled Study for Treatment of FemoropopliTEal In-Stent Restenosis). JACC Cardiovasc Interv. 2015;8(1 Pt A):92–101.

3 Diabetic Neuropathy

Changsik John Pak

3.1 Introduction

Diabetic neuropathy (DN) is a common complication of diabetes that typically presents symmetrically in both lower limbs. It affects both the sensory and motor nerves and is a significant cause of lower extremity amputation. DN is an uncontrollable complication of diabetes, and its prevalence within 1 year of diagnosis ranges from 7 to 50% in diabetics 25 years and older. The presence of cardiovascular autonomic neuropathy (CAN) dramatically shortens a patient's lifespan and increases mortality [1]. Complete loss of sensation in the lower extremities occurs in 1–2% of patients with diabetes, which therefore increases the risk of amputation. Despite efforts to make an early diagnosis and prevent the progression of DN, there is no effective treatment currently available except for the strict control of blood glucose.

3.2 Classification

Many different types of neuropathies have been reported in diabetes mellitus. As a result of DN being a group of heterogeneous states, the clinical classification of various syndromes has proven difficult. Most classifications of DNs are oversimplified due to the inability to explain the variability and duplication of etiologies, clinical manifestations, natural histories, and prognoses. The clinical manifestations and somatic neuropathy measurements were the subject of a recent technical review with an in-depth discussion and relevant references to the literature. Table 3.1 shows the recent recommended comprehensive classification scheme for DN [2].

Table 3.1 Type of neuropathies in diabetes mellitus

Focal
Mononeuritis
Compressive
Upper extremity: Carpal and cubital tunnel syndrome
Lower extremity: Fibular and tarsal tunnel syndrome
Autonomic
Gastroparesis
Cardiac
Vascular
Cranial nerve: VI palsy, III palsy
Amotropy
Mononeuritis multiplex
Diffuse
Large or mixed fiber
Small fiber

C. J. Pak (✉)
Seoul Asan Medical Center, Seoul, South Korea
e-mail: iloveps@amc.seoul.kr

J. P. Hong, H. Suh (eds.), *Diabetic Foot Reconstruction*,
https://doi.org/10.1007/978-981-16-9816-3_3

3.3 Clinical Progress

DN progresses slowly and is overlooked in about 50% with no abnormal initial symptoms or symptoms. Symptoms are often worse in the early stages. Numbness of the foot can increase the risk of developing diabetic foot ulcers. Symptoms and signs of neuropathy include pathophysiologically thick nerve fiber symptoms (muscle weakness, muscle atrophy, etc.) and thin nerve fiber symptoms (loss of sweat, pain and decreased temperature sensation, dry skin, decreased blood flow). On the other hand, it can be classified into benign sensory symptoms (paresthesias: prickling, tingling, "pins and needles," burning, crawling, itching, abnormal sensation to temperature, pain) and negative paresthesias (numbness, insensitivity). Pain is the most common complaint. Symmetrical symptoms on the toes gradually rise to the feet over time, causing symptoms on the fingers and hands (in the form of stocking and glove). Benign symptoms are predominantly more common at night, and some patients may complain of pain just by receiving a duvet or clothing (allodynia). In some patients, the symptoms may progress and the typical sensory ataxia form of gait may be seen due to proprioceptive sensory nerve injury in the sole of the foot. The earliest clinical aspect of motor nerve lesions in DN patients is weakening of the anterior renal muscles of the toes. As a result, local overpressure is applied to the metatarsal head and toe sites when a typical nail toe deformation occurs, and ulcers are likely to occur [3].

In diabetic patients, DN is usually easily diagnosed, but in the case of severe motor neuropathy, polyneuropathy caused by other causes, especially chronic inflammatory demyelinating polyneuropathy (CIDP) or POEMS syndrome (polyneuropathy, organomegaly, endocrinopathy, M protein, skin changes), etc., and peripheral neuropathy caused by hypothyroidism or vitamin B12 deficiency. In addition, care should be taken not to be diagnosed as pseudopolyneuropathy even if it is not polyneuropathy by classifying other accompanying neurological diseases (e.g., spinal diseases).

3.4 Diagnosis

For diagnosis of DN during outpatient treatment, neurological examination for touch, pain, temperature, pressure, and vibration angles, along with clinical symptoms, and examination and examination for muscle weakness and muscle atrophy should be performed. Vibration sensory testing can be performed using a 128 Hz tuning fork. Among several tests, the pressure test using 5.07 Semmes Weinstein monofilament, which can apply a pressure of 10 g, is known as the most straightforward, cheapest, and most reliable method, so it is being performed as a guideline for the prediction of the high-risk group for ulceration. However, the results of previous studies on the sensitivity and specificity of the test are so diverse that some suggest that there is a problem in diagnosing DPN with this test alone. Quantitative sensory test (QST), which objectively evaluates vibration sensation, pressure sensation, and temperature sensory threshold, is considered as a useful tool for DPN diagnosis in both clinical and research fields, as it can detect nerve fiber problems that cannot be confirmed by neuroelectromyography. In particular, the vibration sensory threshold test is the most commonly used alone in clinical practice. However, there is a recent report that QST is not a completely objective test and is influenced by several subjective factors such as age and concentration [4].

Neuroelectromyography is an objective standard guideline for diagnosing DN, determining the current level, type, and worsening, and distinguishing it from other diseases. A decrease in the amplitude of a sensory nerve evoked potential (below 6 μV) due to a decrease in the gastrocnemius axon is considered the earliest reliable change. The decrease in gastro-gastric nerve conduction velocity and peroneal motor nerve conduction velocity due to changes in demyelination is also recognized as a significant initial variable [5].

The American Association of Neurology (AAN) suggested five diagnostic criteria for DN. This refers to the symptoms, neurophysical examination, neuroelectromyography, QST, and autonomic function test areas.

3.5 Treatment

3.5.1 Medical Treatment

3.5.1.1 General Principle

Depending on the patient, DN can range from asymptomatic to severe, with pain and foot ulcers that interfere with daily activities. Treatment of diabetic peripheral neuropathy, including painful neuropathy, is arguably essential to clinicians and is one of the most challenging problems. Consultation with various clinical departments is necessary, and patient education is considered critical. The primary purpose of treatment for diabetic peripheral neuropathy is to prevent nerve regression, support regeneration, improve the quality of life, prevent serious complications, and reduce the burden of medical costs. The treatment of diabetic peripheral neuropathy can be broadly divided into three types: first, treatments that control glycemic control and risk factors that correspond to the underlying causes of DN; second, treatments based on etiologic studies of the development of DN; and third, treatment of symptoms related to pain caused by diabetic peripheral neuropathy [6].

3.5.1.2 Glycemic Control

Glycemic control can have a primary preventive effect on DN, relieve symptoms, and prevent progression. Hyperglycemia and glucose fluctuations are known to affect the exacerbation of symptoms. According to a large epidemiological study (EURODIAB IDDM Complications Study) conducted in Europe, the pathogenesis of DN is smoking, a history of cardiovascular disease, vascularity hypertension, and hyperlipidemia. This shows that the risk factors are closely related to the pathogenesis. When treating diabetic peripheral neuropathy, it is essential to actively regulate the blood glucose level, as it is the leading cause of neuropathy. Prospective and retrospective studies have shown that hyperglycemia and the severity of diabetic peripheral neuropathy are closely correlated and that active regulation of blood glucose is therefore an essential therapeutic factor [7].

3.5.1.3 Symptomatic Treatment

Pain in DN and damaged peripheral nerves causes altered nociception transmission to the central nervous system which can result in functional and structural changes that exacerbate the experience of pain. Painful DN is observed in 10–20% of all diabetic patients and in 40–50% of DN patients. Neuropathic pain requires early treatment, as it can lead to severe symptoms such as sleep disturbance, depression, anxiety, and loss of appetite, resulting in a decreased quality of life for diabetic patients.

Tricyclic antidepressants (TCAs) alone or in combination with phenothiazine fluphenazine (amitriptyline and nortriptyline, etc.), with initial small doses of 10–25 mg at night, can improve symptoms. The dosage can be increased while observing the potential side effects, such as deep vein thrombosis, urinary congestion, and glaucoma.

Antiepileptic drugs such as carbamazepine are widely used, with the initial dosage starting at 100 mg twice daily. The dose is then gradually increased after observing the reported effects and side effects. Leukopenia may occur within 3 months of use, and frequent blood cell testing should therefore be performed.

Gabapentin is another antiepileptic drug that has recently been used to relieve acute mild neuropathic pain. The initial dosage of 300 mg daily can be gradually increased while observing its effectiveness and side effects, with a maximum daily dosage of 2400 mg.

The use of topical capsaicin ointment (0.075%) has been reported in a case of typical c-fiber neuropathy with dysesthesia, such as explosive passage dysfunction and ovulation. It can be applied four times a day. The pain was reported to be worsened initially, but relieved after several days.

A local anesthetic ointment, lidocaine, is best used when there is no response to other pain treatments and for the spontaneous recovery of diseases. Its analgesic effects last for 3–21 days. If the reported therapeutic effect is good, orally administered mexiletine can be administered in combination. The drug has also been effective in clinical studies, with initial daily doses starting at 150 mg and increasing to 600–900 mg [8].

3.6 Surgical Treatment

The traditional medical approach to the treatment of DN is an attempt to achieve a euglycemic state and obtain regular care of the feet. Regular care includes daily foot inspection for the presence of erythema, yearly sensory testing to detect neuropathy, and provision of special protective footwear. If there is a painful neuropathy component, burning, or dysesthetic feet, then the traditional medical approach includes both non-narcotic and narcotic medications, which are often ineffective in relieving pain. Since there is no known cure for DN, the disease inevitably progresses with time. Sensory loss in neuropathy increases the risk for infection, ulceration, and amputation.

Due to the nature of the neurological disease and the ambiguity of the symptoms, surgeons may also miss the opportunity for surgical intervention. Surgical decompression of peripheral nerves is not recommended in all patients with DN but can be performed to reduce pain and prevent complications when local compression of peripheral nerves is considered critical. The most common chronic compression site in the lower extremities of diabetic patients is the tibial nerve in the tarsal tunnel and the common peroneal nerve near the fibular head. DN and chronic compression symptoms are similar to those of carpal tunnel and tarsal tunnel syndromes.

Thus, if a DN patient has local symptoms of nerve compression, symptomatic treatment focused on reducing local edema, inflammation, and pressure with physical therapy and shoe calibration is preferred to surgery. Injecting a mixture of corticosteroids and lidocaine under ultrasound guidance can also be used for both diagnosis and treatment. It is essential to consider and provide alternative treatment options and the clinician can assist in the planning and provision of these options. Finally, if there is a strong suspicion of capture neuropathy due to local nerve compression showing abnormalities, such as Tinel's sign, then decompression surgery should be performed. Therefore, the drug treatment must be maintained [9].

3.6.1 Surgical Approach to Peroneal and Tibial Nerve

3.6.1.1 Common Peroneal Nerve Entrapment

The surgical approach regarding the common peroneal nerve is common, as this nerve can be injured concomitantly with knee and ankle joint injuries. A comparison study of 29 bilateral cadaver dissections and 65 unilateral clinical decompressions was undertaken to identify the anatomic variations of the common peroneal nerve at the fibular neck. This study demonstrated that while the fibrous band deep to the peroneus longus muscle was present in only 30% of cadavers, it was present in 78.5% of cadavers with clinical symptoms of nerve compression that would require neurolysis of the common peroneal nerve. Additional findings were that the lateral gastrocnemius muscle might have a thick fascial origin deep to the common peroneal nerve that requires division. The common peroneal nerve entrance into the anterior and lateral compartments of the leg may be tight because of the proximal origin of the soleus muscle (Fig. 3.1). Therefore, these observations require a surgical approach for neurolysis of this nerve to search for each of these variations [10].

3.6.1.2 Superficial Peroneal Nerve Entrapment

The superficial peroneal nerve (SPN) is located in the lateral compartment of the lower leg, although in 25% of people it can also be found in the anterior compartment and can sometimes be found in both compartments. The SPN exits the fascia of the lateral compartment, on average, approximately 10–12 cm proximal to the lateral malleolus. The incision for neurolysis of the SPN is made anterior to and in parallel with the fibula to permit access to both the anterior and lateral compartments. The incision may be more proximal or distal depending on the

Fig. 3.1 Peroneal innervation of the lower leg

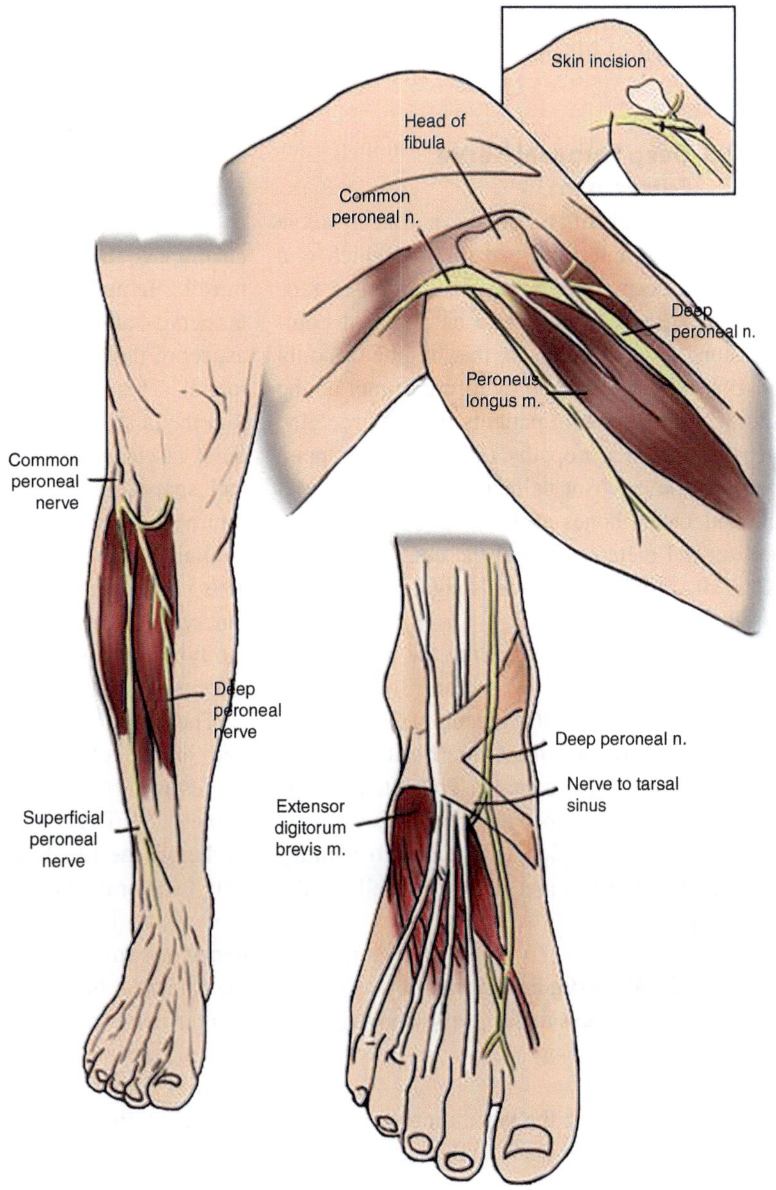

patient's height and the location of the positive Tinel's sign. The incision should be made with caution to the subcutaneous space, to avoid damage to the SPN, which is sometimes found in this space. A slight elevation in the fascia, accompanied by a small blood vessel and some fat, often marks the location of nerve entrapment as the SPN travels from deep toward the superficial fascia to enter the subcutaneous space. An incision of approximately 15 cm is made to ensure the SPN is free from constriction and to avoid a new small muscle herniation through a small fascial window [11].

Both the anterior and lateral compartments should be evaluated, even if the SPN is found in the first compartment entered. If the SPN cannot be found in either, it would lie within the septum itself. The septum should be opened carefully to avoid injury to the SPN or one of its branches. The incised fascial edges is then cauterized, as the fascia is well-vascularized and can cause a postoperative hematoma or seroma. The skin is then sutured with an interrupted intradermal 4–0 monocryl and continuous interrupted 5–0 nylon sutures.

3.6.1.3 Deep Peroneal Nerve Entrapment

The entrapment of the deep peroneal nerve (DPN) in the anterior tarsal tunnel, which is a broad and deep space beneath the extensor retinaculum, has been described as a site of compression. Compression in this region is only possible with trauma and therefore cannot be the site of compression in patients with neuropathy. In patients with neuropathy, the DPN is entrapped between the extensor hallucis brevis tendon and the underlying bones at the juncture of the first and second metatarsals and the cuneiform. This is the site at which the Tinel's sign radiates pain distally [12].

To release this entrapment, the incision is made obliquely across this region. Blunt dissection should be used in the subcutaneous tissue to identify and retract the superficial peroneal branches and prevent damage. The extensor hallucis brevis tendon is then unambiguously identified, and a 2-cm section is resected to identify whether the DPN sits medially or laterally to the dorsalis pedis artery.

3.6.1.4 Tibial Nerve Entrapment

There are four tunnels to decompress in the ankle joint:

1. The tibial nerve in the tarsal tunnel
2. The medial plantar nerve in the medial plantar tunnel
3. The lateral plantar nerve in the lateral plantar tunnel
4. The calcaneal nerve in one or more calcaneal tunnels

The tibial nerve in the tarsal tunnel is approached through an incision that is posterior to the medial malleolus and midway to the Achilles tendon. The tunnel begins immediately proximal to the medial malleolus. The flexor retinaculum is opened and its edges are cauterized to prevent them from re-attaching postoperatively. The tarsal tunnel is usually not a site of chronic compression. This exposure permits the rest of the decompressions to proceed safely and if present permits decompression of intraneural pressure within the tibial nerve. The tarsal tunnel ends when the flexor retinaculum divides to encompass the abductor hallucis brevis (AHB) muscle. To approach the medial and lateral plantar nerves, an incision is made toward the plantar aspect of the foot at the site of the lateral plantar tunnel. This incision is brought proximally to join the tarsal tunnel release incision. The superficial fascia of the AHB muscle is then incised and spread gently. Care must be taken not to injure the small (<1 mm) nerve that goes from the medial plantar nerve superficially to the vessels. This nerve then enters the fascia and emerges to innervate the medial ankle skin at the site where the typical incision is made for a plantar fascia release (Fig. 3.2).

The medial calcaneal tunnel(s) can be identified in one of two ways. First, the calcaneal nerves arise from the tibial nerve within the tarsal tunnel [13]. These are identified in the posterior fat below the tibial nerve and are followed distally to enter the tunnel. Second, from the fibrous roof of the lateral plantar tunnel, the fascia is traced proximally and is found to form the roof of the calcaneal branches that arise from the lateral plantar nerve before it enters the lateral plantar tunnel. Each of these tunnels is spread gently, and the roof is then carefully divided to avoid injury to one of the small branches of the calcaneal nerve [14].

3.7 Postoperative Management

Postoperatively, the patient will be allowed full weight-bearing immediately and will use a walking frame for 3 weeks. The goal of walking with a walking frame is to permit nerve gliding while minimizing the ankle range of motion so that the sutures do not pull out. The dressing is removed after the seventh day, and the sutures can get wet. Betadine must be applied to the incisions twice a

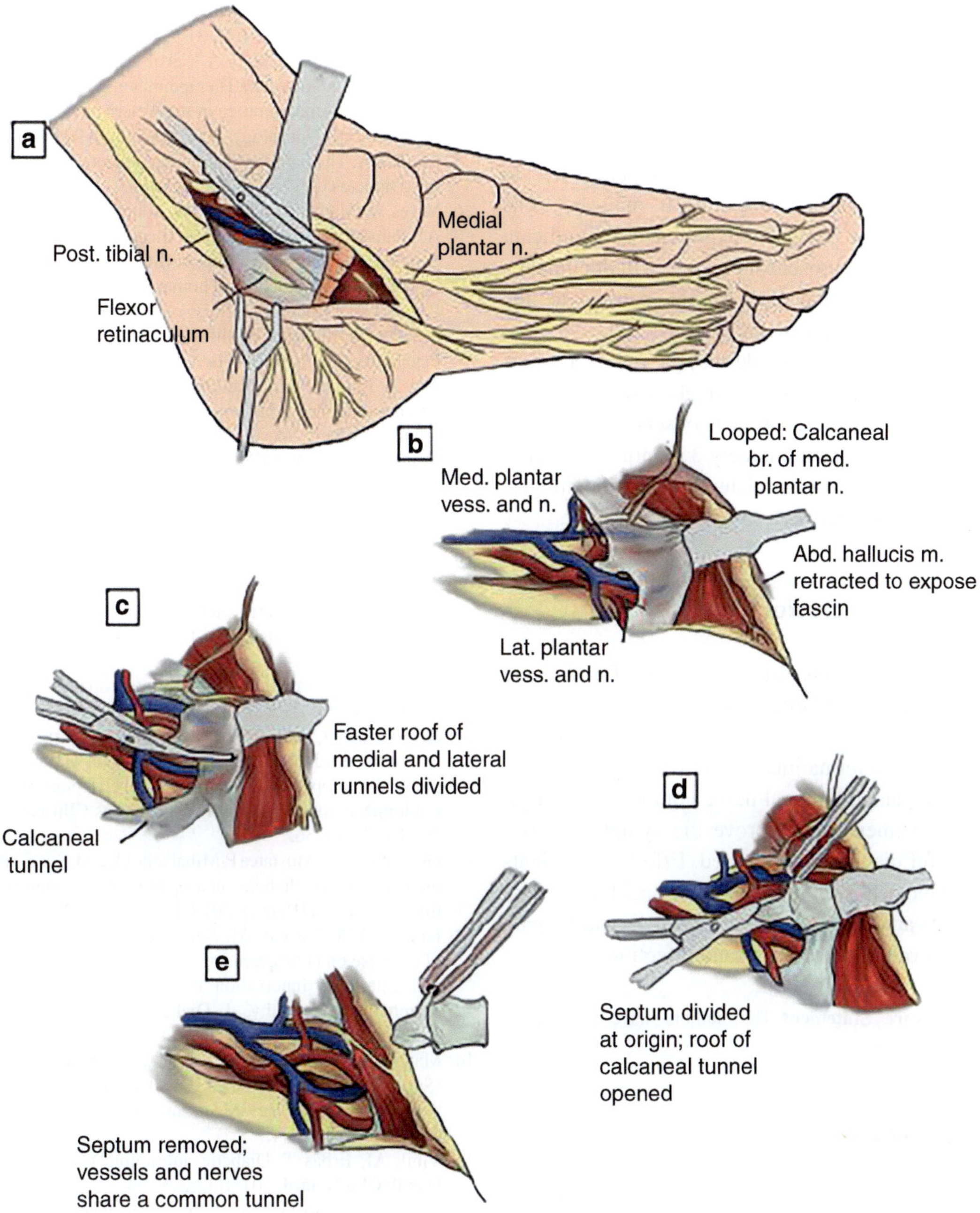

Fig. 3.2 Tibial nerve decompression. (**a**) Incision through flexor retinaculum. (**b**) Identification of calcaneal br. of med. plantar n. (**c**) Division of fascia roof of med. and lat. Tunnels. (**d**) Septum removal. (**e**) Roof of calcaneal tunnel open

day. After removing the sutures, the patient should begin mobilizing in a heated pool as a form of physical therapy. This therapy is preferred three times a week, with twice a week being the minimum. No other therapies are usually necessary. The patient will then progress through increasing degrees of ambulation and activity, as tolerated [15].

Analgesia should be reduced as the pain decreases. In patients who did not complain of pain preoperatively and who experience pain postoperatively due to nerve regeneration, a regimen of neuropathic pain medication can be started, with opioids continued as needed.

Repeat neurosensory testing should be performed at 6–12 weeks postoperatively to document sensory recovery. It may be done sooner if the patient is experiencing significant pain, as the neurosensory testing will document a reassuring nerve regeneration pattern to the patient and the physician [16].

The contralateral side may be operated on as early as 6 weeks postoperatively if sufficient pain relief or sensory recovery is observed. Typically, patients wait approximately 3 months to undergo surgery on the contralateral side. The longest time interval between surgeries was 1 year.

3.8 Conclusion

Although various drug treatments for diabetic neuropathy can relieve pain, symptoms caused by the degeneration of the nerve itself, including sensory abnormalities, do not improve. If it is accompanied by local nerve compression, surgical treatment can improve the symptoms, so a careful diagnosis is required. Efforts by patients and medical staff to maintain normal blood sugar levels are essential, and attention should be paid to preventing foot ulcers and infections.

Disclosure Statement The authors have nothing to disclose.

References

1. Jensen MP, Chodroff MJ, Dworkin RH. The impact of neuropathic pain on health-related quality of life: review and implications. Neurology. 2007;68(15):1178–82.
2. Zochodne DW. Diabetes mellitus and the peripheral nervous system: manifestations and mechanisms. Muscle Nerve. 2007;36(2):144–66.
3. Vinik AI. Diabetic neuropathy: pathogenesis and therapy. Am J Med. 1999;107(2B):17S–26S.
4. Shy ME, Frohman EM, So YT, et al. Quantitative sensory testing: report of the Therapeutics and Technology Assessment Subcommittee of the American Academy of Neurology. Neurology. 2003;60(6):898–904.
5. Malik RA. The pathology of human diabetic neuropathy. Diabetes. 1997;46(Suppl 2):S50–3.
6. Veves A, Manes C, Murray HJ, Young MJ, Boulton AJ. Painful neuropathy and foot ulceration in diabetic patients. Diabetes Care. 1993;16(8):1187–9.
7. Archer AG, Watkins PJ, Thomas PK, Sharma AK, Payan J. The natural history of acute painful neuropathy in diabetes mellitus. J Neurol Neurosurg Psychiatry. 1983;46(6):491–9.
8. Bril V, England JD, Franklin GM, et al. Evidence-based guideline: treatment of painful diabetic neuropathy—report of the American Association of Neuromuscular and Electrodiagnostic Medicine, the American Academy of Neurology, and the American Academy of Physical Medicine & Rehabilitation. Muscle Nerve. 2011;43(6):910–7.
9. Tu Y, Lineaweaver WC, Chen Z, Hu J, Mullins F, Zhang F. Surgical decompression in the treatment of diabetic peripheral neuropathy: a systematic review and meta-analysis. J Reconstr Microsurg. 2017;33(3):151–7.
10. Pinzur MS. Diabetic peripheral neuropathy. Foot Ankle Clin. 2011;16(2):345–9.
11. Best TJ, Best CA, Best AA, Fera LA. Surgical peripheral nerve decompression for the treatment of painful diabetic neuropathy of the foot—a level 1 pragmatic randomized controlled trial. Diabetes Res Clin Pract. 2019;147:149–56.
12. Georgescu DE, Mustatea P, Mihalache O, et al. Surgical management of diabetic neuropathy foot complications. Chirurgia (Bucur). 2018;113(5):634–43.
13. Kluding PM, Pasnoor M, Singh R, et al. The effect of exercise on neuropathic symptoms, nerve function, and cutaneous innervation in people with diabetic peripheral neuropathy. J Diabetes Complications. 2012;26(5):424–9.
14. Mazilu G, Budurca RA, Graur M, Stamate T. [Surgical treatment of tarsal tunnel syndrome in diabetic neuropathy]. Rev Med Chir Soc Med Nat Iasi 2012;116(1):128–34.
15. Vinik AI, Erbas T. Diabetic autonomic neuropathy. Handb Clin Neurol. 2013;117:279–94.
16. Dellon AL. Diabetic neuropathy: medical and surgical approaches. Clin Podiatr Med Surg. 2007;24(3):425–448, viii.

4 Understanding Infection

Felix W. A. Waibel and İlker Uçkay

Key Points

- The diagnosis of infection in the diabetic foot is based on clinical aspects (with eventually radiology for osteomyelitis), not on the microbiology of superficial swabs or serum inflammatory markers.
- The treatment of diabetic foot infections is multidisciplinary, of which iterative debridement and wound care, systemic antibiotic therapies, and adequate off-loading are the cornerstones.
- Most antibiotic therapies can be administered orally and for relatively short periods (approximately 10 days for soft tissue infections, 4–6 weeks for unresected bone).
- The risk for therapy failures and long-term recurrences is high. Therefore, the prevention of infection, corrective and reconstructive surgeries of the altered foot anatomy, and the overall improvement of the patient's compliance is more important than single therapeutic approaches.

4.1 Introduction

Diabetic foot infections (DFI), including diabetic foot osteomyelitis (DFO), are frequent entities with a lifetime risk of 25% among all adult patients with diabetes mellitus [1]. Being almost always the consequence of ulcers secondary to neuro- and vasculopathy, they have a high risk of lower extremity amputation (due to vascular reasons) [2]. Soft tissue closure is important to protect underlying structures from infection, while a persisting infection leads to flap failure. Hence, the reconstruction should be performed without persisting infection [3]. There have been many new insights on the microbiology, diagnosis, and treatment of DFIs, although the implementation of this knowledge into clinical practice has been suboptimal. Today, employing evidence-based guidelines, multidisciplinary teams, and institution-specific clinical pathways helps guide optimal care of this multifaceted problem. Patients are more often treated in the ambulatory setting, with antibiotic regimens that are more targeted, oral and shorter course, and with more conservative (but earlier) surgical interventions.

F. W. A. Waibel
Department of Orthopedic Surgery, Balgrist University Hospital, Zürich, Switzerland
e-mail: felix.waibel@balgrist.ch

İ. Uçkay (✉)
Infectiology, Clinical Research UCAR, Balgrist University Hospital, Zürich, Switzerland
e-mail: ilker.uckay@balgrist.ch

J. P. Hong, H. Suh (eds.), *Diabetic Foot Reconstruction*,
https://doi.org/10.1007/978-981-16-9816-3_4

New diagnostic and therapeutic methods are being developed at an accelerating pace [4]. This chapter reviews the diagnosis and treatment of DFI, including for DFO.

4.2 Infection Matters Regarding Diabetic Foot Reconstruction

Plastic reconstruction in diabetic feet is linked to DFI in mutual ways. On the prevention side, surgeons reconstruct to restore an intact skin barrier that ultimately protects deep structures from infection [3]. The functioning diabetic flap may significantly increase the overall 5-year survival of the affected diabetic foot, when compared to patients with direct major amputations from the start [5, 6]. On the therapeutic side, the absence of an underlying infection is of paramount importance for graft survival [3]. Hence, the first step in the diabetic foot reconstruction is infection control [7, 8]. Any infected soft tissue or bone must be removed [7, 9, 10]. A systematic review of 18 studies identified infection as the main cause for early flap loss [11] in contrast to non-infected flaps, for which anastomotic failures, local thromboses, and local arteriopathies [12] remain the main causes of flap failure [11].

4.3 Diagnosing Infection

A variety of classifications has been proposed for DFIs, mostly being part of broader classifications for diabetic foot ulcers [1, 13, 14]. The Infectious Diseases Society of America (IDSA) and the International Working Group on the Diabetic Foot (IWGDF) developed guidelines specifically aimed to define and classify DFI, and thereby and guide therapy. The IWGDF-PEDIS-classification (an acronym standing for perfusion, extent [size], depth, infection, and sensation/neuropathy) suggests a semi-quantitative four-point scale to describe infection that can be used for including patients in research studies but also appears to help predict the outcome of a DFI [13].

Of note, superficial microbiological culture results alone do not define infection, because all open wounds are colonized with microorganisms. Even quantitative microbiological results such as the presence of $\geq 10^5$ colony forming units/gram of tissue do not define DFI. In consequence, the diagnosis of DFI must base on clinical findings: new or progressive redness, warmth, induration, pain, tenderness and/or purulence (see Fig. 4.1). Some authors suggest to add findings like wound friability, undermining or poor granulation tissue, foul odor or unexpectedly slow healing as signs of infection. Of note, many of these signs are subjective and can be provoked by other non-infectious differential diagnoses such as acute gout, acute ischemia, or acute Charcot neuro-arthropathy [15, 16]. Contrary to many soft tissue infections outside of the diabetic foot, systemic inflammatory signs (fever, chills, hypotension, delirium), elevated serum inflammatory markers (leukocytosis, sedimentation rate (ESR), C-protein, pro-calcitonin) and positive blood cultures are unusual in (chronic) DFI [16, 17]. Microbiological tests from deep infected tissues, bone, or franc pus depict the cornerstone in diagnosis and guidance of DFI treatment. In order to avoid false-positive results due to colonizing species, only deep (intraoperative) samples should be taken after cleaning and the debriding the wound. The best material would be non-necrotic tissue or even pus from deep.

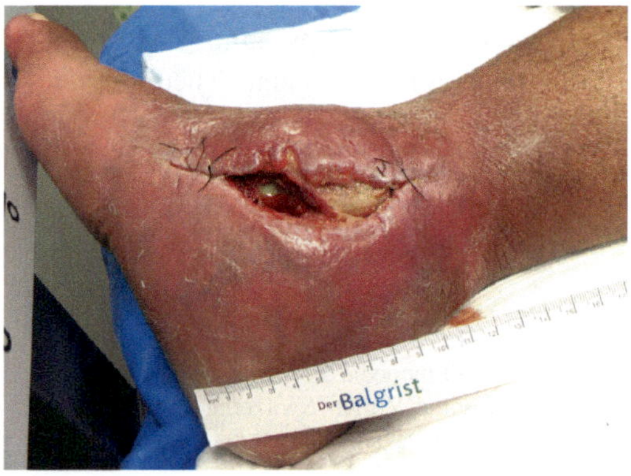

Fig. 4.1 Right foot of a 62-year-old male patient with a diabetic Charcot foot. Soft tissue infection and underlying osteomyelitis. Please note the large wound over the medial hindfoot with frayed wound borders. At the bottom of the wound, a cement spacer can be seen. Image published with the permission of the patient

Superficial microbiological swabs are futile [16], as they reveal more different bacteria (contamination or colonizing bacteria most likely) than deep tissue samples and miss many pathogens like anaerobic bacteria [16, 18].

The only virtually pathognomonic clinical sign for the diagnosis of DFO is the presence of fragments of bone discharging from a wound. This is only possible in advanced infections related to ulcers; and rare. Usually, a DFO is suspected and later confirmed. Blood tests have little value in diagnosing DFO. Large, deep, or chronic wounds (persisting for ≥3 months) or red and swollen toes ("sausage toe") should raise the suspicion of DFO. A simple diagnostic approach is the probe-to-bone test. The clinician uses a sterile blunt metal probe to determine, whether bone can be palpated through the diabetic foot ulcer. A negative test does not completely rule out DFO, while a positive test has high predictive value for bone infection [19, 20]. Although needle puncture of deep soft tissue near bone does not reliably predict the results of bone cultures, puncture of the bone itself may be an easy way to obtain bone culture at the bedside [21]. When DFO is suspected, two separate positive deep bony microbiological samples showing the same bacteria may sometimes confirm the DFO [22]. One or two weeks of "antibiotic free window" before biopsy or surgery are recommended to avoid false-negative results if chronic DFO is suspected [23]. Of note, the microbiological confirmation of DFO is not necessary when the infected area is amputated in toto [24].

Concerning imaging, plain radiographs should be the first imaging modality for every DFI and DFO. Erosions of the osseous borders are characteristic for DFO [25]. Further signs are periosteal reactions or elevations, regional osteopenia or trabecular bone patterns, especially in the calcaneum [26]. Sensitivity of the plain radiography in diagnosing DFO is low, with one review citing a pooled sensitivity of 0.54 and a specificity of 0.68 [27]. Computed tomography (CT) can guide surgical planning and combine a good sensitivity and better prize-quality ratio than Magnetic Resonance Imaging (MRI) [28]. MRI has a good sensitivity (93%) and a high specificity (79%) for diagnosing DFO prior to surgical treatment [29], but is less easily available than standard X-rays, and relatively expensive. Nuclear medicine techniques are less used since the MRI gained momentum throughout the world [30].

4.3.1 Main Pathogens

Aerobic gram-positive cocci (*Staphylococcus aureus* or β-streptococci) remain the main pathogens of community-acquired DFI in temperate areas such as Central Europe or North America [16, 31]. Depending on geographical location, prevalence of distinct pathogens is different. In many arid and tropical areas, *S. aureus* is less prevalent and gram-negative rods like *Pseudomonas aeruginosa* prevail [16]. The reasons for this geographical difference have not been elucidated, but may be related to differences in specimen types, laboratory techniques, prior antibiotic use, availability of non-prescription (over-the-counter) antibiotic agents, foot sweating and washing or reporting bias. Of note, most of these reports emanate from countries in arid and hot areas, especially India [16]. Chronic infected wounds demonstrate polymicrobial infection. An increasing likelihood has been observed for multidrug resistant organisms (MDROs) in DFI [32–34]. The leading multi-resistant pathogen in this regard has been health care-associated methicillin-resistant *S. aureus* (MRSA) two decades ago in many regions of the world. However, the current literature reports decreasing prevalence of MRSA in most countries [35]. Greater actual concern has been raised by multi-resistant gram-negative organisms that produce extended-spectrum β-lactamases or carbapenemases. The impact of fungi in DFI is anecdotic [33, 36, 37].

4.4 Management of Diabetic Foot Infection

4.4.1 Initial Multidisciplinary Approach

Generally, DFIs require a multidisciplinary approach, of debridement (or professional wound care), systemic antibiotic therapy and off-loading are the minimal cornerstones [38]. Revascularization of macroangiopathic arterial stenoses, before or after the surgical intervention, is frequently needed in up to 20% of DFIs [16]. The vascular assessment is highlighted in Chaps. 2 and 7. A first surgical drainage-debridement is particularly important for abscesses, necrotizing fasciitis and for a substantial proportion of DFO cases [39]. Procedures, such as the correction of foot deformities, arthrodesis [40] or combination of correction and debridement for infection [41], may serve to prevent future DFIs. Chaps. 5 and 6 resumes surgical debridement (Chap. 5) and deformity correction (Chap. 6) in detail. Table 4.1 resumes key aspects in the previous and modern managements of DFI.

4.4.2 Antibiotic Therapies for Soft Tissue Infections of the Diabetic Foot

We need systemic antibiotic therapy for the treatment of DFI. As it may fail as a sole modality, it is usually combined with one or more surgical procedures, off-loading and proper wound care. Initial antibiotic treatment is empirical in most cases. It bases on epidemiological features, knowledge of the local resistance patterns, and the infection severity [38]. Several principles help selecting an appropriately regimen [42]. In case of severe infections, or if the patient has failed to respond to a prior narrower-spectrum antibiotic regimen, therapy could target presumed Gram-negative pathogens as well. In case of gangrenous wounds, antibiotics covering anaerobes are recommended [18, 42]. If cultures grow multiple organisms, it is often sufficient to treat the major pathogens (e.g., *S. aureus*, streptococci, *Enterobacteriaceae*). Skin pathogens (coagulase-negative staphylococci, corynebacteria, or *Bacillus* spp.) can be dismissed in most cases, especially in the absence of osteosynthetic

Table 4.1 Key elements in the management of diabetic foot infections (*authors' personal summary*)

Research field	Established today	Potential developments in the future
Pathogens of concern	*Staphylococcus aureus*, streptococci	Multidrug resistant organisms. Gram-negative pathogens in (sub)tropical climates
Microbiological diagnosis	Standard cultures, usually of swab specimens	No changes, except research of microbioma for academic reasons
Imaging	Plain X-rays	Magnetic resonance imaging for preoperative planification?
Antibiotic agents	Amino-penicillins, cephalosporins, fluoroquinolones	Antibiotic stewardship efforts, carbapenems, rifampicin?
Route of administration	Initial intravenous administration, usually in hospital	Oral (sometimes after brief intravenous course)
Duration of antibiotic therapy	Few weeks for soft tissues; ≥6–12 weeks for bone	1–2 weeks for soft tissue infections, 3–6 weeks for osteomyelitis
Surgical approach	Aggressive (ablative) therapeutic surgery; inpatient	Corrective and reconstructive surgery
Revascularization	Open vascular surgery	More percutaneous angioplasty
Management	Mostly individual, empirical approaches	Guidelines based on systematic reviews. Multidisciplinary teams
Scientific publications	Mostly case series and epidemiological surveys	More prospective randomized trials, multicenter studies

Adapted from reference Uçkay et al. [4]

material [43, 44]. Likewise, skin colonization with health-care-associated MRSA does not necessitate empiric coverage of this organism, even in the presence of foreign material [45, 46].

As most DFI go along with some degree of peripheral arterial disease, the question remains whether antibiotic agents penetrate sufficiently. Standard doses of most β-lactam antibiotics achieve relatively low but likely therapeutic tissue levels. Clindamycin, fluoroquinolones, linezolid, rifampin, and to some degree, tetracyclines and co-trimoxazole offer good oral bioavailability together with an acceptable penetration in bone, synovia, biofilm, and necrotic tissue [22, 43]. In consequence, oral absorption of commonly used antibiotics is usually sufficient for oral antibiotic therapy in mild to moderate DFIs [47]. Randomized trials in DFI have failed to show superiority of one particular antibiotic agent or route of administration [48–50]. Today, the evidence is too weak to recommend any particular antimicrobial agent [51] or any particular route of delivery or duration of antibiotic therapy [52, 53]. Currently, the authors of this Chapter lead two randomized trials investigating shorter durations in DFI and DFO [54]. Table 4.2 displays suggested antibiotic regimens based on the IDSA guidelines [55].

4.4.3 Topical Anti-infective Wound Care for Soft Tissue Infections of the Diabetic Foot

Many studies have assessed topical disinfectants or antiseptics for the treatment of DFI, including compounds with silver, povidone, or hypochlorite [4]. The majority of these studies used ulcer healing, rather than resolution or prevention of infection, as the primary outcome. None of these agents has demonstrated superior outcomes compared to non-antiseptic dressings. Likewise, recent systematic reviews have found that various other dressings, such as foam, hydrocolloid, or alginate, offer no advantage over other dressings for ulcer healing or resolution of infection [4]. Thus, as was true three decades ago, dressing changes with simple gauze and saline solution alone appears to be sufficient for most patients.

4.4.4 Management of Necrotizing Fasciitis of the Diabetic Foot

Usually, DFI soft tissue infections evolve during several days before becoming dangerous [56]. In contrast, a special clinical entity among the groups of soft tissue DFI is "necrotizing fasciitis"

Table 4.2 Suggested antibiotic regimens (*author's choices*)

Severity of infection	Expected pathogens	(Empirical) antibiotic agents	Administration route
Mild	*S. aureus*, Streptococci	Cephalosporins, clindamycin, co-amoxiclav	Oral
Moderate	*S. aureus*, Streptococci *Enterobacteriaceae*	Co-amoxiclav	Oral or parenteral (to start)
Severe	All pathogens,	Co-amoxiclav, piperacillin-tazobactam, carbapenem	Parenteral, with later oral switch when stable
Bacteremic	No empiric therapy, since pathogen known	Based on culture and sensitivity results	Parenteral
Chronic osteomyelitis	All pathogens	Based on bone culture	Oral

Inspired from the reference Lipsky et al. [55]

(NF). NF is an hyper-acute soft tissue infection. We have never witnessed a NF issuing from a chronic DFO. Plastic surgery is particularly involved with reconstruction in the aftermath of infection. The rapid tissue necrosis often leads to systemic sepsis, toxic-shock-like syndrome and multi-organ failure. NF in diabetic patients is usually polymicrobial and most often involves both aerobic organisms (especially *Streptococcus pyogenes*) [57]. Using multivariable analysis, one study of patients with NF found that the presence of diabetes was associated with a significantly increased risk of amputation [57]. Treatment of NF requires rapid fluid and electrolyte corrections, hemodynamic stabilization, support for failing organ systems and appropriate parenteral antibiotic therapy. Several different regimens of antibiotics have been recommended, and the choice may be institution dependent. In general, we consider broad-spectrum agents, such as piperacillin-tazobactam, or carbapenems, or vancomycin MRSA is suspected. In addition, early aggressive surgical debridement (often repeated to ensure all necrotic tissue has been removed) is usually necessary. Various adjunctive treatments, including hyperbaric oxygen therapy or intravenous immunoglobulins, have been used, but the efficacy of each is unclear [57].

4.4.5 Antibiotic Treatment for Non-amputated Diabetic Foot Osteomyelitis

As non-resected DFOs genuinely require long antibiotic treatments, it is important to identify the underlying pathogen(s). The optimal duration of antibiotic therapy for DFO is uncertain. A systematic review of chronic osteomyelitis in adult patients, with and without diabetes, found no evidence for a better outcome with antibiotic therapies for more than 4–6 weeks compared with shorter regimens, including for the diabetic foot [58]. In the diabetic foot, a recent single-center evaluation with 1018 episodes of DFI and DFO equally failed to determine an optimal duration of systemic antibiotic administration in terms of remission of infection [59]. A small, randomized-controlled study found that 6 weeks compared with 12 weeks of treatment of diabetic foot osteomyelitis produced similar results [60].

There are hundreds of reports of apparently successful treatment without surgery. Thus, when the patient or the medical team prefers to avoid surgery, a trial of exclusively antibiotic therapy is reasonable. But, the advantages of surgical therapy (especially in case of toe amputations), including the relatively short lengths of hospital stay, reduced antibiotic consumption and likely higher remission rates, should be weighed against the potential risks. The risk of clinical and radiological failures of the conservative approach for DFO is around 30–40% [61], albeit if the proportion of microbiological recurrences (with the same pathogens as in the index episode) is lower with approximately 20% [61]. In case with concomitant severe ischemia it might be higher.

Ideally, the treatment of DFO contains surgical debridement, or the resection of necrotic and infected bone (total amputation). A study of 50 patients with chronic toe DFO showed that patients with surgical resections had a significantly lower relapse rate [62]. This was also witnessed in the aforementioned single-center survey with partial amputations [59]. In well-selected patients and neuropathic DFO cases without progressive ischemia, other studies report successful treatment without surgery, with selected remission rates of 60–70% [63, 64]. When surgery is avoided for different reasons, a trial of exclusively antibiotic therapy may be reasonable. But generally, the advantages of concomitant surgical therapy, such as the reduced antibiotic consumption and higher remission rates in the average DFI patient, should be weighed against the potential risks. Of note, the proportion of antibiotic-related side effects in randomized-controlled DFI trials during a week-long therapy may compromise up to 20–30% of all DFO regimens [65]. Lastly and most importantly, in the wake of persisting underlying osteomyelitis as the main identified reason for flap failure [11], a definitive surgical removal of infected bone is paramount when reconstructive plastic surgery is planned.

4.4.6 Antibiotic Management Before and After Reconstruction

The different antibiotic approaches around the timing of elective plastic reconstruction are not evidence-based and should be subject of future research. Today, this antibiotic policy depends on the preference of the treating plastic surgeon. Some reconstruct under current antibiotic therapy and continue the therapy afterwards. Others swab the ulcer surface (often several times) to ensure the near-absence of potential pathogens colonizing the future site, and frequently postpone the elective surgery. A third group of surgeons stop eventual therapeutic antibiotics before elective reconstruction and re-start therapy after reconstruction; with the opportunity to perform intraoperative samples non-selected by ongoing antibiotic therapies.

The authors of this chapter have the following opinion: We avoid superficial sampling of future reconstruction sites before elective surgery, unless there is real, clinical, infection. The presence of bacteria in superficial samples of skin breakdowns depends on the laboratory and the localization of swabbing, and is influenced by chance. All chronic lesions are colonized with various bacteria that can just differ by the localization. This colonization does not correlate with the microorganisms of eventual future surgical site infections. Moreover, such a blind swabbing policy postpones surgery in case of positive findings which is costly and cumbersome for the hospital and patients. Instead, we propose an "antibiotic-free window" of several days before elective surgery, to sample 2–4 deep tissue specimens (not swabs) during reconstruction, and to start an empirical antibiotic therapy (if clinically necessary). This therapy can be switched to oral antibiotic regimens targeted on the intraoperative findings. The widespread intravenous administration is not necessary in the absence of franc infection (pus, cellulitis, etc.).

The post-reconstruction antibiotic therapy is justified in case of massive contamination of the surgical site, of which the duration depends on the intraoperative visual aspects, the chronicity of the problem and the past history of local and recurrent infection. The minimal post-reconstruction antibiotic duration relies on the experience of the surgeon. It can be as short as 3 days (in analogy to acute open fractures [66]) or prolonged for some days. In any case and according to current knowledge, the utmost duration is 6 weeks (unless the infection is due to mycobacteria, actinomyces, or fungi). In osteoarticular infectiology, any antibiotic administration beyond 6 weeks for usual pyogenic bacteria is futile [67]. Because after this time, chemistry alone will not heal the problem without new surgical debridement. This utmost limit of 6 weeks is valid for every plastic surgery, even for sacral osteomyelitis coverage with higher risks of recurrence than for diabetic foot plastic surgery [68].

4.5 Adjunctive Treatments

4.5.1 Hyperbaric Oxygen Therapy

The value of hyperbaric oxygen therapy (HBOT) for DFI continues to be hotly debated. A 2012 Cochrane systematic review concluded that HBOT significantly increased ulcer healing in the short term, but not the long term; because of the flawed trials, however, they were not confident in the results [69]. Some studies suggest that HBOT facilitates wound healing and decreases rates of lower extremity amputation in diabetic patients with a foot ulcer or postsurgical amputation wound, but most experience is retrospective and non-comparative. There are, however, no published data directly related to the effect of HBOT for infectious aspects (either soft tissue or bone) of the diabetic foot [4].

4.5.2 Off-Loading

Off-loading pressure from an ulcer is critical to getting it to heal, including those that are infected [4]. This was, is, and will be the cornerstone of both treatment and secondary prevention. The criterion standard method for off-loading, the total contact cast, leads to ulcer healing in over 90% of cases, and has been available for decades. For patients with little or no foot deformity, prefabricated extra depth footwear with a stiff rocker bottom walking sole is usually sufficient. Cases with moderate deformity may require custom-made shoes with custom-molded, full contact insoles. Off-loading can be partial and surgical, e.g., performing a flexor-tenotomy in a patient with claw toes. An elective surgical approach may be right when conservative therapy has failed to prevent severe deformity or joint instability or in the presence of ulcerating hammer and claw toes. Clinicians should generally explain to the patient the benefit of off-loading [4].

4.6 Conclusion

The diagnosis of DFI is based on clinical aspects (with additional radiology for DFO); not on the microbiology of superficial swabs or serum inflammatory markers. The microbiology identifies the pathogens and is of confirmatory nature regarding the diagnosis in the soft tissues, but decisive for the bone. The treatment is multidisciplinary resuming iterative debridement, surgery in its multiple forms, professional wound care, antibiotic therapy, strict off-loading, and eventual revascularization. Most antibiotics can be given orally for approximately 1–2 weeks for soft tissue infection, and during 4–6 weeks for unresected DFO. The risk for treatment failures and infectious recurrences is high. Prevention of infection, as well as reconstructive surgeries of the altered foot, is very important.

Disclosure Statement We have nothing to disclose and no conflict of interests. There is no funding for this chapter.

References

1. Singh N, Armstrong DG, Lipsky BA. Preventing foot ulcers in patients with diabetes. JAMA. 2005;293:217–28.
2. Zingg M, Nicodème JD, Uçkay I, Ray A, Suva D. Lower limb amputation: indication, preoperative workup and complications. Rev Med Suisse. 2015;10:2409–13.
3. Clemens MW, Attinger CE. Functional reconstruction of the diabetic foot. Semin Plast Surg. 2010;24:43–56.
4. Uçkay I, Aragón-Sánchez J, Lew D, Lipsky BA. Diabetic foot infections: what have we learned in the last 30 years? Int J Infect Dis. 2015;40:81–91.
5. Oh TS, Lee HS, Hong JP. Diabetic foot reconstruction using free flaps increases 5-year-survival rate. J Plast Reconstr Aesthet Surg. 2013;66:243–50.
6. Sato T, Yana Y, Ichioka S. Free flap reconstruction for diabetic foot limb salvage. J Plast Surg Hand Surg. 2017;51:399–404.
7. Suh HS, Oh TS, Hong JP. Innovations in diabetic foot reconstruction using super-microsurgery. Diabetes Metab Res Rev. 2016;32:275–80.
8. Attinger CE, Bulan EJ. Débridement. The key initial first step in wound healing. Foot Ankle Clin. 2001;6:627–60.
9. Gonzalez MH, Weinzweig N. Muscle flaps in the treatment of osteomyelitis of the lower extremity. J Trauma. 2005;58:1019–23.
10. Ha Van G, Siney H, Danan J-P, Sachon C, Grimaldi A. Treatment of osteomyelitis in the diabetic foot: contribution of conservative surgery. Diabetes Care. 1996;19:1257–60.
11. Fitzgerald O'Connor EJ, Vesely M, Holt PJ, Jones KG, Thompson MM, Hinchliffe RJ. A systematic review of free tissue transfer in the management of non-traumatic lower extremity wounds in patients with diabetes. Eur J Vasc Endovasc Surg. 2011;41:391–9.
12. Kim HB, Altıparmak M, Pak CJ, Suh HP, Hong JP. Reconstruction using free flaps for diabetic heel defects: outcomes and risk factor analysis. J Reconstr Microsurg. 2020;36:494–500.
13. Schaper NC. Diabetic foot ulcer classification system for research purposes: a progress report on criteria for including patients in research studies. Diabetes Metab Res Rev. 2004;20:90–5.
14. Chuan F, Tang K, Jiang P, Zhou B, He X. Reliability and validity of the perfusion, extent, depth, infection and sensation (PEDIS) classification system and score in patients with diabetic foot ulcer. PLoS One. 2015;10:0124739.
15. Berli M, Vlachopoulos L, Leupi S, Böni T, Baltin C. Treatment of Charcot Neuroarthropathy and osteomyelitis of the same foot: a retrospective cohort study. BMC Musculoskelet Disord. 2017;18:460.
16. Uçkay I, Gariani K, Pataky Z, Lipsky BA. Diabetic foot infections: state-of-the-art. Diabetes Obes Metab. 2014;16:305–16.
17. Uçkay I, Garzoni C, Ferry T, Harbarth S, Stern R, Assal M, et al. Postoperative serum pro-calcitonin and C-reactive protein levels in patients with orthopedic infections. Swiss Med Wkly. 2010;140:13124.
18. Charles PG, Uçkay I, Kressmann B, Emonet S, Lipsky BA. The role of anaerobes in diabetic foot infections. Anaerobe. 2015;34:8–13.
19. Butalia S, Palda VA, Sargeant RJ, Detsky AS, Mourad O. Does this patient with diabetes have osteomyelitis of the lower extremity? JAMA. 2008;299:806–13.

20. Aragón-Sánchez J, Lipsky BA, Lázaro-Martínez JL. Diagnosing diabetic foot osteomyelitis: is the combination of probe-to-bone test and plain radiography sufficient for high-risk inpatients? Diabet Med. 2011;28:191–4.
21. Senneville E, Morant H, Descamps D, Dekeyser S, Beltrand E, Singer B, et al. Needle puncture and transcutaneous bone biopsy cultures are inconsistent in patients with diabetes and suspected osteomyelitis of the foot. Clin Infect Dis. 2009;48:888–93.
22. Bernard L, Assal M, Garzoni C, Uçkay I. Predicting the pathogen of diabetic toe osteomyelitis by two consecutive ulcer cultures with bone contact. Eur J Clin Microbiol Infect Dis. 2011;30:279–81.
23. Govaert GAM, Kuehl R, Atkins BL, Trampuz A, Morgenstern M, Obremskey WT, et al. Diagnosing fracture-related infection: current concepts and recommendations. J Orthop Trauma. 2020;34:8–17.
24. Rossel A, Lebowitz D, Gariani K, Abbas M, Kressmann B, Assal M, et al. Stopping antibiotics after surgical amputation in diabetic foot and ankle infections—a daily practice cohort. Endocrinol Diabetes Metab. 2019;2:00059.
25. Álvaro-Afonso FJ, Lázaro-Martínez JL, Aragón-Sánchez J, García-Morales E, Cecilia-Matilla A, Beneit-Montesinos JV. Interobserver and intraobserver reproducibility of plain X-rays in the diagnosis of diabetic foot osteomyelitis. Int J Low Extrem Wounds. 2013;12:12–5.
26. Waibel FWA, Uçkay I, Sairanen K, Waibel L, Berli MC, Boni T, et al. Diabetic calcaneal osteomyelitis. Infez Med. 2019;27(3):225–38.
27. Newman LG, Waller J, Palestro CJ, Schwartz M, Klein MJ, Hermann G, et al. Unsuspected osteomyelitis in diabetic foot ulcers. Diagnosis and monitoring by leukocyte scanning with indium in 111 oxyquinoline. JAMA. 1991;266(9):1246–51.
28. Pineda C, Espinosa R, Pena A. Radiographic imaging in osteomyelitis: the role of plain radiography, computed tomography, ultrasonography, magnetic resonance imaging, and scintigraphy. Semin Plast Surg. 2009;23:80–9.
29. Lauri C, Tamminga M, Glaudemans A, Juarez Orozco LE, Erba PA, Jutte PC, et al. Detection of osteomyelitis in the diabetic foot by imaging techniques: a systematic review and meta-analysis comparing MRI, white blood cell scintigraphy, and FDG-PET. Diabetes Care. 2017;40:1111–20.
30. Glaudemans AW, Uçkay I, Lipsky BA. Challenges in diagnosing infection in the diabetic foot. Diabet Med. 2015;32:748–59.
31. Gardner SE, Hillis SL, Heilmann K, Segre JA, Grice EA. The neuropathic diabetic foot ulcer microbiome is associated with clinical factors. Diabetes. 2013;62:923–30.
32. Byren I, Peters EJ, Hoey C, Berendt A, Lipsky BA. Pharmacotherapy of diabetic foot osteomyelitis. Expert Opin Pharmacother. 2009;10:3033–47.
33. Boyanova L, Mitov I. Antibiotic resistance rates in causative agents of infections in diabetic patients: rising concerns. Expert Rev Anti-Infect Ther. 2013;11:411–20.
34. Djahmi N, Messad N, Nedjai S, Moussaoui A, Mazouz D, Richard JL, et al. Molecular epidemiology of *Staphylococcus aureus* strains isolated from inpatients with infected diabetic foot ulcers in an Algerian University Hospital. Clin Microbiol Infect. 2013;19:398–404.
35. Zenelaj B, Bouvet C, Lipsky BA, Uçkay I. Do diabetic foot infections with methicillin-resistant *Staphylococcus aureus* differ from those with other pathogens? Int J Low Extrem Wounds. 2014;13:263–72.
36. Bader M, Jafri AK, Krueger T, Kumar V. Fusarium Osteomyelitis of the Foot in a Patient with Diabetes Mellitus. Scand J Infect Dis. 2003;35:895–7.
37. Missoni EM, Kalenić S, Vukelić M, De Syo D, Belicza M, Kern J, et al. [Role of yeasts in diabetic foot ulcer infection]. Acta Med Croatica 2006;60:43–50.
38. Ertuğrul B, Uçkay I, Schöni M, Peter-Riesch B, Lipsky BA. Management of diabetic foot infections in the light of recent literature and new international guidelines. Expert Rev Anti-Infect Ther. 2020;18:293–305.
39. Widatalla AH, Mahadi SE, Shawer MA, Mahmoud SM, Abdelmageed AE, Ahmed ME. Diabetic foot infections with osteomyelitis: efficacy of combined surgical and medical treatment. Diabet Foot Ankle. 2012;3 https://doi.org/10.3402/dfa.v3i0.18809.
40. Assal M, Stern R. Realignment and extended fusion with use of a medial column screw for midfoot deformities secondary to diabetic neuropathy. J Bone Joint Surg Am. 2009;91:812–20.
41. Wirth SH, Viehofer AF, Tondelli T, Hartmann R, Berli MC, Böni T, et al. Mid-term walking ability after Charcot foot reconstruction using the Ilizarov ring fixator. Arch Orthop Trauma Surg. 2020;140(12):1909–17. https://doi.org/10.1007/s00402-020-03407-5.
42. Lipsky BA. Empirical therapy for diabetic foot infections: are there clinical clues to guide antibiotic selection? Clin Microbiol Infect. 2007;13:351–3.
43. Uçkay I, Pittet D, Vaudaux P, Sax H, Lew D, Waldvogel F. Foreign body infections due to *Staphylococcus epidermidis*. Ann Med. 2009;41:109–19.
44. Richard JL, Sotto A, Jourdan N, Combescure C, Vannereau D, Rodier M, et al. Risk factors and healing impact of multidrug-resistant bacteria in diabetic foot ulcers. Diabetes Metab. 2008;34:363–9.
45. Reber A, Moldovan A, Dunkel N, Emonet S, Rohner P, Tahintzi P, et al. Should the methicillin-resistant *Staphylococcus aureus* carriage status be used as a guide to treatment for skin and soft tissue infections? J Infect. 2012;64:513–9.
46. Uçkay I, Teterycz D, Ferry T, Harbarth S, Lübbeke A, Emonet S, et al. Poor utility of MRSA screening to predict staphylococcal species in orthopaedic implant infections. J Hosp Infect. 2009;73:89–91.
47. Gariani K, Lebowitz D, Kressmann B, von Dach E, Sendi P, Waibel F, et al. Oral amoxicillin-clavulanate

for treating diabetic foot infections. Diabetes Obes Metab. 2019;21:1483–6.
48. Schaper NC, Dryden M, Kujath P, Nathwani D, Arvis P, Reimnitz P, et al. Efficacy and safety of IV/PO moxifloxacin and IV piperacillin/tazobactam followed by PO amoxicillin/clavulanic acid in the treatment of diabetic foot infections: results of the RELIEF study. Infection. 2013;41:175–86.
49. Lipsky BA, Armstrong DG, Citron DM, Tice AD, Morgenstern DE, Abramson MA. Ertapenem versus piperacillin/tazobactam for diabetic foot infections (SIDESTEP): prospective, randomised, controlled, double-blinded, multicentre trial. Lancet. 2005;366:1695–703.
50. Lipsky BA, Stoutenburgh U. Daptomycin for treating infected diabetic foot ulcers: evidence from a randomized, controlled trial comparing daptomycin with vancomycin or semi-synthetic penicillins for complicated skin and skin-structure infections. J Antimicrob Chemother. 2005;55:240–5.
51. Nelson EA, O'Meara S, Golder S, Dalton J, Craig D, Iglesias C. Systematic review of antimicrobial treatments for diabetic foot ulcers. Diabet Med. 2006;23:348–59.
52. Embil JM, Rose G, Trepman E, Math MC, Duerksen F, Simonsen JN, et al. Oral antimicrobial therapy for diabetic foot osteomyelitis. Foot Ankle Int. 2006;27:771–9.
53. Spellberg B, Lipsky BA. Systemic antibiotic therapy for chronic osteomyelitis in adults. Clin Infect Dis. 2012;54:393–407.
54. Waibel F, Berli M, Catanzaro S, Sairanen K, Schoni M, Boni T, et al. Optimization of the antibiotic management of diabetic foot infections: protocol for two randomized controlled trials. Trials. 2020;21:54.
55. Lipsky BA, Berendt AR, Cornia PB, Pile JC, Peters EJ, Armstrong DG, et al. 2012 Infectious Diseases Society of America clinical practice guideline for the diagnosis and treatment of diabetic foot infections. Clin Infect Dis. 2012;54:132–73.
56. Tobalem M, Uçkay I. Evolution of a diabetic foot infection. New Engl J Med. 2013;369:2252.
57. Dworkin MS, Westercamp MD, Park L, McIntyre A. The epidemiology of necrotizing fasciitis including factors associated with death and amputation. Epidemiol Infect. 2009;137:1609–14.
58. Lazzarini L, Lipsky BA, Mader JT. Antibiotic treatment of osteomyelitis: what have we learned from 30 years of clinical trials? Int J Infect Dis. 2005;9:127–38.
59. Gariani K, Lebowitz D, von Dach E, Kressmann B, Lipsky BA, Uçkay I. Remission in diabetic foot infections: duration of antibiotic therapy and other possible associated factors. Diabetes Obes Metab. 2019;21:244–51.
60. Tone A, Nguyen S, Devemy F, Topolinski H, Valette M, Cazaubiel M, et al. Six-week versus twelve-week antibiotic therapy for nonsurgically treated diabetic foot osteomyelitis: a multicenter open-label controlled randomized study. Diabetes Care. 2015;38:302–7.
61. Lebowitz D, Gariani K, Kressmann B, Dach EV, Huttner B, Bartolone P, et al. Are antibiotic-resistant pathogens more common in subsequent episodes of diabetic foot infection? Int J Infect Dis. 2017;59:61–4.
62. Simpson AH, Deakin M, Latham JM. Chronic osteomyelitis. The effect of the extent of surgical resection on infection-free survival. J Bone Joint Surg Br. 2001;83:403–7.
63. Pittet D, Wyssa B, Herter-Clavel C, Kursteiner K, Vaucher J, Lew PD. Outcome of diabetic foot infections treated conservatively: a retrospective cohort study with long-term follow-up. Arch Intern Med. 1999;159:851–6.
64. Jeffcoate WJ, Lipsky BA. Controversies in diagnosing and managing osteomyelitis of the foot in diabetes. Clin Infect Dis. 2004;39:115–22.
65. Uçkay I, Kressmann B, Malacarne S, Toumanova A, Jaafar J, Lew D, et al. A randomized, controlled study to investigate the efficacy and safety of a topical gentamicin-collagen sponge in combination with systemic antibiotic therapy in diabetic patients with a moderate or severe foot ulcer infection. BMC Infect Dis. 2018;18:361.
66. Dunkel N, Pittet D, Tovmirzaeva L, Suvà D, Bernard L, Lew D, et al. Short duration of antibiotic prophylaxis in open fractures does not enhance risk of subsequent infection. Bone Joint J. 2013;95-B:831–7.
67. Bernard L, Legout L, Zürcher-Pfund L, Stern R, Rohner P, Peter R, et al. Six weeks of antibiotic treatment is sufficient following surgery for septic arthroplasty. J Infect. 2010;61:125–32.
68. Jugun K, Richard JC, Lipsky BA, Kressmann B, Pittet-Cuenod B, Suvà D, et al. Factors associated with treatment failure of infected pressure sores. Ann Surg. 2016;264:399–403.
69. Kranke P, Bennett MH, Martyn-St James M, Schnabel A, Debus SE, Weibel S. Hyperbaric oxygen therapy for chronic wounds. Cochrane Database Syst Rev. 2015;2015:004123.

Understanding Wound Bed Preparation

5

Paul J. Kim

Key Points

- Proper wound bed preparation is fundamental in achieving wound healing.
- The primary goal of wound bed preparation is to support a positive healing trajectory or to support a graft or flap.
- There are a variety of techniques, devices, and biologics available that can accelerate wound bed preparation.
- Excisional debridement is fundamental to wound bed preparation.

5.1 Introduction

Wound bed preparation is essential for the next stage of wound healing. This next stage may include an application of a bioengineered alternative tissue, primary closure, autologous skin graft, local flap, or free tissue transfer. In some instances, the wound may be left to heal through secondary intention. A wound bed must be maximally perfused with low bioburden to increase the odds of success. This may include vascular intervention, the use of negative pressure wound therapy (NPWT) with or without instillation, antibiosis, or the use of topical antiseptics. The use of classification systems is helpful to assess and describe the wound, and there are a variety of ulcer classification systems utilized (Table 5.1) [1–3]. These systems include descriptions of aspects of the wound including depth, infection, and ischemia. None of the currently utilized classification systems are all encompassing and do not describe the impact of biomechanical influences or make treatment recommendations. In addition to local factors, the patient's comorbidities must be addressed. For example, a diabetic patient must have blood glucose control to decrease complication rates including surgical site infections [4, 5]. Nutrition must also be addressed to support a healing environment [6]. The goal is to achieve a wound bed that is ready to support ultimate healing.

Appropriate wound bed preparation can be achieved through a variety of methods including serial clinic-based sharp debridement, surgical excisional debridement in the operating room, use of negative pressure wound therapy with or without instillation, or application of a bioengineered alternative tissue to create a neodermis.

Supplementary Information The online version contains supplementary material available at [https://doi.org/10.1007/978-981-16-9816-3_5].

P. J. Kim (✉)
Department of Plastic Surgery and Department of Orthopedic Surgery, Wound Program, University of Texas Southwestern, Dallas, TX, USA
e-mail: Paul.Kim@UTSouthwestern.edu

J. P. Hong, H. Suh (eds.), *Diabetic Foot Reconstruction*,
https://doi.org/10.1007/978-981-16-9816-3_5

Table 5.1 Diabetic foot ulcer classifications

Wagner and Meggitt	
Grade 0	Intact skin; hyperkeratotic lesion around or under bony deformity
Grade 1	Superficial ulcer; base may be necrotic or viable with early granulation tissue
Grade 2	Deep lesion extending to bone, ligament, tendon, joint capsule, or deep fascia; no abscess or osteomyelitis
Grade 3	Deep abscess, osteitis, or osteomyelitis
Grade 4	Portion of the toes or forefoot is gangrenous (moist or dry)
Grade 5	Complete involvement of foot; no foot healing or local procedure possible

The University of Texas at San Antonio Ulcer Classification				
	Grade 0	Grade 1	Grade 2	Grade 3
Stage A	Pre- or post-ulcerative lesions completely epithelialized	Superficial wound not involving tendon, capsule, or bone	Wound penetrating to tendon or capsule	Wound penetrating to bone or joint
Stage B	Infected	Infected	Infected	Infected
Stage C	Ischemic	Ischemic	Ischemic	Ischemic
Stage D	Infected and ischemic	Infected and ischemic	Infected and ischemic	Infected and ischemic

The Society for Vascular Surgery Lower Extremity Threatened Limb Classification System: Risk Stratification Based on Wound, Ischemia, and foot Infection (WIfI)			
Wound	Ulcer	Gangrene	Clinical description
Grade 0	No ulcer	No gangrene	Ischemic rest pain (requires typical symptoms + ischemia grade 3); no wound
Grade 1	Small, shallow ulcer(s) on distal leg or foot; no exposed bone, unless limited to distal phalanx	No gangrene	Minor tissue loss. Salvageable with simple digital amputation (1 or 2 digits) or skin coverage
Grade 2	Deeper ulcer with exposed bone, joint, or tendon; generally not involving the heel; shallow heel ulcer without calcaneal involvement	Gangrenous changes limited to digits	Major tissue loss salvageable with multiple (≥3) digital amputation or standard TMA ± skin coverage
Grade 3	Extensive, deep ulcer involving forefoot and/or midfoot; deep, full thickness heel ulcer ± calcaneal involvement	Extensive gangrene involving forefoot and/or midfoot; full thickness heel necrosis ± calcaneal involvement	Extensive tissue loss salvageable only with a complex foot reconstruction or nontraditional TMA (Chopart or LisFranc); flap coverage or complex wound management needed for large soft tissue defect
Ischemia	ABI	Ankle systolic pressure	TP, $TcPO_2$
Grade 0	≥0.80	>100 mmHg	≥60 mmHg
Grade 1	0.6–0.79	70–100 mmHg	40–59 mmHg
Grade 2	0.4–0.59	50–70 mmHg	30–39 mmHg
Grade 3	≤0.39	<50 mmHg	<30 mmHg
Foot infection	Clinical manifestation of infection	SVS	IDSA/PEDIS infection severity
No symptoms or signs of infection		0	Uninfected

Table 5.1 (continued)

The Society for Vascular Surgery Lower Extremity Threatened Limb Classification System: Risk Stratification Based on Wound, Ischemia, and foot Infection (WIfI)			
Wound	Ulcer	Gangrene	Clinical description
Infection present, as defined by the presence of at least 2 of the following items: • Local swelling or induration • Erythema >0.5 to ≤2 cm around the ulcer • Local tenderness or pain • Local warmth • Purulent discharge (thick, opaque to white, or serosanguinous) Local infection involving only the skin and the subcutaneous tissue (without involvement of deeper tissues or without systemic signs described below) Exclude other causes of an inflammatory response of the skin (e.g., trauma, gout, acute Charcot neuro-arthropathy, fracture, thrombosis, venous stasis)		1	Mild
Local infection(as described above) with erythema >2 cm, or involving structures deeper than skin and subcutaneous tissues (e.g., abscess, osteomyelitis, septic arthritis, fasciitis) No systemic inflammatory response signs (as described below)		2	Moderate
Local infection (as described above with the signs of SIRS, manifested by two or more of the following: • Temperature > 38° or < 36 °C. • Heart rate > 90 beats/min • Respiratory rate > 20 breaths/min or $PaCO_2$ < 32 mmHg • White blood cell count >12,000 or < 4000 cu/mm or 10% immature (band) forms		3	Severe

TMA transmetatarsal amputation, *ABI* ankle-brachial index, *PVR* pulse volume recording, *SPP* skin perfusion pressure, *TP* toe pressure, *tcPO₂* transcutaneous oximetry, *SVS* Society for Vascular Surgery, *IDSA* Infectious Disease Society of America, *IWGDF* International Working Group on the Diabetic Foot, *PEDIS* perfusion, extent/size, depth/tissue loss, infection, sensation, *$PACO_2$* partial pressure of arterial carbon dioxide, *SIRS* systemic inflammatory response syndrome

There are more conservative methods for wound bed preparation including the use of collagenases, maggot therapy, or wet-to-dry dressing changes [7]. A novel perforated foam design for negative pressure wound therapy with instillation has also been introduced to accelerate removal of nonviable tissue [8]. All these approaches attempt to remove nonviable tissue, decrease bacterial bioburden, increase local perfusion, and release prohealing cells and proteins. The focus of this chapter will be on the surgical approach to wound bed preparation.

There are key indicators that allow the surgeon to identify whether or not the wound has been sufficiently prepared for the next stage. Infection is a key indicator that the wound is not sufficiently prepared. The surrounding tissue must not have signs of infection which include increased drainage, purulence, malodor, erythema, edema, calor, or dolor. In an immunocompromised host, these classic signs or symptoms (including malaise, flu-like symptoms, fever, nausea, vomiting) may not be present. It is especially concerning when, for example, a diabetic patient with peripheral neuropathy and an infected foot ulcer presents with pain or their blood glucose elevates significantly. In this population it is often malodor that may signal the presence of an infection. All wounds have some degree of serous drainage (except in cases of dry gangrene); however, frank purulence, liquified tissue, or a sudden increase in the amount of drainage may indicate an infection. The wound is deemed appropriately prepared when there is visible evidence of granulation tissue and the absence of necrotic or nonviable tissue as well as the absence of the above. A bed of granulation tissue should not be thought of as a goal but rather as an indicator that the wound bed has low bioburden and is adequately perfused.

Laboratory markers may not be a good indicator of infection in the immunocompromised host. The white blood cell count may not be elevated until later stages of infection. Further, markers of inflammation including C-reactive protein and erythrocyte sedimentation rate may not be helpful in infection diagnosis, but down-trending of these markers can indicate waning infection. Radiographic markers of gas and bone destruction on plain films are clear and unambiguous indicators. Advanced imaging utilizing computer tomography, magnetic resonance imaging, and indium-labeled scan can be helpful but often is unnecessary. A gestalt approach that includes assessing the clinical signs and symptoms, laboratory makers, radiographic findings, and the patient's wound and medical history should be utilized to ensure that wound bed is sufficiently prepared.

5.2 Pre-operative Evaluation and Special Considerations

Maximizing perfusion to the wound bed is critical. Both global and regional/local perfusion should be assessed. This may include the assessment and optimization of cardiac function. Regional/local perfusion assessment should be performed that escalates from a hand-held doppler to contrast angiography. Chronic lower extremity wounds often have compromised perfusion to the wound and surrounding tissue. Diagnostic angiography can assist in determining the areas of ischemia. If intervention via open bypass or angioplasty is not possible, then the diagnostic angiogram will still provide vital information necessary in planning soft tissue reconstruction. Optimally, if revascularization is possible, the target should be to the affected angiosome [9]. There is no consensus as to the timing of wound bed closure or coverage after vascular intervention [10, 11]. In the author's opinion, generally, if an angioplasty is performed it is recommended to delay closure or coverage for a period of 3–7 days. Further, it is recommended to perform wound coverage or closure as soon as possible after this initial period in order to maximize the window of arterial intervention patency. Venous disease can also contribute to nonhealing ulcers in the lower extremity. An obstruction in the venous system or incompetent valves can contribute to retarding the conversion of a wound to a healthier state. Thus, a complete venous system work-up that includes ultrasonography with appropriate intervention including venous ablation as well as compression therapy may be needed.

Vascular intervention is a reliable method of improving arterial flow for larger vessels. However, in some instances (e.g., diabetes) small vessels are also compromised. This is important because of the arterioles and capillaries that directly feed the wound bed. It is true that opening larger vessels can assist in opening the smaller vessels by increasing the velocity of flow to the smaller vessels and opening up of choke vessels. However, this may not be sufficient. Other methods have been proposed that can enhance local perfusion such as hyperbaric oxygen therapy (HBO). There is some evidence to support the use of HBO to increase flap survival post free tissue transfer [12, 13]. It can also be used in preparation of wound closure or coverage including in areas of irradiated tissue [14]. The efficacy of HBO in healing diabetic foot ulcers remains controversial [15]. There are limitations to HBO therapy including narrow indications, contraindications, the need for multiple serial treatments, and potential adverse effects.

Bacterial contamination/infection in the form of biofilm and planktonic bacteria can delay wound bed conversion to a healthy state as well as cause complications post closure or coverage. The use of antibiotics is effective against planktonic bacteria but has limited efficacy on biofilm due to the biofilm's decreased metabolic state [16]. Further, if there is arterial compromise the antibiotic may not be able to reach the target tissue. There are also other limitations in identifying and speciating the offending bacteria. Classic swab culturing methods may not accurately represent the offending bacteria [17]. Sampling should include tissue obtained from the deepest margins of the wound which may provide more accurate representation of the offending bacteria. Further, biofilm cannot be captured utilizing the standard agar culturing technique. More advanced culturing methods utilizing quantitative polymerase chain reaction (qPCR) can capture and identify bacteria in biofilm form. This technique also has limitations including its limited availability and the results may provide excessive information with identifying hundreds of species of bacteria that may not be relevant to the clinical scenario.

Topical antimicrobials can be used to decrease the amount of bacteria counts on the surface of the wound. This includes the use of neomycin/polymyxin, gentamycin, mupirocin, and compounds including polyhexanide. The effectiveness/efficacy of these products in chronic wounds is unclear [18]. The topical antibiotic formulations still have the same limitations as oral or parenteral antibiotics in its inability to impact biofilm due to their mechanism of action. Further, the majority of topical antibiotics are petrolatum base which acts as a barrier to exudate release into the dressing which can cause periwound maceration and subsequent loss of skin integrity. The use of antiseptic solutions can impact both planktonic bacteria and surface biofilm (Table 5.2). Antiseptics are often used as wound washes via irrigating the solution over the wound for a short period. However, to maximize the effects of antiseptics a longer contact time is needed through a soaked gauze medium placed or packed onto/into the wound for greater than 10 min [19–21]. Antiseptics typically lyse cells and require contact with differing levels of efficacy depending on the type of bacteria. For example, dilute acetic acid is more effective against gram-negative bacteria than gram-positive bacteria [22], whereas Dakins solution has a long history and has demonstrated efficacy against a broad spectrum of microbes [23]. Biofilm can be deeply embedded into the tissue. Thus, antiseptics cannot reach the biofilm without debridement. Further, long-term antiseptic use can have deleterious effects on healthy tissue and can delay healing [24].

Table 5.2 Examples of commonly used antiseptic solutions

Solution	Formulation and typical concentrations
Chlorhexidine	Chlorhexidine gluconate (0.005–0.05%)
Dakin's solution	Dilute sodium hypochlorite (0.025–0.05%)
Dilute vinegar	Dilute acetic acid (0.25–1%)
Dilute betadine	Povidone-iodine (0.5–1%)
Hypochlorous acid	Water 99.57%, sodium chloride 0.4%, Hypochlorous acid 0.025%, sodium chlorate 0.001%
Polyhexanide with betaine	Polyaminopropyl biguanide 0.1% and undecylenamidopropyl betaine 0.1%

Medical optimization is critical for wound bed preparation. Beyond better blood glucose management in diabetic patients, often patients with chronic diseases are nutritionally compromised. Specifically, protein deficiency can have significant deleterious effect on wound healing. Classic markers of malnutrition such as prealbumin, albumin, and total protein may not accurately reflect a patient's nutritional state [25, 26]. These laboratory markers are often diluted if the patient is in an inflammatory state. Thus, these laboratory markers can be used to track trends which assists in timing for surgical planning.

5.3 Approach to Wound Bed Preparation

Excisional debridement is fundamental to wound healing [27]. Excisional debridement removes surface contaminants and nonviable tissue and activates the coagulation cascade which mobilizes proteins and growth factors that converts the wound from a chronic state into an acute state (Table 5.3). A surgical approach to wound care differs from that of nonsurgical approach. A nonsurgical approach includes serial clinic-based sharp wound debridement and the reliance on topical therapies and dressings [28]. Generally, the nonsurgical goal is healing through secondary intension, although a referral to a surgeon for final closure or coverage is sometimes conducted. Alternatively, a surgeon may perform the above activities but also includes an operating room-based approach of one-stage or multi-staged excisional debridement that terminates in closure or coverage of the wound. There are advantages and limitations to both approaches (Table 5.4) (Fig. 5.1). The surgical approach is preferred for larger, deeper, or more complex wounds. However, a patient may not be a surgical candidate due to a variety of reasons including the risk of anesthesia or the patient declines surgical intervention. Other factors include practical matters including limited availability to the operating room or limited access to qualified surgeons.

The algorithm for a surgically based approach varies from surgeon to surgeon and institution to institution. There is no widely adopted singular approach. Multiple factors may dictate the algorithm utilized and should

Table 5.3 Goals of debridement

Removal of inhibitory healing factors (matrix metalloproteinases)
Growth factor activation
Removal of fibrotic/indurated tissue
Removal of tissue *likely* to become infected
Removal of infected tissue
Disruption of biofilm
Pressure relief- edge effect

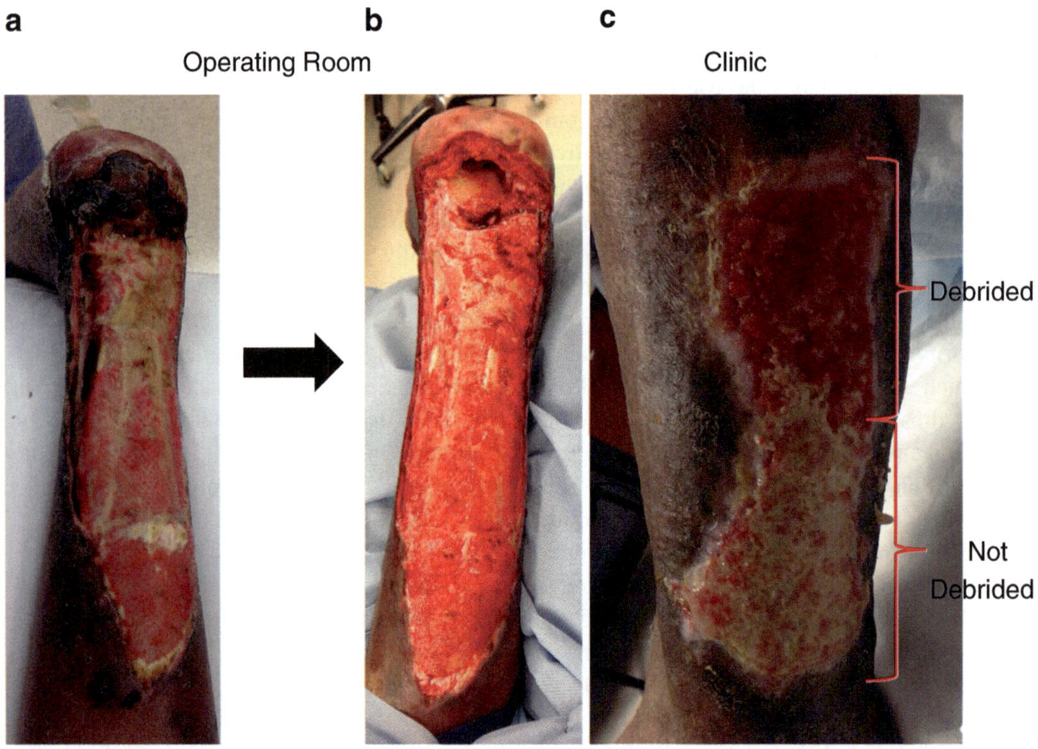

Fig. 5.1 (**a**) depicts a posterior leg wound prior to excisional debridement in the operating room. Note the necrotic tissue around the posterior heel as well as the necrotic tendon on the lateral border. (**b**) shows the wound after excisional debridement is performed. Note the absence of nonviable tissue and the appearance of healthy tissue. (**c**) depicts a chronic lateral leg wound managed in the clinic setting. The inferior portion depicts the nondebrided portion of the wound with significant bioburden. The superior portion has been sharply debrided. However, note the remaining islands of nonviable tissue that still remain

be individualized for the needs of the patient. In general, wounds have bacterial contamination and are perhaps acutely infected. Thus, a staged approach is a prudent to reduce or eliminate bacteria prior to closure or coverage (Fig. 5.2). The initial stage involves eliminating or reducing the amount of bacteria through decompression and excision of all nonviable tissue. The appearance of the wound, culture results, radiographic findings, as well as laboratory values should guide the surgeon as to the necessity of additional excisional debridement in the operating room. Once the wound bed is sufficiently prepared and the patient is medically optimized, the final operation is used to close or cover the wound.

Table 5.4 Advantages and limitations of clinic-based vs. surgery-based wound bed debridement

	Advantages	Limitations
Clinic-based	No regional or general anesthesia risk Nonsterile environment Convenience for the patient	Cannot be as aggressive in debridement due to limited pain management capabilities as well as risk of blood loss Nonsterile environment
Surgery-based	Can be aggressive in excisional debridement technique due to anesthesia and the ability to control bleeding Sterile environment Availability of equipment	Patient not a surgical candidate due to underlying medical condition(s) Risk of anesthesia complications Patients may elect not to undergo surgery

Generally, the technique for excisional debridement is uncomplicated. Again, the goal is to remove all infected, contaminated, as well as nonviable tissue. Nonviable tissue is defined as tissue that is necrotic, liquefied, fibrinous, and/or nonvascularized. It is important that the wound bed and the wound perimeter be excised. The approach should be conducted as if the wound is a soft tissue tumor. This mandates an aggressive

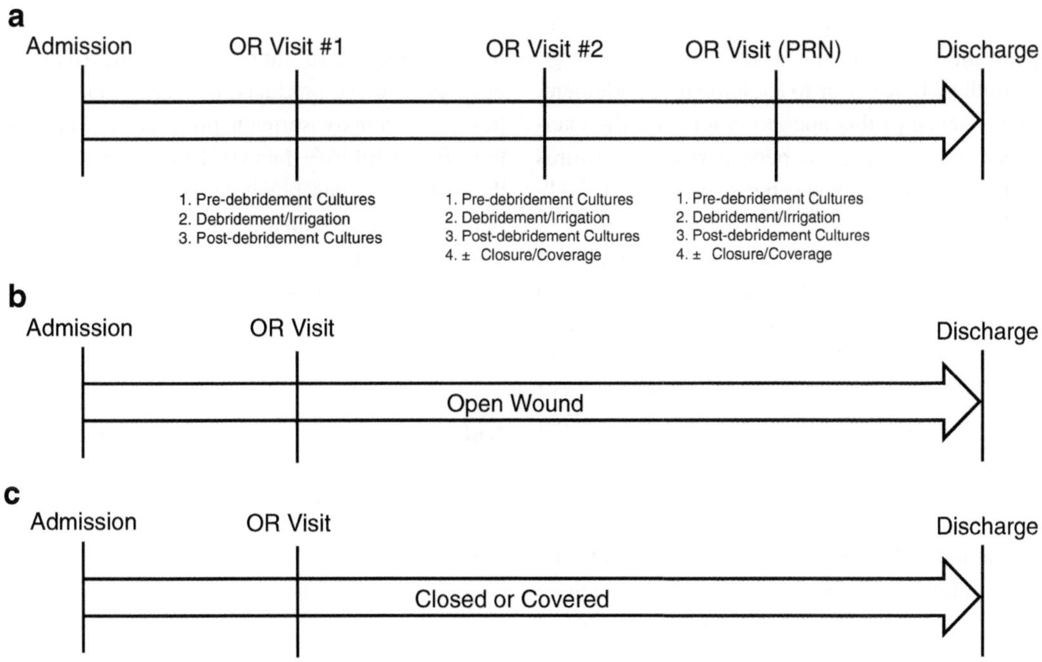

Fig. 5.2 (**a**) depicts a suggested algorithm for and infected wound. (**b**) depicts an algorithm when an initial excisional debridement is performed and the wound is not closed or covered before discharge. The patient can then have the definitive wound at a later date. (**c**) depicts an algorithm where a one stage of excisional debridement and wound closure or coverage is performed

approach with complete excision of the wound and its margins. This excision should penetrate several millimeters in depth as well as encompass several millimeters of the wound perimeter. The typical sharp instruments of a scalpel, scissors, curettes, and rongeur are utilized, but additional devices may be helpful. Contact ultrasound or a hydrosurgical scalpel can be helpful to expedite excisional debridement. These devices may have the added advantage of more precise and efficient removal of tissue. However, with both of the above devices the visual field may become obscured as well as the potential for aerosolizing bacteria during the procedure. Further, these devices may lull the surgeon into a false sense of comprehensive excision. Punctate bleeding, healthy appearing tissue, and lack of odor are cues that excisional debridement has been adequately performed. Absence or presence of certain colors can denote healthy appearing tissue. A general rule is to remove all the tissue that is not red, yellow, or white. Blue tissue can also indicate nonviable tissue unless it is identified as a vein. Another technique that may assist in confirming complete excisional debridement is to paint the surface of the wound with a dye (e.g., methylene blue) prior to excisional debridement. The absence of this applied color after the excisional debridement has been performed ensures that all surfaces have been comprehensively addressed.

The use of NPWT has been utilized for decades to accelerate wound healing to terminal epithelialization [29]. NPWT can also be used to expedite wound bed preparation for surgical coverage or closure by decreasing the dimensions of the wound as well as to build tissue over deeper exposed structures. NPWT is also used for a staged surgical approach during hospitalization in between operating room visits, after the initial excisional debridement, or at the time of discharge. Innovations to traditional NPWT include the use of intermittent installation of a topical solution which can decrease bacterial counts as well as promote greater granulation tissue growth [30–32]. Essentially, this device provides the benefits of standard NPWT combined with irrigation in a programmed fashion. Normal saline or an antiseptic can be used as the choice on solution [33]. The cycling of negative pressure and dwelling of a solution on the wound bed allows for cleansing of the wound bed between surgical debridement procedures as well as for preparation of the wound for closure or coverage. A novel foam dressing used in conjunction with NPWT with instillation encompasses large perforations in the foam dressing that can expedite removal of nonviable tissue for more efficient wound bed preparation [34].

Bioengineered alternative tissue (BAT) are products that can assist in wound bed preparation [35]. There are many categories of BATs with the class of dermoconductive agents (scaffolds) playing the most prominent role from the surgical perspective. Dermoconductive agents are acellular tissues including allografts and bioengineered animal-derived tissues (Table 5.5). These scaffolds typically produce a neodermis to cover deeper structures with planned staging to cover the area with a local flap, free tissue transfer, or autologous skin graft. These are unlike the classic xenografts used in burn surgery which is typically used as a biological dressing. There are no robust comparative studies of the effectiveness/efficacy of these products; hence, product selection is driven by surgeon preference. The cost may be prohibitive factor. However, the use of these products can preclude the need for a local flap or free tissue transfer [36]. After the neodermis is formed an autologous skin graft can be applied or the wound can be left to heal through secondary intention. The neodermis should be pink in color without any necrosis. The disadvan-

Table 5.5 Examples of commonly utilized bioengineered alternative tissues: dermoconductive agents

Tissue type	Composition
Human dermis	Acellular cadaver dermis
Bovine derived	Adult type 1 collagen ± shark chondroitin-6-sulfate Fetal type 1 and type 3 collagen
Porcine derived	Small intestine submucosa Basement membrane and subjacent lamina propria of urinary bladder
Marine derived	Acellular dermal matrix

tage of this approach is the delay between the time of application of the dermoconductive agent and the application of the flap or autologous skin graft. It takes several weeks for neodermis to form which places the wound at risk of an infection or further tissue loss may ensue during this period. A single-stage approach with application of these products in addition to an autologous skin graft has been reported but is largely relegated to clinical observations and case reports. The surgeon must ensure that bacterial count is low to ensure neodermis formation. This approach places significant demand on the wound bed for vascularization to occur; thus, adequate wound bed preparation is vitally important.

5.4 Discussion

The formation of granulation tissue is often an indicator for achieving the goal of appropriate wound bed preparation. Thus, there is hesitation of removing granulation tissue at the time of closure or coverage. It is important to understand that granulation tissue is marker of wound health and not necessarily a primary goal. There is a high likelihood that if granulation tissue developed once, it will develop again. There may be bacteria deeply imbedded in the underlying granulation tissue that must be uncovered and removed. Thus, excision of granulation tissue is recommended every time excisional debridement procedures are performed and at the time of closure or coverage.

5.5 Conclusion

Wound bed preparation is necessary for the next stage of wound healing whether it is to advance secondary healing or for closure or coverage. Wound bed preparation encompasses impacting both local and host factors. Optimization of medical comorbidities, maximizing perfusion, and minimizing bacterial burden is critical for appropriate wound bed preparation.

Disclosure Statement I am a consultant for 3M Inc. (St. Paul, MN) and Integra LifeSciences Inc. (Plainsboro NJ).

References

1. Wagner FW Jr. The dysvascular foot: a system for diagnosis and treatment. Foot Ankle. 1981;2(2):64–122.
2. Lavery LA, Armstrong DG, Harkless LB. Classification of diabetic foot wounds. J Foot Ankle Surg. 1996;35(6):528–31.
3. Mills JL Sr, Conte MS, Armstrong DG, Pomposelli FB, Schanzer A, Sidawy AN, et al. The Society for Vascular Surgery Lower Extremity Threatened Limb Classification System: risk stratification based on wound, ischemia, and foot infection (WIfI). J Vasc Surg. 2014;59(1):220–34.e1–2.
4. de Vries FE, Gans SL, Solomkin JS, Allegranzi B, Egger M, Dellinger EP, et al. Meta-analysis of lower perioperative blood glucose target levels for reduction of surgical-site infection. Br J Surg. 2017;104(2):e95–e105.
5. Hasan R, Firwana B, Elraiyah T, Domecq JP, Prutsky G, Nabhan M, et al. A systematic review and meta-analysis of glycemic control for the prevention of diabetic foot syndrome. J Vasc Surg. 2016;63(2 Suppl):22S–8S.e1–2.
6. Armstrong DG, Hanft JR, Driver VR, Smith AP, Lazaro-Martinez JL, Reyzelman AM, et al. Effect of oral nutritional supplementation on wound healing in diabetic foot ulcers: a prospective randomized controlled trial. Diabet Med. 2014;31(9):1069–77.
7. Game FL, Apelqvist J, Attinger C, Hartemann A, Hinchliffe RJ, Londahl M, et al. Effectiveness of interventions to enhance healing of chronic ulcers of the foot in diabetes: a systematic review. Diabetes Metab Res Rev. 2016;32(Suppl 1):154–68.
8. Kim PJ, Applewhite A, Dardano AN, Fernandez L, Hall K, McElroy E, et al. Use of a novel foam dressing with negative pressure wound therapy and instillation: recommendations and clinical experience. Wounds. 2018;30(3 suppl):S1–S17.
9. Neville RF, Attinger CE, Bulan EJ, Ducic I, Thomassen M, Sidawy AN. Revascularization of a specific angiosome for limb salvage: does the target artery matter? Ann Vasc Surg. 2009;23(3):367–73.
10. Steel MW, DeOrio JK. Forefoot amputation with limb revascularization: the effects of amputation, timing, and wound closure on the peripheral vascular bypass graft site. Foot Ankle Int. 2007;28(6):690–4.
11. Doyle MD, Hastings G, Dontsi M, Dionisopoulos SB, Kane LA, Pollard JD. The effects of endovascular timing and in-line flow on the success of pedal amputations. J Foot Ankle Surg. 2020;59(5):964–8.
12. Baynosa RC, Zamboni WA. The effect of hyperbaric oxygen on compromised grafts and flaps. Undersea Hyperb Med. 2012;39(4):857–65.
13. Larson JV, Steensma EA, Flikkema RM, Norman EM. The application of hyperbaric oxygen therapy in the management of compromised flaps. Undersea Hyperb Med. 2013;40(6):499–504.
14. Borab Z, Mirmanesh MD, Gantz M, Cusano A, Pu LL. Systematic review of hyperbaric oxygen therapy for the treatment of radiation-induced skin necrosis. J Plast Reconstr Aesthet Surg. 2017;70(4):529–38.

15. Zhao D, Luo S, Xu W, Hu J, Lin S, Wang N. Efficacy and safety of hyperbaric oxygen therapy used in patients with diabetic foot: a meta-analysis of randomized clinical trials. Clin Ther. 2017;39(10):2088–94 e2.
16. Wolcott R, Dowd S. The role of biofilms: are we hitting the right target? Plast Reconstr Surg. 2011;127(Suppl 1):28S–35S.
17. Wolcott RD, Cox SB, Dowd SE. Healing and healing rates of chronic wounds in the age of molecular pathogen diagnostics. J Wound Care. 2010;19(7):272–8, 0–1.
18. Peters EJ, Lipsky BA, Aragon-Sanchez J, Boyko EJ, Diggle M, Embil JM, et al. Interventions in the management of infection in the foot in diabetes: a systematic review. Diabetes Metab Res Rev. 2016;32(Suppl 1):145–53.
19. Fabry WH, Kock HJ, Vahlensieck W. Activity of the antiseptic polyhexanide against gram-negative bacteria. Microb Drug Resist. 2014;20(2):138–43.
20. Minnich KE, Stolarick R, Wilkins RG, Chilson G, Pritt SL, Unverdorben M. The effect of a wound care solution containing polyhexanide and betaine on bacterial counts: results of an in vitro study. Ostomy Wound Manage. 2012;58(10):32–6.
21. Muller G, Kramer A. Biocompatibility index of antiseptic agents by parallel assessment of antimicrobial activity and cellular cytotoxicity. J Antimicrob Chemother. 2008;61(6):1281–7.
22. Madhusudhan VL. Efficacy of 1% acetic acid in the treatment of chronic wounds infected with Pseudomonas aeruginosa: prospective randomised controlled clinical trial. Int Wound J. 2016;13(6):1129–36.
23. McCullough M, Carlson GW. Dakin's solution: historical perspective and current practice. Ann Plast Surg. 2014;73(3):254–6.
24. Punjataewakupt A, Napavichayanun S, Aramwit P. The downside of antimicrobial agents for wound healing. Eur J Clin Microbiol Infect Dis. 2019;38(1):39–54.
25. Bharadwaj S, Ginoya S, Tandon P, Gohel TD, Guirguis J, Vallabh H, et al. Malnutrition: laboratory markers vs nutritional assessment. Gastroenterol Rep (Oxf). 2016;4(4):272–80.
26. Keller U. Nutritional laboratory markers in malnutrition. J Clin Med. 2019;8(6):775.
27. Attinger CE, Bulan EJ. Debridement. The key initial first step in wound healing. Foot Ankle Clin. 2001;6(4):627–60.
28. Attinger CE, Janis JE, Steinberg J, Schwartz J, Al-Attar A, Couch K. Clinical approach to wounds: debridement and wound bed preparation including the use of dressings and wound-healing adjuvants. Plast Reconstr Surg. 2006;117(7 Suppl):72S–109S.
29. Liu Z, Dumville JC, Hinchliffe RJ, Cullum N, Game F, Stubbs N, et al. Negative pressure wound therapy for treating foot wounds in people with diabetes mellitus. Cochrane Database Syst Rev. 2018;10:CD010318.
30. Kim PJ, Silverman R, Attinger CE, Griffin L. Comparison of negative pressure wound therapy with and without instillation of saline in the management of infected wounds. Cureus. 2020;12(7):e9047.
31. Kim PJ, Lavery LA, Galiano RD, Salgado CJ, Orgill DP, Kovach SJ, et al. The impact of negative-pressure wound therapy with instillation on wounds requiring operative debridement: pilot randomised, controlled trial. Int Wound J. 2020;17(5):1194–208.
32. Rycerz AM, Allen D, Lessing MC. Science supporting negative pressure wound therapy with instillation. Int Wound J. 2013;10(Suppl 1):20–4.
33. Kim PJ, Attinger CE, Oliver N, Garwood C, Evans KK, Steinberg JS, et al. Comparison of outcomes for normal saline and an antiseptic solution for negative-pressure wound therapy with instillation. Plast Reconstr Surg. 2015;136(5):657e–64e.
34. Teot L, Boissiere F, Fluieraru S. Novel foam dressing using negative pressure wound therapy with instillation to remove thick exudate. Int Wound J. 2017;14(5):842–8.
35. Garwood CS, Steinberg JS, Kim PJ. Bioengineered alternative tissues in diabetic wound healing. Clin Podiatr Med Surg. 2015;32(1):121–33.
36. Kim PJ, Attinger CE, Orgill D, Galiano RD, Steinberg JS, Evans KK, et al. Complex lower extremity wound in the complex host: results from a multicenter registry. Plast Reconstr Surg Glob Open. 2019;7(4):e2129.

Elective Surgery in the Diabetic Foot to Heal Foot Ulcerations and Prevent Re-ulceration

6

Lawrence A. Lavery, Katerina Grigoropoulos, Amanda L. Killeen, and Javier La Fontaine

6.1 The Etiology of Diabetic Foot Ulcerations

Understanding the etiology of diabetic foot ulcerations is essential to understanding treatments and prevention strategies. There is a combination of factors that contribute to the development of foot ulceration in people with diabetes including peripheral neuropathy, macro and micro peripheral arterial disease, structural foot deformity, limited joint mobility, and pressure and shear on the foot. People with diabetes are also prone to traumatic injuries such as puncture wounds and painless fractures and dislocations. The assessment of these variables is largely based on history and physical examination of the foot and ankle.

People with diabetes often develop Diabetic Symmetrical Polyneuropathy (DSPN), motor neuropathy, and autonomic neuropathy. In a position statement by the American Diabetes Association, DSPN was defined as the presence of symptoms and/or signs of peripheral nerve dysfunction in people with diabetes after the exclusion of other causes [1]. This is a very broad definition and may not be useful to identify people that are at high risk of ulceration. Many of the tests in clinical practice are done to identify the extent of sensory neuropathy with loss of protective sensation, or enough sensory loss that the subject can injury themselves and not feel the injury.

Diabetic symmetrical polyneuropathy is one of the most important factors in the development of ulceration. However, it is often not evaluated by primary care physicians, even though it is one of the most common diabetes-related complications. Sensory loss is commonly due to large fiber peripheral neuropathy that patients describe as their feet feeling numb, asleep, tingling, or with sensations of formication. Patients will say that their feet feel cold, even when their spouse feels their feet and tells them they are warm. Patients sometime say they feel like they have mud caked on the bottom of their foot or they are wearing a thick stocking. In contrast to large fiber neuropathy, small fiber neuropathy is associated with symptoms of burning, allodynia, and electrical shooting pain. Clinical testing is usually accomplished by evaluating the ability to identify temperature sensation. Painful neuropathy is often identified with large fiber neuropathy. Motor neuropathy often affects the intrinsic muscles in the feet and hands and can be identified clinically by muscle atrophy of the abductor hallucis muscle and hollow areas between the metatarsal bones where intrinsic muscles have wasted. Autonomic

L. A. Lavery (✉) · K. Grigoropoulos · A. L. Killeen
J. La Fontaine
Department of Plastic Surgery, University of Texas Southwestern Medical Center, Dallas, TX, USA
e-mail: larry.lavery@utsouthwestern.edu

J. P. Hong, H. Suh (eds.), *Diabetic Foot Reconstruction*,
https://doi.org/10.1007/978-981-16-9816-3_6

neuropathy contributes to dry skin and arteriovenous shunting.

Simple screening questions are an accurate means to identify DSPN [2]. For instance, the diabetic neuropathy symptom score is a four-item validated tool that asks about postural instability in gait, numbness, paresthesias, and neuropathic pain symptoms [3]. These types of screening questions can be obtained during intake processing by a nurse and are often sufficient to make an initial diagnosis.

Testing for sensory neuropathy is fast, inexpensive and can be performed by a trained medical assistant or a nurse. A 128 Hz tuning fork should be struck to make the ends clang and then applied to a bony prominence such as the first metatarsal head or the distal tip of the great toe. The patients are asked if they feel the vibration and then to indicate when the vibration stops [4]. Normally, patients should feel the vibration for 20 s. The average time diabetic patients feel the vibration is 8 s. In addition to vibration perception, the 10-gram Semmes Weinstein monofilament is often used to screen for sensory loss. The monofilament measures pressure sensation. The instrument is applied perpendicular to the skin until the monofilament bends and held for about 1 s. Investigators have evaluated using as many as ten sites on the foot. Other techniques such as pin prick and Achilles deep tendon reflex have been described to assess large fiber neuropathy, but are not as widely used or reported in the medical literature [5].

Diabetic symmetrical polyneuropathy (DSPN) with loss of protective sensation provides an environment in which the patient can experience injury to the foot that is painless and unrecognized [6]. It is not uncommon for a patient to step on a nail through the sole of their shoe and only identify the injury because they cannot take their shoe off. Another common scenario is for a patient to identify a foot ulcer because of blood on their stockings or on the floor and not because of pain at the site of the ulcer. DSPN is one of the most common underlying causes of diabetic foot ulcerations (DFU) [2, 7, 8]. DSPN is easy to evaluate from symptoms and with clinical examination.

6.2 The Role of Biomechanics, Deformity, Pressure, and Shear

Abnormal biomechanics have been associated with elevated foot pressures and shear forces on the sole of the foot. Ulcerations on the sides of the feet are often due to constant, low pressures and high shear from ill-fitting shoes, tight hose, or dressings. Ulcers on the sole of the foot are usually associated with moderate to high pressure and shear forces on the ball of the foot or toes [9–11].

Abnormal biomechanics are usually associated with structural foot deformity and limited joint mobility. The most common structural deformities include hammer toe deformities, subluxed, or dislocated metatarsophalangeal joints, and hallux valgus deformity. Diabetic motor neuropathy causes wasting of the intrinsic muscles in the foot. Because diabetic neuropathy progress from distal to proximal, motor neuropathy affects intrinsic foot muscles (lumbricales, flexor hallucis brevis, abductor hallucis, abductor digiti minimi, quadratus plantae) before extrinsic muscles [12]. This creates an imbalance. Intrinsic muscles function to stabilize the toes against the metatarsal heads and to maintain alignment of the toes. When there is an imbalance because the intrinsic and short flexors are weak, the long flexor tendons overpower the extensors. This contributes to the development of hammer toe deformities and subluxed and dislocated metatarsophalangeal joints [13, 14]. At the extreme, intrinsic motor wasting causes the development of the "intrinsic minus foot (Fig. 6.1)" [15]. The foot appears to have a high arch because of the wasting of the abductor hallucis muscle, tightening of the plantar fascia and the dorsal subluxation of the toes on the metatarsal heads. When there is subluxation and dislocation at the metatarsophalangeal joints, the toes contract, and the fat pad displaces anteriorly. As the metatarsophalangeal joints sublux, there is retrograde bucking. The toes hammer or claw and the metatarsophalangeal joints sublux and then dislocate, so the base of the proximal phalanx sits on the dorsal surface of the metatarsal head (Fig. 6.2). As the toes sublux, the

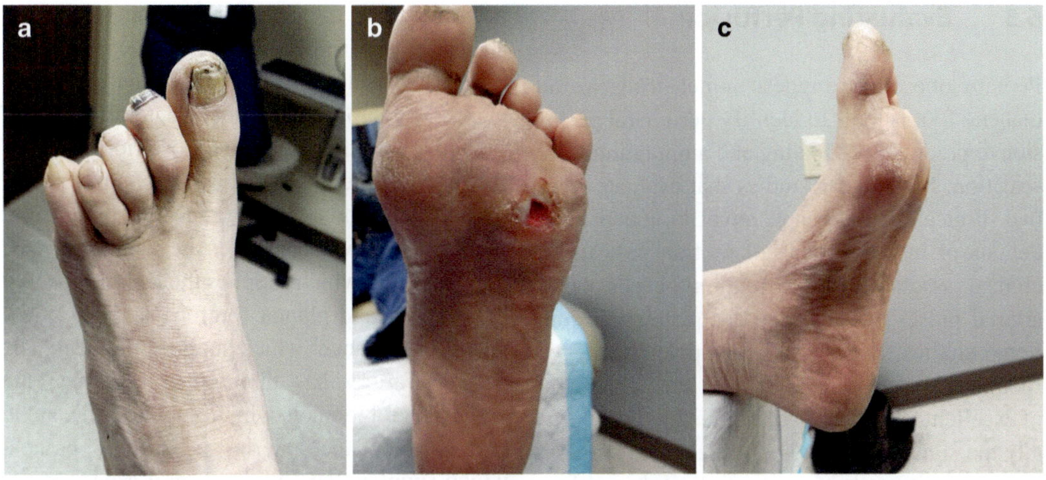

Fig. 6.1 Clinical features of the intrinsic minus foot. There is (**a**) hammering of the digits, (**b**) subluxation of the metatarsophalangeal joints, and (**c**) wasting of the abductor hallucis muscle belly

fat pad that is normally under the ball of the foot is anteriorly displaced, so it rests in the sulcus of the toes and is no longer in a weigh bearing area. The heads of the metatarsals are often literally driven through the sole of the foot in patients with DSPN.

Several studies have shown severe intrinsic muscle wasting in people with DSPN compared to age-matched controls [12, 16, 17]. Muscle is replaced with adipose tissue. Intrinsic muscle wasting has been associated with limited ankle joint range of motion and metatarsophalangeal joint deformity [14]. Limited joint mobility has also been associated with advanced glycation end products that reduce the elasticity of tendons in people with diabetes. Advanced glycation end products affect collagen crosslinking in joint capsule and tendons. This changes the biomechanical properties and increases the stiffness of the involved structures [18]. Clinically, limited joint mobility is observed in reduced ankle joint motion (equinus deformity), limited motion of the first metatarsophalangeal joint (hallux rigidus), and reduced motion in the hand (adhesive capsulitis) [19, 20]. Limited joint motion usually translates into changes in gait patterns, altered loading patterns of the foot, and increased pressure and shear forces on the sole of the foot.

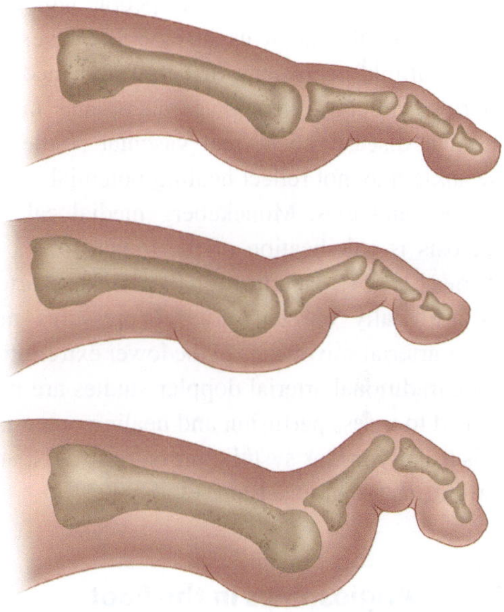

Fig. 6.2 The illustrations show the progression of deformity at the metatarsophalangeal joint and proximal interphalangeal joint and distal interphalangeal joint. The normal view demonstrates normal alignment with congruous joints. As the deformity progresses, only half of the base of the proximal phalanx articulates with the articular cartilage of the metatarsal head, and there contracture of the proximal interphalangeal joint. The last illustration demonstrates dislocation of the metatarsophalangeal joint and contracture of the proximal interphalangeal joint and distal interphalangeal joint

6.3 Evaluating Perfusion

Perhaps one of the biggest unmet needs in the diabetic foot is tools to identify peripheral perfusion to predict ulcer healing and amputation level selection. Most of the studies that evaluate elective surgical procedures to repair biomechanical deficits or increase range of motion only use a clinical assessment of palpation of peripheral arterial pulses to determine adequate perfusion. Some studies obtain arterial Doppler studies if foot pulses are absent. However, even at centers of excellent, advanced vascular testing is not usually the standard of care before elective surgery. The reliability and accuracy of clinical examination to determine PAD are notoriously poor [21, 22]. Despite these important limitations, complications are not common.

Peripheral arterial disease in people with diabetes classically involves infrapopliteal vessels with multiple occlusions of small and medium arteries. Patients often have macro and micro vascular disease, so normal vascular studies at the ankle may not reflect healing potential in the forefoot and toes. Monckeberg medial calcific sclerosis is calcification of the tunica media of arteries [23, 24]. Calcification of peripheral arteries artificially elevates arterial pressures and blunts arterial waveforms in the lower extremities when traditional arterial doppler studies are performed to assess perfusion and healing potential. This usually means systolic pressures, ABIs, and waveforms are of uncertain reliably [25].

6.4 Angiosomes in the Foot

Diabetic foot and ankle wounds are often challenging to heal secondarily. The concept of angiosomes may be helpful when planning elective or emergent surgeries in the diabetic foot. The foot and ankle are composed of six distinct angiosomes that include connections between muscle, fascia, and skin with their source of blood flow from arteries with functional vascular connections [26]. The six angiosomes originate from the posterior tibial artery, anterior tibial artery, and peroneal artery. Anatomically, the posterior tibial artery supplies the medial ankle and the plantar foot, the anterior tibial artery supplies the dorsal aspect of the foot, and the peroneal artery supplies the antero-lateral aspect of the ankle and the lateral and posterior aspect of the foot. Furthermore, the posterior tibial artery divides into three main branches: the medial plantar artery, which supplies the central arch, the plantar artery, which supplies the lateral aspect of the midfoot and plantar forefoot, and the calcaneal artery branch, which supplies the heel. The peroneal artery has three main branches: the antero-lateral branch which supplies the ankle and rearfoot, the anterior perforating branch, which supplies the anterior lateral aspect of the superior ankle, and the calcaneal branch, which supplies the lateral and plantar heel. Finally, the anterior tibial artery supplies the anterior ankle, and the dorsum of the foot via its extension of the dorsalis pedis artery.

In general, each of the angiosomes has multiple branches that extend to the distal aspect of the foot and the digits. The clinical application of angiosomes depends on detailed understanding of the vascular anatomy. One of the most important aspects of utilizing angiosomes is the arterial-arterial connections that allow blood flow to the foot despite the occlusion of one or more arteries. Understanding the anatomy of these connections will allow the surgeon to appreciate the surgical applications in foot and ankle surgery.

Incision placement is an important factor in any surgical procedure of the foot and ankle. There are several factors to consider when deciding placement of the incision, when the procedure is elective. First, the incision should allow for adequate exposure. Secondly, the best healing will occur with adequate blood supply on both sides of the incision. Thirdly, the incision should avoid damage to structures such as nerves, vessels, and tendons. Lastly, an incision placement should be done along joint line to avoid scar contracture. In an ideal situation, the best incision is the one placed between two angiosomes because blood flow from both angiosomes will supply the incision. However, in many instances, blood flow to any of the angiosomes may be disrupted. In those cases, the placement of the incision will need to be reconsidered and adapted for what the priority of the procedure is. For example, a lateral foot infection will need to be approached with a lateral incision despite knowing the lateral foot angiosome might be vascularly compromised, but the incision will allow better access to address the infection.

Choke vessels are vascular anastomoses between adjacent angiosome which play an important role in flap expansion and survival [27]. They also have capacity to dilate and increase the local blood flow. In instances where one angiosome's vascular supply is disrupted, the ischemic angiosome depends on the blood flow from the choke vessels. This type of vessel requires 4–10 days to become patent during an ischemic event to the angiosomes [28]. An incision made during the period of acute ischemia will run the risk of necrosis.

When performing a planned surgery, the concept of angiosomes becomes an important one. Creativity may be required, based on the procedure to be performed.

Amputations: On many occasions, when performing some sort of foot amputation, surgeons are at the mercy of the initial presentation of the patient. Often, the remaining skin flap, soft tissue and muscles are not enough to cover or close a wound. However, knowing the vascular anatomy will help in deciding between a complex closure vs. revising the amputation. If possible, incisions should be designed to be between 2 angiosomes to optimize blood flow. Undermining should be limited—when is necessary—to avoid devascularization of viable tissue. When compromised blood flow exists, the review of the previous angiogram might be helpful in planning the best procedure to do. In lieu of an angiogram, a detailed noninvasive evaluation of arterial blood flow could be done as described by Attinger et al. [29]. Care must be taken to protect the arterial connections between the dorsal and plantar aspects of the foot (Fig. 6.3). For instance, the vascular supply to the dorsum of the foot could be antegrade from the peroneal artery via the lateral malleolar artery alone when an occlusion exists at the proximal aspect of the anterior tibial artery.

Heel Wounds: The initial incision depends on the location of the ulcer and the amount of excisional debridement to be performed. When the wound is free of nonviable tissue, the final wound closure can be designed if primary closure is the goal and the blood flow is adequate. For wounds in the posterior aspect of the heel, a linear incision along the midline of the calcaneus is ideal [30] as it is located between the medial and lateral angiosomes, supplied by the posterior tibial and peroneal arteries, respectively (Fig. 6.4). If an incision is made along the glabrous junction of the posterior heel, care should be taken with the medial portion of the incision to protect medical calcaneal neurovascular structures. If the wound is in the lateral aspect of the calcaneus, the safest incision is along the glabrous junction between the lateral heel and the plantar heel. This location

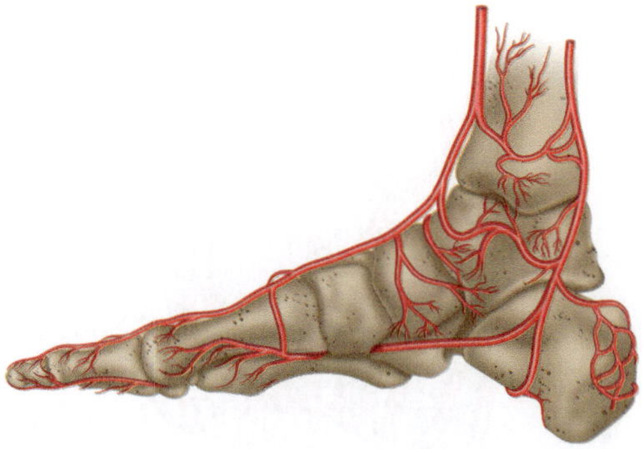

Fig. 6.3 Dorsalis Pedis and Posterior Tibial arteries with their branches. Notice the perforating branch connecting from Dorsalis Pedis artery to the Medial Plantar artery at the base of the first metatarsal bone

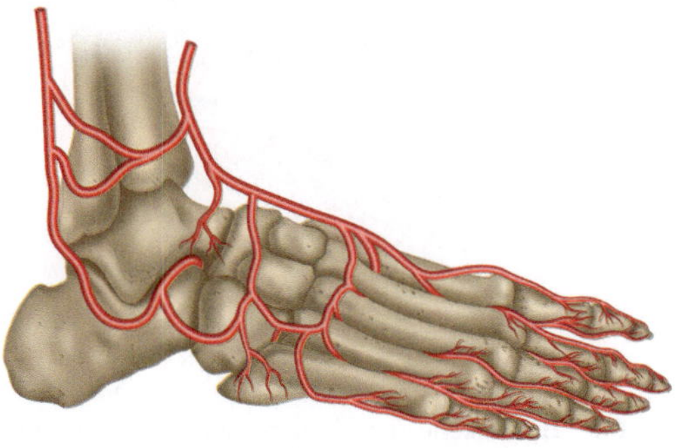

Fig. 6.4 The Peroneal artery and Anterior Tibial artery with arterial to arterial connections

will avoid damage to either the calcaneal branch of the peroneal artery or the lateral branch of the posterior tibial artery.

Ulcerations on the sole of the foot are common and can be especially challenging. The plantar aspect of the foot is vascularized by the medial and lateral plantar arteries. The lateral plantar artery turns medially forming the deep plantar arch (Fig. 6.5). It anastomoses with the dorsalis pedis artery in the first proximal interspace (Fig. 6.6). This is an important concept to understand because an occluded lateral plantar artery can only perfuse the plantar foot if retrograde flow from the dorsalis pedis and/or medial plantar artery occurs. The best incision placement

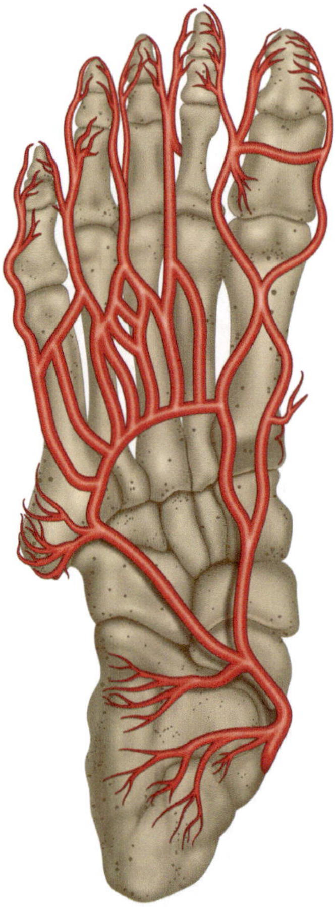

Fig. 6.5 The Posterior Tibial artery divides plantarly into Medial Plantar artery and Lateral Plantar artery. The Lateral Plantar artery turns in the midfoot to form the plantar arch

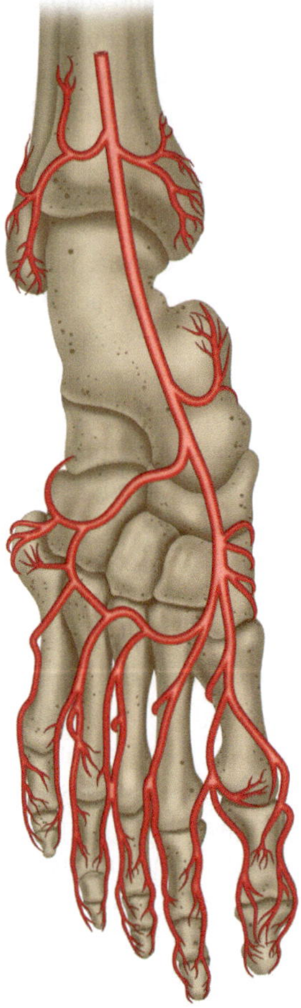

Fig. 6.6 The Dorsalis Pedis artery extends and give off the digital arteries. Notice perforating arteries at the midfoot that connect with plantar arch

when there is no occlusion of the plantar arteries is at the midline of the plantar arch of the foot. Fortunately, this incision will allow the surgeon the best visualization of the plantar space of the foot [31]. This incision is located at the junction of the medial and lateral angiosomes. However, a plantar space infection located in the medial or lateral plantar space of the foot could be approached with a medial or lateral incision at the level of the glabrous skin. Both incisions will be located at the junction of the dorsal and plantar angiosomes of the medial or lateral plantar arteries.

Toe Ulcers: The vascular supply to the toes arises from the dorsalis pedis and posterior plantar artery. Dorsally, the dorsalis pedis artery has three lateral branches and two medial branches. The most distal lateral branch is the arcuate artery, which provides metatarsal arteries to lesser toes. After giving off the arcuate artery, the dorsalis pedis is buried through the first interspace, gives off the first dorsal metatarsal artery, and connects plantarly to the lateral plantar artery. The dorsal to plantar connection between these two arteries are very important to understand for revascularization of the foot when occlusion exists in either artery. Antegrade or retrograde flow can be attained with revascularization via these arterial interconnections. At the metatarsal heads, each dorsal metatarsal artery divides medially and laterally to supply each toe, and then travel to the plantar region via the distal perforating arteries. This connection allows each toe to receive dorsal and plantar blood flow from the dorsalis pedis artery and the lateral plantar artery.

6.5 Surgery to Heal DFUs

There is a growing body of work that reports the effectiveness and safety of elective surgical procedures to correct structural deformities or increase limited joint mobility in diabetic patients with neuropathic foot ulcerations. The literature concerning elective surgery to heal foot ulcerations is predominantly retrospective cohort studies. There are only three randomized controlled trials (RCTs). The studies' sample sizes are very small. For instance, the two RCTs that evaluate Achilles tendon lengthening include 64 and 29 subjects [32, 33]. Cohort studies include 10–287 subjects.

Studies have demonstrated fewer infections, fewer amputations, faster healing, and fewer recurrent ulcers after surgical intervention compared to patients with diabetic foot ulcers that are treated with standard local wound care. The key to understanding the risks and benefits of elective foot surgery is having an understanding of the results of traditional diabetic foot ulcer treatments, so patients have a reference standard. The results of standard ulcer treatments are poor. Patients with diabetic foot ulcers experience a protracted course of healing, a high incidence of infection and amputations, as well as a high rate of re-ulceration.

The rate of healing is often low, and the time to heal prolonged for patients with diabetic foot ulcerations. In many diabetic foot ulcer randomized clinical trials, the proportion of ulcers that heal in the standard of care arm ranges from 17 to 49% in 12-week studies. However, the median proportion of ulcers that heal is only about 30% [34–37]. Among the small proportion of patients that heal ulcers with traditional ulcer care in randomized clinical trials, the median time to heal is long (48–90 days). The poor healing response is one of the main reasons for significantly higher infection and amputation rates in the standard of care arm of these randomized clinical trials. Non-healing diabetic foot ulcers simply have a longer exposure with an open portal for bacterial infection.

The risk of foot infection and amputation is very high in patients with diabetic foot ulcerations. Wukich and colleagues reported results from a prospective registry that demonstrated the risk of infection attributed to diabetes and neuropathy. Wukich reported that the incidence of infection in elective foot and ankle surgery in patients without diabetes was 1.7% compared to 7.0% in non-diabetics with neuropathy, 3.0% in diabetics without neuropathy, and 10.4% in diabetics with neuropathy [38]. In contrast, the incidence of infection in patients with DFUs is much higher than in people that have elective foot surgery. In diabetic foot ulcer randomized clinical trials, 0–36% of patients that receive standard wound care have infections during a 12-week evaluation period. However, DFU randomized clinical trials are highly selective, so the highest risk subjects are usually systematically eliminated. Randomized clinical trials usually exclude high-risk people with end stage renal disease, poor glucose control (glycated hemoglobin >12%), and moderate and severe peripheral arterial disease. In addition, moderate and severe ulcers are often excluded, such as wounds that are deep with exposed tendon, capsule, or bone, wounds that are large (>10–15 cm^2) and wounds that have been present for more than a year. Even though the incidence of infection seems very high in randomized clinical trials, in clinical practice, the incidence is much higher because very high-risk people cannot be eliminated. For instance, in prospective cohort studies of patients with DFUs that were followed longitudinally, 40–60% of patients develop foot infections [39, 40].

Amputation is common in patients with foot ulcerations and infections. The incidence of amputation and the level of amputation is higher in persons with peripheral arterial disease (PAD) and end stage renal disease (ESRD). The incidence of lower extremity amputations ranges from 2.1 to 13.7 per 1000 person years [41, 42]. However, when the need for repeated amputations is evaluated the rates are higher. Lavery and colleagues reported a cumulative amputation incidence of 13.3 per 1000 person years and an ulcer to amputation ratio of 15.8; however, among dialysis patients, the cumulative amputation incidence was 72.0 per 1000 person years, and the ulcer to amputation ratio was only 4.4 [43].

The rate of ulcer recurrence once a patient with a foot ulcer heals is high [44]. When high-risk patients do not receive education, regular foot care and bespoke shoes and insoles, 50–83% develop another ulcer in the next year [45, 46]. However, when prevention services are provided, the rate of re-ulceration is reduced by half (Table 6.1). However, even with very good prevention services, the rate of re-ulceration continues to be very high. One of the most dramatic benefits in studies of elective surgery to heal DFUs is the very low rate of re-ulceration. Once a key component of the underlying etiology is corrected, the risk of re-injury is reduced.

6.6 Percutaneous Achilles Tendon Lengthening

Decreased dorsiflexion of the ankle joint has been associated with increased forefoot pressures and ulceration [52]. It is thought that at least 10° of ankle joint dorsiflexion is required for normal gait; however, in most studies that evaluate these procedures, patients have no dorsiflexion after surgery or their foot is just perpendicular to the leg [32]. Range of motion of the ankle should be evaluated with the knee flexed and fully extended.

There is a growing body of work that supports the effectiveness of both percutaneous Achilles tendon lengthening (ATL) and gastrocnemius recession (GR) to treated equinus deformity in patients with diabetic foot ulcers. Both approaches increase ankle joint range of motion; however, only ATL has been studied and demonstrated to change gait parameters. Mueller and colleagues compared barefoot pressures before and after ATL and showed a 27% reduction in peak pressure, a 42% reduction in pressure time integral, 53% reduction in plantar flexor moment and 65% reduction in plantar flexor power in people with diabetes. On average, patients had an 11° increase in ankle joint dorsiflexion [52].

Table 6.1 Diabetic foot ulcer recurrence with bespoke shoes and insoles

	Pressure-based insole $N = 130$	Custom made insoles $N = 171$	Custom made insoles $N = 298$	Manufactured shoes $N = 64$	Rocker shoes and insole $N = 51$
Author	Ulbrecht 2014 [47]	Bus 2013 [48]	Rizzo 2012 [49]	Uccioli 1995 [50]	Busch 2003 [51]
Study design	RCT	RCT	RCT	RCT	Prospective cohort
Study duration	18 months	18 months	12 months	12 months	12 months
Treatment group (%) healing	Pressure-based insole 9.1%	Custom insole 38.8%	Custom insole 11.5%	Manufactured shoe and insole 27.7%	Rocker shoe and insole 15.0%
Control group (%) healing	Standard of care Therapeutic shoes and insoles 45.3%	Standard of care Therapeutic shoes and insoles 44.2%	Standard of care Therapeutic shoes and insoles 38.6%	Self-selected Shoes 58.3%	Self-selected Shoes 60.0%

RCT Randomized Controlled Trial

There are two RCTs and five retrospective cohort studies (Table 6.2) that evaluate the risks and benefits of surgery to lengthen the Achilles tendon to heal foot ulcers and prevent re-ulceration. The results of percutaneous Achilles tendon lengthening procedures and gastrocnemius recession (Table 6.3) appear to be similar, although there are no head-to-head comparisons. The advantage of the percutaneous ATL procedure is that it is easy to perform. The procedure

Table 6.2 Achilles tendon lengthening

Author	Subjects	PAD assessment	Healed	Time to heal (days)	Re-ulceration	Infection	Amputation
Mueller 2003 [32]	64 subjects 31 ATL 33 TCC	Palpated pulses	100% ATL 88% TCC	ATL 57.5 ± 47.0 TCC 40.8 ± 28.1	ATL 15% TCC 59%	ATL 3.2% TCC 0%	None
Allam 2006 [33]	29 subjects 15 ATL 14 TCC	Palpated pulses	93.3% ATL 78.6% TCC	ATL 30 TCC 49	Recurrence ATL 16.7% TCC 22.2%	None	None
Lin 1996 [53]	Surgical 15 TCC 21	ABIs Pulse volume recording	93.3% ATL 100% TCC	Surgical 39.4 TCC 43.5	Recurrence Surgical 0% TCC 19%	None	None
Colen 2013 [54]	Surgical: 138 subjects 145 ulcers Non-surgical: 149 subjects 179 ulcers	Palpated pulses ABIs	Not reported	Not reported	Surgical: Recurrence 2% Transfer ulcer 4% Non-surgical: Recurrence 25% Transfer ulcer 12%	Not reported	Surgical 5.7% Non-surg 4.6%
Holstein 2004 [55]	68 subjects 75 ulcers	Palpated pulses If non-palpable: ABIs TBIs	91%	90	Recurrence 50% Transfer ulcer 54.5%	Not reported	2.9%
La Fontaine 2008 [56]	28 subjects	ABI > 0.8	86%	65.8	Recurrence 35.7% Transfer ulcer 21%	None	None
Meshkin 2020 [57]	91 subjects 84 ulcers 7 subjects without ulcer	Not reported	78.6%	90.3	Recurrence 43.9% Transfer ulcer 13%	None	None

RCT Randomized Controlled Trial, *ATL* Achilles Tendon Lengthening, *TCC* Total Contact Cast, *PAD* Peripheral Arterial Disease, *ABI* Ankle Brachial Index

Table 6.3 Gastrocnemius recession

Author	Subjects	PAD assessment	Healed	Time to heal (days)	Re-ulceration	Infection	Amputation
Laborde 2008 [58]	17 subjects 20 ulcers	Palpated pulses	95%	Not reported	Not reported	None	5.8%
Laborde 2009 [59]	11 subjects	Palpated pulses	91%	Not reported	Recurrence 9%	None	9%

PAD Peripheral Arterial Disease

can be done under a local block in a few minutes, and it is easy to evaluate the amount of correction that has been achieved intraoperatively. On the other hand, gastrocnemius aponeurosis requires a larger surgical incision. Patients usually require general endotracheal anesthesia because they must be positioned prone. Unfortunately, there is very little published concerning gastrocnemius recession as an isolated procedure, so clinical outcomes and safety data are very limited.

When compared to patients with DFUs that receive "best practices," the proportion and time to heal ulcers is very similar. For instance, Mueller and colleagues reported the results of an RCT that compared people treated with total contact casts and ATL. A high proportion of ulcers healed (TCC 88% vs. ATL 100%), and the time of healing was similar (TCC 40.8 vs. ATL 57.5 days). Likewise, Allam and colleagues [33] compared ATL, with both percutaneous procedures and GR, to TCC and found similar results to Mueller. There was no difference in the proportion of ulcers that healed and faster healing (TCC 90.0 vs. ATL 75.5 days).

As expected, patients treated with total contact casts in these studies had very high rates of healing. In retrospective cohort studies and randomized clinical trials of TCCs about 90% of ulcers heal in 42 days [60, 61]. Diabetic foot ulcer randomized clinical trials that evaluate drugs or devices for healing do not use TCCs as part of the standard of care. That is why phase 3 and 4 randomized clinical trials have a low incidence of healed ulcers and a much longer median and mean time to heal. Selection of the "standard of care" is critical to evaluate the effectiveness of Achilles tendon surgery. If ATL procedures had used another, less rigorous and effective standard of care, such as healing sandals or felt and foam dressings [62, 63], the studies would have likely shown a threefold improvement in healing and half the time to heal in subjects treated with ATL surgeries. In the USA, even in specialty wound centers, TCCs are not a standard treatment. Only 1.7% of centers use this treatment [64]. The very high incidence of healing and the faster time to heal in ATL procedures may be misrepresented because total contact casts were used as the control.

A common complication with Achilles tendon lengthening is transfer ulcers or pressure lesions on the heel. In a gait laboratory study, Maluf and colleagues reported reduction in forefoot pressure parameters with an increase in rear foot peak pressure of 34% and pressure time integral of 48% [52]. In Mueller's RCT, during the follow-up 13% of ATL subjects developed a heel ulcer [32], and in Allam's RCT, 20% of subjects developed a transfer ulcer and 16.7% experienced tendon rupture [33]. In retrospective cohort studies, heel transfer ulcers are a common complication and have been reported in 1.3%, 13.2% and 14.7% of subjects [54, 55, 57]. Holstein reported a tendon rupture rate of 10%. Heel ulcers are probably more common in people that have more than >15° of dorsiflexion. Among patients treated with gastrocnemius recession transfer ulcers to the heel seem to be less common. Only 0–5% of patients develop heel ulcers and 16.7% have tendon rupture [58, 59].

The incidence of infection and amputation is very low in ATL surgeries. Most authors report no surgery-related infections or ulcer-related infections of the study foot. Only a few studies identify these complications. For instance, Mueller reported one infection (3.0%) [32], and Laborde reported one above the knee amputation (5.0%) [58].

One of the most significant outcomes of ATL procedures is the reduction in recurrent foot ulcerations. Consistently, the incidence of re-ulceration is lower than would be expected with standard prevention services. Mueller reported ulcer recurrence of 15% in the ATL group and 58% in the TCC group at 7 months and 38% and 81%, respectively, in these groups after 2 years [32]. In contrast, Allam and colleagues reported no difference in re-ulceration (16.7 vs. 22.2%) in surgery and TCC treatment arms. In a retrospective study, Colen reported 2.0% re-ulceration in 145 patients with ATL and 25% re-ulceration in 179 people without ATL [54]. Other retrospective cohort studies of percutaneous ATL report recurrence rates of 0 [53], 8% [65], 13.3% [55], 43.9% [57]. In gastroc recession surgery, ulcer recurrence is also low (0 and 9.0%) [58, 59]. Unfortunately, none of the published studies specifies if study patients receive bespoke shoes and insoles, education or regular diabetic foot care as part of ulcer prevention.

6.6.1 Surgical Technique

A gastrocnemius aponeurosis recession is performed with the patient in the prone position. To identify the gastrocnemius aponeurosis, the foot is dorsiflexed with the knee extended and the aponeurosis is palpated. An incision is made medial to midline and below the heads of the gastrocnemius muscle. Dissection is performed to identify the gastrocnemius (superficial) and soleus aponeurosis as they merge to form the Achilles tendon. The gastrocnemius aponeurosis is surgical incised and lengthened. The soleus muscle is deeper, and it is left intact. When the aponeurosis is incised, tension should be placed on the structures by dorsiflexing the foot with the knee in extension (Fig. 6.7).

Percutaneous Achilles tendon lengthening can be performed with the patient prone or in a frog leg lateral position. The foot should be dorsiflexed to keep the tendon under tension, so the surgeon can feel the "give" with each incision and assess the surgical correction. First, the surgeon should identify the boundary of the Achilles tendon to properly mark the incision. The procedure entails three percutaneous partial sections of the Achilles tendon. Two medial incisions and one lateral incision are made (Fig. 6.8). The first incision is made approximately 1–2 cm proximal to the superior portion of the calcaneus based on the overall length of the Achilles tendon. Using an 11 blade, a small incision is made through the skin and through the medial one-third of the tendon. The second incision is made 1–2 cm proximal from the first, and lateral one-third of the tendon is incised. The third incision, once again, is made about 1–2 cm proximal from the second incision, and one-third of the tendon is incised [66]. The traditional approach is a hemisection at

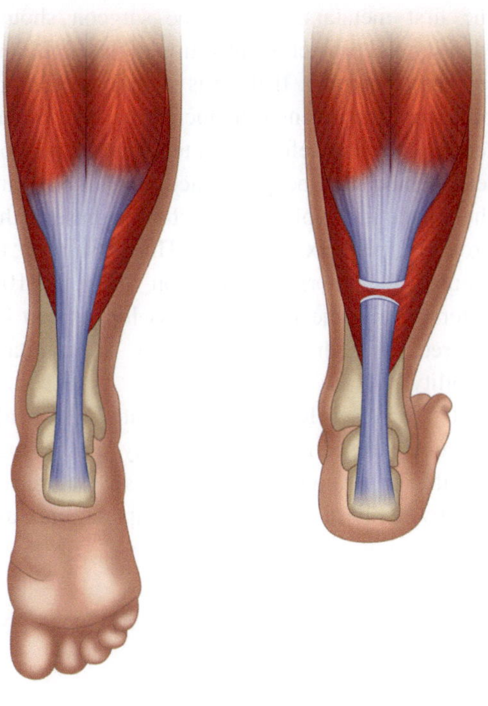

Fig. 6.7 Surgical approach for gastrocnemius aponeurosis recession

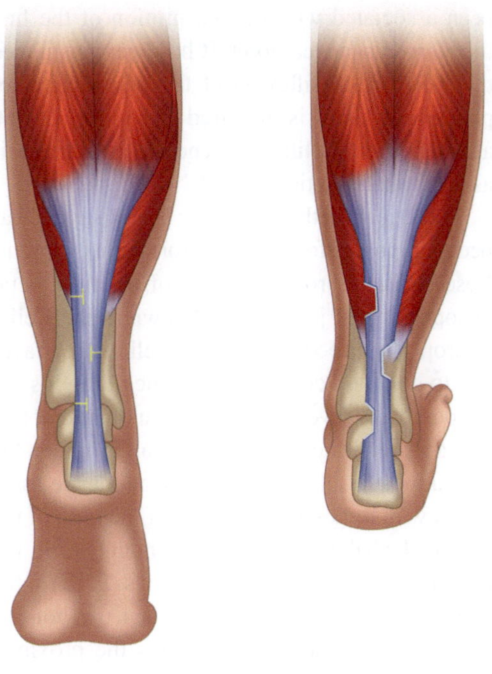

Fig. 6.8 Surgical approach for percutaneous Achilles tendon lengthening

each site, or 50% of the width of the tendon is incised. Our approach to only incise a third of the tendon at each site with the goal of <10° of ankle joint dorsiflexion to avoid tendon rupture and heel ulcers. If the desired amount of correction is achieved after the first two incisions, the third incision is not needed. If more lengthening is needed, the procedure can be repeated to incise more of the tendon. Postoperative management is critical to avoid tendon rupture or overlengthening the tendon. Since the vast majority of patients cannot safely use crutches or remain non-weightbearing, patients are casted for 3–4 weeks followed by off-loading with a removable cast boot for 3–4 weeks. Patients are encouraged to use a knee scooter or wheelchair.

6.7 Resectional Arthroplasty of the Great Toe

Ulcers on the plantar surface of the great toe at the interphalangeal joint are very common, often refractory to standard therapies, and have a very high rate of re-ulceration. Ulcers at this site have been associated with limited motion of the first metatarsophalangeal joint. It has been postulated that >50° of dorsiflexion of the first metatarsophalangeal joint is required for normal gait, although there is little evidence to establish this as a "normal functional level."

Resectional arthroplasty for hallux rigidus has been proposed for decades for hallux rigidus. Resectional arthroplasty (RA) of the first metatarsophalangeal joint is also known as the Keller arthroplasty procedure [67]. It fell out of favor due to common complications, including loss of toe purchase, development of hallux hammer toe, and transfer lesion and metatarsalgia under the lateral metatarsal heads. Complications are associated with removing too much of the base of the proximal phalanx [68] and not maintaining the insertion of the flexor hallucis brevis (FHB) at the plantar base of the great toe when the bone is resected [69]. The FHB stabilizes the proximal phalanx against the head of the first metatarsal in gait, so the medial column can act as a rigid lever during propulsion. If the flexor hallucis brevis insertion is cut during the procedure, the sesamoids retract, and the imbalance from stronger extensor halluces brevis and longus causes dorsiflexion at the metatarsophalangeal joint and plantar flexion of the interphalangeal joint.

6.7.1 Surgical Technique

A dorsal medial incision is made directly over the first metatarsophalangeal joint to the level of capsule. A capsulotomy is performed to expose the first metatarsal head and the base of the proximal phalanx. If there is an exostosis of the head of the first metatarsal, a cheilectomy is performed. Next, about 20% of the base of the proximal phalanx is resected (Fig. 6.9). The landmark for resecting an adequate amount of bone is the dorsal tubercle for the insertion of the extensor hallucis brevis at the base of the proximal phalanx. The joint should be put through a range of motion to determine if more bone should be removed. A burr is then used to contour of the residual base of the proximal phalanx, so it matches the head of the first metatarsal bone The surgeon should identify and protect the insertion of the FHB during the osteotomy. If there is significant enough pull from the extensor hallucis brevis or longus tendon to cause deformity, a tenotomy or tendon lengthening can be performed. Drill holes are then made in the plantar aspect of the base of the proximal phalanx, and the FHB is sutured to secure the normal insertion (Fig. 6.10). Alternatively, the flexor hallucis longus can be sutured through the drill hole to maintain stability.

There are no RCTs that evaluate DFU healing using resectional arthroplasty of the first metatarsophalangeal joint. There are two retrospective cohort studies that compare this sur-

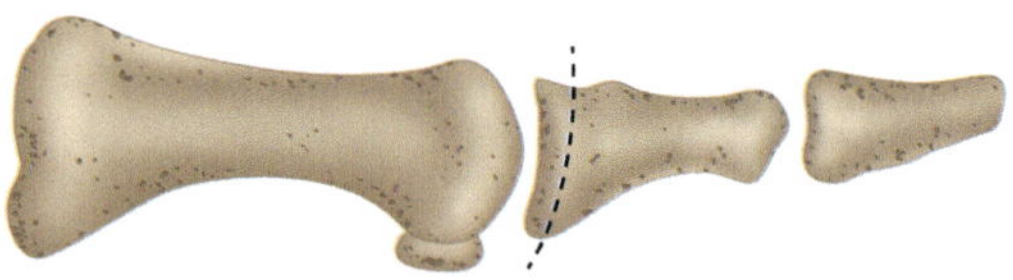

Fig. 6.9 Lateral view of the foot that demonstrates resection of the base of the proximal phalanx

gery to a standard of care group, and there are two retrospective cohort studies that are purely descriptive (Table 6.4). The healing rate and time to heal after resectional arthroplasty surgery is high. Tamir reported that 78.5% of 28 DFUs of the great toe healed, and Lin, Armstrong and Berner reported that 100% of their patient healed after resectional arthroplasty of the proximal phalanx. The mean time to heal was 21.7–24 days.

The incidence of infection and amputation is very low after resectional arthroplasty surgery of the first metatarsophalangeal joint. In Lin's comparison study, there were no infections or amputation in either treatment group. In Armstrong's comparative study the incidence of infection was similar in patients that had surgery and standard of care (40.0 vs. 38.1%). Tamir and Berner reported 21.4 and 24.7% infection and no amputations.

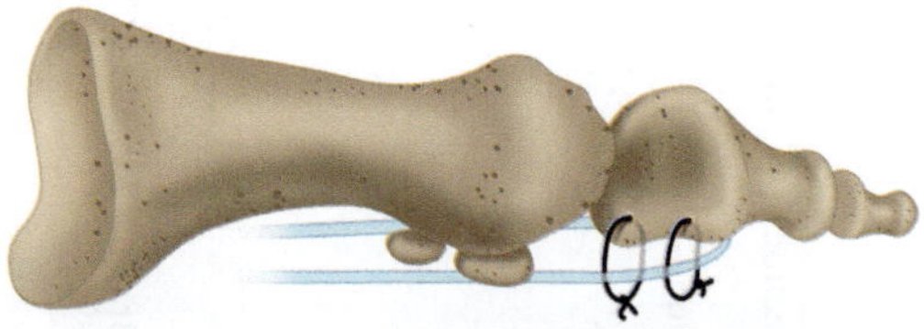

Fig. 6.10 Two drill holes are placed on in the base of the proximal phalanx the both heads of the flexor hallucis tendon are sutured to the base of the proximal phalanx

After RA surgery of the first metatarsophalangeal joint, there is a low rate of re-ulceration and transfer ulcers. The yearly incidence of re-ulceration ranged from 4.8 to 38.5%. Both Armstrong and Lin reported a 4.8% re-ulceration incidence rate after surgery, a 10 and 35% re-ulceration with non-surgical standard care. Tamir and Berner reported 22.0 and 38.5% after 1 year. As with other studies involving surgical procedures, none of these studies specifies if standard prevention services were provided.

6.8 Isolated Metatarsal Head Resection

Metatarsal head resection is a common surgical procedure to treat diabetic foot ulcers (Table 6.5). The common wisdom would suggest that the risk of transfer lesions and foot re-ulcerations is expected to be high because the adjacent metatarsal bone will be required to bear more pressure. Most of the work in this area combines results of different metatarsal head resections. There is one study that specifically addresses fifth metatarsal head resection [75].

The surgical approach can include either a dorsal or a plantar incision. When a plantar incision is used, the ulcer is excised completely. The flexor tendons are retracted, and a capsulotomy is

Table 6.4 Resectional arthroplasty of the first metatarsophalangeal joint

Author	Subjects	PAD assessment	Healed	Time to heal (days)	Re-ulceration	Infection	Amputation
Armstrong 2003 [70]	21 surgical 20 non-surg	Palpated pulses	Not reported	Surgical 24.2 ± 9.9 Non-surg 67.1 ± 17.1	Recurrence: Surgical 33% Non-surg 35%	Surgical 42.8% Non-surgical 40%	Surgical 4.8% Non-surg 10%
Lin 2000 [71]	14 surgical 15 TCC	ABIs TBI > 0.65	Surg 100% TCC 100%	Surgical 24.0 TCC 47.0	Surgical 0% TCC 0%	None	None
Berner 2005 [72]	11 subjects 13 ft	Palpated pulses ABIs	100%	Not reported	Recurrence 38.5%	23%	None
Tamir 2015 [73]	20 subjects 28 ft	Palpated pulses ABIs	78.5%	21.7 ± 11.9	Not reported	21.4%	None

TCC Total Contact Cast, *PAD* Peripheral Arterial Disease, *ABI* Ankle Brachial Index, *TBI* Toe Brachial Index

Table 6.5 Isolated metatarsal head resection

Author	Subjects	PAD assessment	Healed	Time to heal (days)	Re-ulceration	Infection	Amputation
Tardaguila-Garcia 2019 [74]	108 subjects 53 plantar approach 55 dorsal approach	Palpated pulses ABIs TBIs TCOM	100%	Plantar 100 ± 58 Dorsal 97 ± 84	Recurrence Plantar 52.8% Dorsal 42.6%	Plantar 22.6% Dorsal 21.8%	Plantar 13.2% Dorsal 32.7%
Armstrong 2005 [75]	40 subjects 22 surgical 18 non-surgical	Palpated pulses ABIs	100%	Surgical 40.6 ± 20.3 Non-surg 60.9 ± 30.1	Recurrence Surgical 4.5% Non-surgical 27.8%	Surgical 18.2% Non-surgical 22.2%	Surgical 4.5% Non-surg 11.7%
Elbarbary 2020 [76]	70 subjects 35 head resections 35 CAM boot	Palpated pulses ABIs	Surgical 88.6% Non-surg 67.6%	Surgical 20 ± 18 Non-surg 25 ± 14	Recurrence Surgical 5.7% Non-surgical 14.3%	Surgical 0% Non-surgical 5.7%	Surgical 11.4% Non-surg 5.7%
Kalantar Motamedi 2017 [77]	40 subjects 24 surgical ulcers evaluated 25 non-surgical ulcers evaluated	None reported	Surgical 100% Non-surg 60%	Surgical 37 ± 32 Non-surg 384 ± 329	Recurrence Surgical 0% Non-surgical 16%	Surgical 0% Non-surgical 56%	None
Faglia 2012 [78]	207 subjects 110 bone resection group 97 toe/ray amputation group	Palpated pulses ABIs TCOM	Bone resection: 86.4% Amputation: 89.9%	Not reported	*Recurrence* Bone resection 15.5% Amputation 17.3% *Transfer ulcer* Bone resection 10.3% Amputation 12.7%	Bone resection 13.6% Amputation 3%	None from bone resection group
Kalantar Motamedi 2020 [79]	30 subjects	None	96.60%	35	Recurrence 3.3% Transfer ulcer 10%	10%	None
Molines-Barroso 2013 [80]	101 subjects	Palpated pulses ABIs TCOM	100%	Not reported	Recurrence 41%	None	None
Wieman 1998 [81]	101 subjects 162 ulcers	Not reported	88%	84	Recurrence 52.3%	10.50%	11.8%

CAM Controlled Ankle Motion, *PAD* Peripheral Arterial Disease, *ABI* Ankle Brachial Index, *TBI* Toe Brachial Index, *TCOM* Transcutaneous Oxygen Measurement performed to expose the metatarsal head. Then, the metatarsal head is resected using a sagittal saw. The same steps are used with a dorsal excision, except of course the ulcer is not excised. When Tardguila-Garcia and colleagues used this approach, there was no difference in the incidence of healing, the time to heal or incidence of re-ulceration based on the site of the surgical incision [74].

There is a large and growing body of work that reports clinical outcomes of patients with diabetes with metatarsal head resection, and while most of the available literature is comprised of small retrospective cohort studies, there is consistency across studies. In general, the incidence of healing is high, the time to heal is short and complications such as infection, amputation and re-ulceration are lower than expected with non-surgical diabetic foot ulcer treatments. The results are best illustrated by the studies that used a comparison group. We identified three studies that had a non-surgical comparison group in retrospective studies of isolated metatarsal head resection [75–77, 82].

Armstrong and colleagues evaluate clinical outcomes of patients that required an isolated uninfected fifth metatarsal head resection compared to standard non-surgical treatment. All of the patients healed in both treatment groups, but the time to heal was significantly faster in the surgery group (40.6 vs. 60.9 days), and the incidence of re-ulceration was significantly lower (4.5 vs. 27.8%). However, there were no differences in infections (18.2 vs. 22.2%) and amputations (4.5 vs. 11.7%) in the surgical and non-surgical treatment groups. Elbarbary and colleagues compared a removable cast boot to metatarsal head resection surgery and reported similar results to Armstrong and colleagues. The surgery group had a significantly higher incidence of healing (88.6 vs. 67.6%) and faster time to heal (84 vs. 108 days). There were no differences in infections (14.2 vs. 11.4%), minor amputations, (5.7 vs. 11.4%), and re-ulcerations (5.7 vs. 14.3%). Likewise, Kalantar Motamedi compared surgical and non-surgical treatment and showed a significantly higher incidence of healing (100 vs. 60%), faster healing (37.3 vs. 384.1 days), fewer infections (0 vs. 56%), and fewer re-ulcerations (0 vs. 16%) [77].

6.9 Metatarsal Osteotomies

Metatarsal osteotomies have been advocated to treat metatarsalgia for many years. The approach reported elevates the metatarsal head to reduce forefoot pressures and heal neuropathic foot ulcerations. Distal Metatarsal Diaphyseal Osteotomy (DMDO) with and without internal fixation has been reported by several authors to heal diabetic foot ulcerations. The main concerns with the procedure are overcorrection, causing the metatarsal to be elevated, which leads to transfer ulcers. In addition, non-unions and Charcot arthropathy are more common in patients with diabetes and sensory neuropathy.

There is a growing body of work to report clinical outcomes of metatarsal osteotomies to heal diabetic foot ulcers (Table 6.6). We identified one prospective study and five retrospective studies that used this surgical approach. Mehlhorn and colleagues reported the results a prospective study of 26 patients that had failed non-surgical treatments. Patients had Distal Metatarsal Diaphyseal Osteotomy (DMDO) of the 2, 3, and 4 metatarsals unless the ulcer was under the 5 metatarsal head. Then DMDO was performed on just the fifth metatarsal bone. This is the only paper that uses this surgical approach to do surgery on multiple metatarsals. All study subjects healed in an average of 5.0 weeks with no infections, Charcot arthropathy or amputation. Re-ulceration and transfer ulceration incidence was 7.7 and 11.5% [87]. The retrospective studies that evaluated isolated metatarsal osteotomies had similar findings. There was a high rate of healing, (94–100%), short time to heal (35.0–55.3 days), few infections (0–5.0%) and fewer transfer ulcers (0–25%) than would be expected with non-surgical care [85, 88, 89].

Table 6.6 Metatarsal osteotomy

Author	Subjects	PAD assessment	Healed	Time to heal (days)	Re-ulceration	Infection	Amputation
Tamir 2020 [83]	32 subjects Osteotomy without fixation	Palpated pulses or ABI > 0.7	100%	25 ± 29	Recurrence 3.1% Transfer lesion 12.5%	6.2%	None
Tamir 2020 [84]	21 subjects Osteotomy without fixation	Palpated pulses or ABI > 0.9	90.4%	26	Recurrence 85% Transfer ulcers 23%	14%	4.7%
Biz 2018 [85]	30 subjects 35 ulcers Osteotomy with fixation	Palpated pulses TCOM	100%	55 ± 28	None	None	None
Fleischli 1999 [86]	20 subjects 22 osteotomies Osteotomy with fixation	Palpated pulses If non-palpable: Arterial dopplers TCOM	95%	40	Recurrence 13.6% Transfer ulcers 9.0%	14%	5%

TCOM Transcutaneous Oxygen Measurement, *ABI* Ankle Brachial Index

6.10 Pan Metatarsal Head Resection

Pan metatarsal head resection is commonly done in patients with advanced rheumatoid arthritis with claw toes and dislocated metatarsophalangeal joints because of chronic joint synovitis [90, 91]. In the advanced intrinsic minus foot, those with diabetic sensory and motor neuropathy, there is similar dislocation of the metatarsophalangeal joints and hammering and clawing of the digits. In order to remove the structural deformity and alleviate pressure on the sole of the foot, a pan metatarsal head resection can be performed. Classically, the Hoffman Clayton procedure included arthrodesis of the first metatarsophalangeal joint, resection of the lesser metatarsal heads and osteoclasis of the proximal interphalangeal joints or resection of the head of the proximal phalanx of the toes to correct hammer toe deformities for people with rheumatoid arthritis [92, 93]. In the diabetic foot, the first metatarsophalangeal joint (MTPJ) is not usually as deformed as in patients with rheumatoid arthritis, so fusion or resection of the first metatarsophalangeal joint may not be needed.

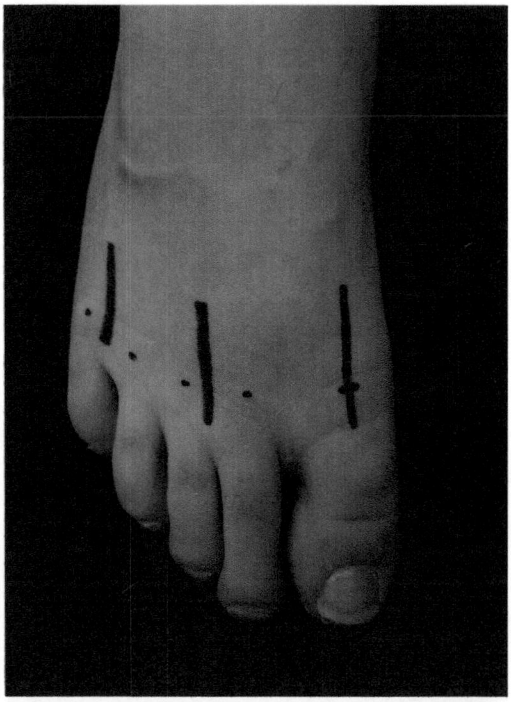

Fig. 6.11 Dorsal incisional approach for pan metatarsal head resection

6.10.1 Surgical Technique

Either three dorsal incisions or a transverse plantar incision is used to expose the metatarsal heads. When using a dorsal approach, the first incision is placed over the first metatarsophalangeal joint. The second incision is placed between the second and third metatarsals, and the third incision is placed between the fourth and fifth metatarsals (Fig. 6.11) [94]. However, when the metatarsophalangeal joints are severely dislocated, access to the lesser metatarsal heads may be easier with a plantar transverse incision place at the base of the proximal phalanges (Fig. 6.12) [95]. Once the metatarsal heads have been exposed, they are resected with a sagittal saw. The normal metatarsal parabola should be maintained (Fig. 6.13). If the patient does not have a history of ulcer under the first metatarsal head, severe hallux valgus or hallux rigidus, the first metatarsophalangeal joint may not require surgery. Alternatively, resectional arthroplasty of the base of the proximal may be needed instead of resecting the head of the first metatarsal. If the patient has a cavus foot structure, all of the metatarsal heads are usually removed.

We identified one study that included a comparison group that received non-surgical DFU care and three retrospective cohort studies that were descriptive (Table 6.7). Patients in the pan metatarsal head surgery group healed faster (39.2 vs. 84.2 days), had fewer infections (35.4 vs. 64.5%), fewer amputations (6.5 vs. 13.0%), and fewer recurrent ulcer events (15.2 vs. 39.1%) compared to the standard of care, non-surgical group. Giurini and colleagues [97] evaluated 34 people with diabetes that required pan metatarsal head resection and reported similar results. All of the surgical sites healed. There were no amputations, and only one patient experienced a re-ulceration. Jacobs reported the results of 12 patients. All of the ulcers healed with no postoperative complications and no amputations [99].

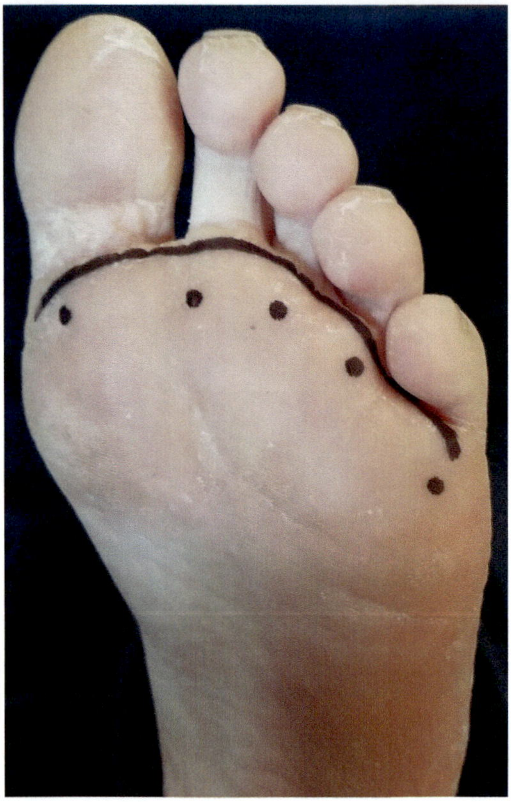

Fig. 6.12 Transverse plantar approach for pan metatarsal head resection

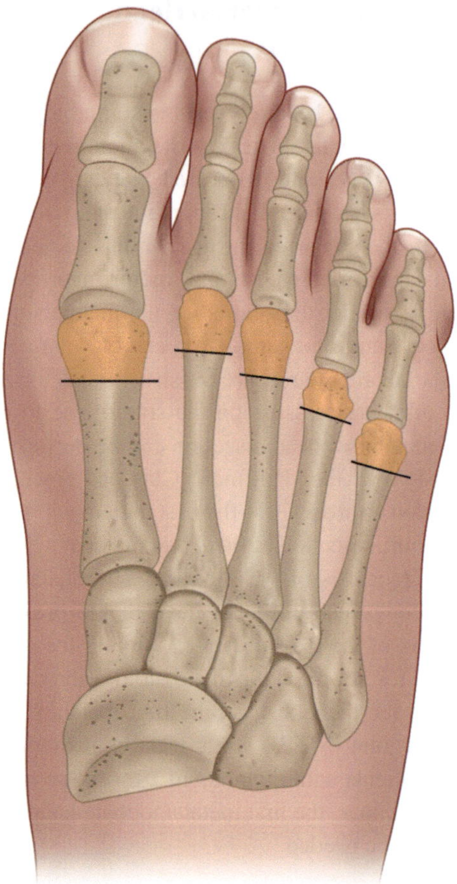

Fig. 6.13 Resection of the lesser metatarsal heads with care to maintain the normal metatarsal parabola

Table 6.7 Pan metatarsal head resection

Author	Subjects	PAD assessment	Healed	Time to heal (days)	Re-ulceration	Infection	Amputation
Armstrong 2012 [96]	92 subjects 46 surgical 46 non-surgical	Palpated pulses ABIs TBIs	Surgical 94% Non-surgical 87%	Surgical 30 ± 28 Non-surgical 84 ± 40	Recurrence Surgical 15.2% Non-surg 39.1%	Surgical 35.5% Non-surg 64.5%	Surgical 6.5% Non-surg 13%
Giurini1993 [97]	34 subjects	Palpated pulses If not palpable ABI	97%	Not reported	Recurrence 2.9%	None	None
Giurini 1987 [98]	15 subjects 16 ft	Palpated pulses If not palpable ABI	93%	Not reported	Not reported	Not reported	None
Jacobs 1982 [99]	12 subjects	ABIs Arterial waveforms	100%	Not reported	Not reported	Not reported	None

PAD Peripheral Arterial Disease, *ABI* Ankle Brachial Index, *TBI* Toe Brachial Index

6.11 Hammer Toe Correction

For patients with ulcers on the tip of the toe, a simple tenotomy of the long flexor tendon is very effective. The toe deformity should be reducible when the toe is manipulated. If there is a rigid bony deformity, a resection arthroplasty of the proximal interphalangeal joint will likely be required. As with other surgical procedures, the results of flexor tenotomies to heal toe ulcers has a very high success rate, and few infections, amputations or ulcer recurrences (Table 6.8).

The surgery is very easy and safe to perform. It can easily be done in the office with a local digital block. The flexor tendon can be cut with an 18-gauge needle, so there is only a small puncture site to heal. The needle is inserted on the plantar aspect of the digit distal to the proximal interphalangeal joint. The toe is straightened, so the flexor longus tendon is under tension and the sharp side of the needle is used to perform a tenotomy across the entire tendon. The clawing of the deformity is corrected as the tendon is incised (Fig. 6.14). The procedure can also be done with a scalpel, but a larger incision is needed.

When there is a non-reducible, rigid hammer toe deformity, a resectional arthroplasty of the proximal interphalangeal joint can be used to reduce the deformity and heal the ulcer. Armstrong and colleagues reported the results of a retrospective study of 31 patients with diabetes and 33 patients without diabetes that required resectional arthroplasty of the head of the proximal phalanx [109]. The overall re-ulceration rate was 3.7%. Patients with a history of foot ulcer developed infections at a rate of 14.3%, compared to zero infections in people without diabetes and in people with diabetes and neuropathy.

6.12 Summary

There is a growing body of evidence that suggests elective surgery to heal foot ulcers in people with diabetes is effective and safe. Postoperative infection is less common than the infections rate of receiving standard wound care for an ulceration and re-ulceration is low. There are very few studies that report catastrophic complications such as amputation of the leg or death. However, there are shortcomings in the existing literature. First, there are only a few randomized clinical studies, and the existing randomized clinical trials are small. Additionally, the literature does not codify important risk factors for infection and amputation such as poor glucose control, co-morbidities such as chronic kidney disease [110], medications such as insulin or steroids [111] and adequate perfusion. Many studies only relied on clinical examination of foot pulses to determine adequate perfusion. Some studies obtained arterial doppler studies or transcutaneous oxygen measurements if pulses were abnormal. Even with these limitations, results are quite consistent and support expanded work in the area.

Table 6.8 Flexor tenotomy of the toes

Author	Subjects	PAD assessment	Healed	Time to heal (days)	Re-ulceration	Infection	Amputation
Tamir 2008 [100]	14 subjects 38 digits 3 digits had OM	Palpated pulses	100%	21 without OM 56 with OM	None	None	None
Laborde 2007 [101]	18 subjects 28 ulcers	Palpated pulses	100%	Not reported	None	None	None
Van Netten 2013 [102]	33 subjects 38 ulcers	Palpated pulses ABIs TBIs	92%	13	Recurrence 18.4%	None	7.8%
Rasmussen 2013 [103]	38 subjects 27 ulcers 38 prophylactic	Palpated pulses ABIs TBIs	93%	21	Recurrence 11.1%	None	None
Schmitz 2019 [104]	101 ft 84 ulcers 17 prophylactic	Palpated pulses	95%	27	None	4.7%	1.1%
Smith 2020 [105]	23 subjects 76 tenotomies	Palpated pulses ABIs TBIs	100%	10.2 ± 4.3	None	2.3%	None
Kearney 2010 [106]	48 subjects 58 tenotomies	Palpated pulses	98.30%	40 ± 52	None	5%	1.9%
Tamir 2014 [107]	83 subjects 160 ulcers 160 tenotomies	Palpated pulses ABIs	89%	30	Transfer ulcer 8%	1.2%	None
Anderson 2019 [108]	81 patients 36 ulcers 106 tenotomies	Palpated pulses ABIs TBIs	94%	28	None	None	None

OM Osteomyelitis, *PAD* Peripheral Arterial Disease, *ABI* Ankle Brachial Index, *TBI* Toe Brachial Index

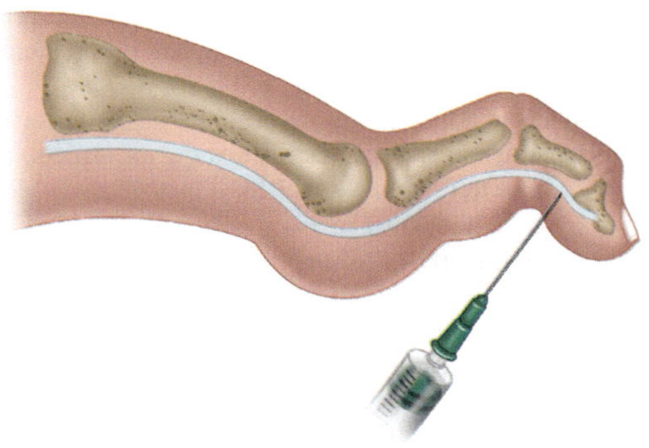

Fig. 6.14 Flexor tenotomy using an 18 gauge needle. The needle can be inserted from the side of the toe or from directly under the distal interphalangeal joint. The sharp edge of the needle is used to transect the long flexor tendon

References

1. Pop-Busui R, et al. Diabetic neuropathy: a position statement by the American Diabetes Association. Diabetes Care. 2017;40(1):136–54.
2. Armstrong DG, et al. Choosing a practical screening instrument to identify patients at risk for diabetic foot ulceration. Arch Intern Med. 1998;158(3):289–92.
3. Yang Z, Chen R, Zhang Y, Huang Y, Hong T, Sun F, Ji L, Zhan S. Scoring systems to screen for diabetic peripheral neuropathy. Cochran Database Syst Rev. 2018;7:CD010974.
4. Oyer DS, Saxon D, Shah A. Quantitative assessment of diabetic peripheral neuropathy with use of the clanging tuning fork test. Endocr Pract. 2007;13(1):5–10.
5. Park JH, Kim DS. The necessity of the simple tests for diabetic peripheral neuropathy in type 2 diabetes mellitus patients without neuropathic symptoms in clinical practice. Diabetes Metab J. 2018;42(5):442–6.
6. Lavery LA, Peters EJ, Armstrong DG. What are the most effective interventions in preventing diabetic foot ulcers? Int Wound J. 2008;5(3):425–33.
7. Reiber GE, et al. Causal pathways for incident lower-extremity ulcers in patients with diabetes from two settings. Diabetes Care. 1999;22(1):157–62.
8. Lavery LA, et al. Practical criteria for screening patients at high risk for diabetic foot ulceration. Arch Intern Med. 1998;158(2):157–62.
9. Fernando M, et al. Biomechanical characteristics of peripheral diabetic neuropathy: a systematic review and meta-analysis of findings from the gait cycle, muscle activity and dynamic barefoot plantar pressure. Clin Biomech (Bristol, Avon). 2013;28(8):831–45.
10. Caselli A, et al. The forefoot-to-rearfoot plantar pressure ratio is increased in severe diabetic neuropathy and can predict foot ulceration. Diabetes Care. 2002;25(6):1066–71.
11. Lott DJ, Zou D, Mueller MJ. Pressure gradient and subsurface shear stress on the neuropathic forefoot. Clin Biomech (Bristol, Avon). 2008;23(3):342–8.
12. Andreassen CS, et al. Accelerated atrophy of lower leg and foot muscles—a follow-up study of long-term diabetic polyneuropathy using magnetic resonance imaging (MRI). Diabetologia. 2009;52(6):1182–91.
13. Cheuy VA, et al. Intrinsic foot muscle deterioration is associated with metatarsophalangeal joint angle in people with diabetes and neuropathy. Clin Biomech (Bristol, Avon). 2013;28(9–10):1055–60.
14. Cheuy VA, et al. Muscle and joint factors associated with forefoot deformity in the diabetic neuropathic foot. Foot Ankle Int. 2016;37(5):514–21.
15. Bernstein RK. Physical signs of the intrinsic minus foot. Diabetes Care. 2003;26(6):1945–6.
16. Kimura T, et al. Neuropathy, claw toes, intrinsic muscle volume, and plantar aponeurosis thickness in diabetic feet. BMC Musculoskelet Disord. 2020;21(1):485.
17. Henderson AD, et al. Early-stage diabetic neuropathy reduces foot strength and intrinsic but not extrinsic foot muscle size. J Diabetes Res. 2020;2020:9536362.
18. Grasa J, et al. Variations in tendon stiffness due to diets with different glycotoxins affect mechanical properties in the muscle-tendon unit. Ann Biomed Eng. 2013;41(3):488–96.
19. Gerrits EG, et al. Limited joint mobility syndrome in diabetes mellitus: a minireview. World J Diabetes. 2015;6(9):1108–12.
20. Alabdali LAS, et al. Awareness of limited joint mobility in type 2 diabetes in general practice in the Netherlands: an online questionnaire survey. BMC Fam Pract. 2019;20(1):98.
21. Forsythe RO, et al. Effectiveness of bedside investigations to diagnose peripheral artery disease among people with diabetes mellitus: a systematic review. Diabetes Metab Res Rev. 2020;36(Suppl 1):e3277.
22. Alvaro-Afonso FJ, et al. Interobserver reliability of the ankle-brachial index, toe-brachial index and distal pulse palpation in patients with diabetes. Diab Vasc Dis Res. 2018;15(4):344–7.
23. Rocha-Singh KJ, Zeller T, Jaff MR. Peripheral arterial calcification: prevalence, mechanism, detection, and clinical implications. Catheter Cardiovasc Interv. 2014;83(6):E212–20.
24. Losurdo F, et al. Association of infrapopliteal medial arterial calcification with lower-limb amputations in high-risk patients: a systematic review and meta-analysis. Vasc Med. 2020;26:1358863X20979738.
25. Potier L, et al. Use and utility of ankle brachial index in patients with diabetes. Eur J Vasc Endovasc Surg. 2011;41(1):110–6.
26. Taylor GI, Palmer JH. The vascular territories (angiosomes) of the body: experimental study and clinical applications. Br J Plast Surg. 1987;40(2):113–41.

27. Dhar SC, Taylor GI. The delay phenomenon: the story unfolds. Plast Reconstr Surg. 1999;104(7):2079–91.
28. Morris SF, Taylor GI. The time sequence of the delay phenomenon: when is a surgical delay effective? An experimental study. Plast Reconstr Surg. 1995;95(3):526–33.
29. Attinger CE, et al. Angiosomes of the foot and ankle and clinical implications for limb salvage: reconstruction, incisions, and revascularization. Plast Reconstr Surg. 2006;117(7 Suppl):261S–93S.
30. Gaenslen FJ. Split heel approach in osteomyelitis of os calcis. J Bone Joint Surg. 1931;13:759.
31. Loeffler RD Jr, Ballard A. Plantar fascial spaces of the foot and a proposed surgical approach. Foot Ankle. 1980;1(1):11–4.
32. Mueller MJ, et al. Effect of Achilles tendon lengthening on neuropathic plantar ulcers. A randomized clinical trial. J Bone Joint Surg Am. 2003;85(8):1436–45.
33. Allam AM. Impact of achilles tendon lengthening (ATL) on the diabetic plantar forefoot ulceration. Egypt J Plast Reconstr Surg. 2006;30:43–8.
34. Driver VR, et al. A prospective, randomized, blinded, controlled trial comparing transdermal continuous oxygen delivery to moist wound therapy for the treatment of diabetic foot ulcers. Ostomy Wound Manage. 2017;63(4):12–28.
35. Reyzelman A, et al. Clinical effectiveness of an acellular dermal regenerative tissue matrix compared to standard wound management in healing diabetic foot ulcers: a prospective, randomised, multicentre study. Int Wound J. 2009;6(3):196–208.
36. Niederauer MQ, et al. Continuous diffusion of oxygen improves diabetic foot ulcer healing when compared with a placebo control: a randomised, double-blind, multicentre study. J Wound Care. 2018;27(Sup9):S30–45.
37. Huang W, et al. Effectiveness and safety of human amnion/chorion membrane therapy for diabetic foot ulcers: an updated meta-analysis of randomized clinical trials. Wound Repair Regen. 2020;28(6):739–50.
38. Wukich DK, et al. Neuropathy and poorly controlled diabetes increase the rate of surgical site infection after foot and ankle surgery. J Bone Joint Surg Am. 2014;96(10):832–9.
39. Lavery LA, et al. Risk factors for foot infections in individuals with diabetes. Diabetes Care. 2006;29(6):1288–93.
40. Jia L, et al. Incidence and risk factors for developing infection in patients presenting with uninfected diabetic foot ulcers. PLoS One. 2017;12(5):e0177916.
41. Bartus CL, Margolis DJ. Reducing the incidence of foot ulceration and amputation in diabetes. Curr Diab Rep. 2004;4(6):413–8.
42. Deruaz-Luyet A, et al. Incidence of lower extremity amputations among patients with type 1 and type 2 diabetes in the United States from 2010 to 2014. Diabetes Obes Metab. 2020;22(7):1132–40.
43. Bast RC Jr, et al. Elevation of serum CA 125 prior to diagnosis of an epithelial ovarian carcinoma. Gynecol Oncol. 1985;22(1):115–20.
44. Petersen BJ, et al. Recurrence rates suggest delayed identification of plantar ulceration for patients in diabetic foot remission. BMJ Open Diabetes Res Care. 2020;8(1):e001697.
45. Edmonds ME, et al. Improved survival of the diabetic foot: the role of a specialized foot clinic. Q J Med. 1986;60(232):763–71.
46. van Netten JJ, et al. Prevention of foot ulcers in the at-risk patient with diabetes: a systematic review. Diabetes Metab Res Rev. 2020;36(Suppl 1):e3270.
47. Ulbrecht JS, et al. Prevention of recurrent foot ulcers with plantar pressure-based in-shoe orthoses: the CareFUL prevention multicenter randomized controlled trial. Diabetes Care. 2014;37(7):1982–9.
48. Bus SA, et al. Effect of custom-made footwear on foot ulcer recurrence in diabetes: a multicenter randomized controlled trial. Diabetes Care. 2013;36(12):4109–16.
49. Rizzo L, et al. Custom-made orthesis and shoes in a structured follow-up program reduces the incidence of neuropathic ulcers in high-risk diabetic foot patients. Int J Low Extrem Wounds. 2012;11(1):59–64.
50. Uccioli L, et al. Manufactured shoes in the prevention of diabetic foot ulcers. Diabetes Care. 1995;18(10):1376–8.
51. Busch K, Chantelau E. Effectiveness of a new brand of stock 'diabetic' shoes to protect against diabetic foot ulcer relapse. A prospective cohort study. Diabet Med. 2003;20(8):665–9.
52. Maluf KS, et al. Tendon Achilles lengthening for the treatment of neuropathic ulcers causes a temporary reduction in forefoot pressure associated with changes in plantar flexor power rather than ankle motion during gait. J Biomech. 2004;37(6):897–906.
53. Lin SS, Lee TH, Wapner KL. Plantar forefoot ulceration with equinus deformity of the ankle in diabetic patients: the effect of tendo-Achilles lengthening and total contact casting. Orthopedics. 1996;19(5):465–75.
54. Colen LB, et al. Achilles tendon lengthening: friend or foe in the diabetic foot? Plast Reconstr Surg. 2013;131(1):37e–43e.
55. Holstein P, et al. Achilles tendon lengthening, the panacea for plantar forefoot ulceration? Diabetes Metab Res Rev. 2004;20(Suppl 1):S37–40.
56. La Fontaine J, et al. New and recurrent ulcerations after percutaneous achilles tendon lengthening in transmetatarsal amputation. J Foot Ankle Surg. 2008;47(3):225–9.
57. Meshkin DH, et al. Plantar foot ulcer recurrence in neuropathic patients undergoing percutaneous tendo-achilles lengthening. J Foot Ankle Surg. 2020;59(6):1177–80.
58. Laborde JM. Neuropathic plantar forefoot ulcers treated with tendon lengthenings. Foot Ankle Int. 2008;29(4):378–84.

59. Laborde JM. Midfoot ulcers treated with gastrocnemius-soleus recession. Foot Ankle Int. 2009;30(9):842–6.
60. Elraiyah T, et al. A systematic review and meta-analysis of off-loading methods for diabetic foot ulcers. J Vasc Surg. 2016;63(2 Suppl):59S–68S. e1–2.
61. Morona JK, et al. Comparison of the clinical effectiveness of different off-loading devices for the treatment of neuropathic foot ulcers in patients with diabetes: a systematic review and meta-analysis. Diabetes Metab Res Rev. 2013;29(3):183–93.
62. Meneses J, et al. The effects of felted foam in diabetic foot treatment: systematic review with meta-analysis. Rev. Esc Enferm USP. 2020;54:e03640.
63. Lewis J, Lipp A. Pressure-relieving interventions for treating diabetic foot ulcers. Cochrane Database Syst Rev. 2013;1:CD002302.
64. Wu SC, et al. Use of pressure offloading devices in diabetic foot ulcers: do we practice what we preach? Diabetes Care. 2008;31(11):2118–9.
65. Batista F, et al. Minimally invasive surgery for diabetic plantar foot ulcerations. Diabet. Foot Ankle. 2011;2 https://doi.org/10.3402/dfa.v2i0.10358.
66. Lin Y, et al. Modified percutaneous achilles tendon lengthening by triple hemisection for achilles tendon contracture. Biomed Res Int. 2019;2019:1491796.
67. Keller WL. The surgical treatment of bunions and hallux valgus. NY Med J. 1904;15:741–2.
68. Wrighton JD. A ten-year review of Keller's operation. Review of Keller's operation at the Princess Elizabeth Orthopaedic Hospital, Exeter. Clin Orthop Relat Res. 1972;89:207–14.
69. Johnson KA. Surgery of the foot and ankle. New York: Raven Press; 1989.
70. Armstrong DG, et al. Clinical efficacy of the first metatarsophalangeal joint arthroplasty as a curative procedure for hallux interphalangeal joint wounds in patients with diabetes. Diabetes Care. 2003;26(12):3284–7.
71. Lin SS, Bono CM, Lee TH. Total contact casting and Keller arthoplasty for diabetic great toe ulceration under the interphalangeal joint. Foot Ankle Int. 2000;21(7):588–93.
72. Berner A, Sage R, Niemela J. Keller procedure for the treatment of resistant plantar ulceration of the hallux. J Foot Ankle Surg. 2005;44(2):133–6.
73. Tamir E, et al. Resection arthroplasty for resistant ulcers underlying the hallux in insensate diabetics. Foot Ankle Int. 2015;36(8):969–75.
74. Tardaguila-Garcia A, et al. Complications associated with the approach to metatarsal head resection in diabetic foot osteomyelitis. Int Wound J. 2019;16(2):467–72.
75. Armstrong DG, Rosales MA, Gashi A. Efficacy of fifth metatarsal head resection for treatment of chronic diabetic foot ulceration. J Am Podiatr Med Assoc. 2005;95(4):353–6.
76. Elbarbary AH, Sallam EM, Ismail AM. Metatarsal head resection versus a removable mechanical device for offloading of the neuropathic diabetic plantar forefoot ulcer. Int J Low Extrem Wounds. 2020:1534734620971106.
77. Kalantar Motamedi A, Ansari M. Comparison of metatarsal head resection versus conservative care in treatment of neuropathic diabetic foot ulcers. J Foot Ankle Surg. 2017;56(3):428–33.
78. Faglia E, et al. Feasibility and effectiveness of internal pedal amputation of phalanx or metatarsal head in diabetic patients with forefoot osteomyelitis. J Foot Ankle Surg. 2012;51(5):593–8.
79. Kalantar Motamedi A, Kalantar Motamedi MA. Determinants of success after metatarsal head resection for the treatment of neuropathic diabetic foot ulcers. J Foot Ankle Surg. 2020;59(5):909–13.
80. Molines-Barroso RJ, et al. Analysis of transfer lesions in patients who underwent surgery for diabetic foot ulcers located on the plantar aspect of the metatarsal heads. Diabet Med. 2013;30(8):973–6.
81. Wieman TJ, et al. Resection of the metatarsal head for diabetic foot ulcers. Am J Surg. 1998;176(5):436–41.
82. Vanlerberghe B, et al. [Conservative surgical treatment for diabetic foot ulcers under the metatarsal heads. A retrospective case-control study]. Ann Chir Plast Esthet. 2014;59(3):161–9.
83. Tamir E, et al. Effect of mini-invasive floating metatarsal osteotomy on plantar pressure in patients with diabetic plantar metatarsal head ulcers. Foot Ankle Int. 2020;42:1071100720976099.
84. Tamir E, et al. Mini invasive floating metatarsal osteotomy for diabetic foot ulcers under the first metatarsal head: a case series. Int J Low Extrem Wounds. 2020:1534734620934579.
85. Biz C, et al. Minimally invasive distal metatarsal diaphyseal osteotomy (DMDO) for chronic plantar diabetic foot ulcers. Foot Ankle Int. 2018;39(1):83–92.
86. Fleischli JE, Anderson RB, Davis WH. Dorsiflexion metatarsal osteotomy for treatment of recalcitrant diabetic neuropathic ulcers. Foot Ankle Int. 1999;20(2):80–5.
87. Mehlhorn AT, Harrasser N, Walther M. [Treatment of plantar, neuropathic and metatarsal ulcers by minimally invasive metatarsal osteotomy]. Orthopade. 2020;49(7): 625–31.
88. Tillo TH, et al. Review of metatarsal osteotomies for the treatment of neuropathic ulcerations. J Am Podiatr Med Assoc. 1990;80(4):211–7.
89. Tamir E, et al. Mini-Invasive floating metatarsal osteotomy for resistant or recurrent neuropathic plantar metatarsal head ulcers. J Orthop Surg Res. 2016;11(1):78.
90. Kadambande S, et al. Rheumatoid forefoot reconstruction: first metatarsophalangeal fusion and excision arthroplasty of lesser metatarsal heads. Acta Orthop Belg. 2007;73(1):88–95.
91. Simon MJK, et al. Forefoot reconstruction following metatarsal head resection arthroplasty with a plantar approach-A 20-year follow-up. Foot Ankle Int. 2019;40(7):769–77.

92. Hoffmann P. An operation for severe grades of contracted or clawed toes. Am J Orthop. 1911;9:441–9.
93. Clayton ML. Surgery of the forefoot in rheumatoid arthritis. Clin Orthop. 1960;16:136–40.
94. Hodor L, Dobbs BM. Pan metatarsal head resection. A review and new approach. J Am Podiatry Assoc. 1983;73(6):287–92.
95. Fowler AW. A method of forefoot reconstruction. J Bone Joint Surg Br. 1959;41-B:507–13.
96. Armstrong DG, et al. Clinical efficacy of the pan metatarsal head resection as a curative procedure in patients with diabetes mellitus and neuropathic forefoot wounds. Foot Ankle Spec. 2012;5(4):235–40.
97. Giurini JM, et al. Panmetatarsal head resection. A viable alternative to the transmetatarsal amputation. J Am Podiatr Med Assoc. 1993;83(2):101–7.
98. Giurini JM, Habershaw GM, Chrzan JS. Panmetatarsal head resection in chronic neuropathic ulceration. J Foot Surg. 1987;26(3):249–52.
99. Jacobs RL. Hoffman procedure in the ulcerated diabetic neuropathic foot. Foot Ankle. 1982;3(3):142–9.
100. Tamir E, et al. Outpatient percutaneous flexor tenotomies for management of diabetic claw toe deformities with ulcers: a preliminary report. Can J Surg. 2008;51(1):41–4.
101. Laborde JM. Neuropathic toe ulcers treated with toe flexor tenotomies. Foot Ankle Int. 2007;28(11):1160–4.
102. van Netten JJ, Bril A, van Baal JG. The effect of flexor tenotomy on healing and prevention of neuropathic diabetic foot ulcers on the distal end of the toe. J Foot Ankle Res. 2013;6(1):3.
103. Rasmussen A, et al. Percutaneous flexor tenotomy for preventing and treating toe ulcers in people with diabetes mellitus. J Tissue Viability. 2013;22(3):68–73.
104. Schmitz P, et al. The effect of percutaneous flexor tenotomy on healing and prevention of foot ulcers in patients with claw deformity of the toe. J Foot Ankle Surg. 2019;58(6):1134–7.
105. Smith SE, Miller J. The safety and effectiveness of the percutaneous flexor tenotomy in healing neuropathic apical toe ulcers in the outpatient setting. Foot Ankle Spec. 2020;13(2):123–31.
106. Kearney TP, Hunt NA, Lavery LA. Safety and effectiveness of flexor tenotomies to heal toe ulcers in persons with diabetes. Diabetes Res Clin Pract. 2010;89(3):224–6.
107. Tamir E, et al. Percutaneous tenotomy for the treatment of diabetic toe ulcers. Foot Ankle Int. 2014;35(1):38–43.
108. Hedegaard Andersen J, et al. The effect of needle tenotomy on hammer, mallet and claw toe deformities in patients with diabetes, a retrospective study. J Clin Transl Endocrinol. 2019;18:100208.
109. Armstrong DG, et al. Is prophylactic diabetic foot surgery dangerous? J Foot Ankle Surg. 1996;35(6):585–9.
110. Naqvi SB, Collins AJ. Infectious complications in chronic kidney disease. Adv Chronic Kidney Dis. 2006;13(3):199–204.
111. Lavery LA, et al. Increased risk of nonunion and charcot arthropathy after ankle fracture in people with diabetes. J Foot Ankle Surg. 2020;59(4):653–6.

When and How to Prepare for Surgery

7

Paige K. Dekker, Kevin G. Kim, Kenneth L. Fan, and Karen K. Evans

Key Points

- Thorough preoperative evaluation not only allows for effective surgical planning but also allows the surgeon to identify and proactively manage conditions that may otherwise predispose a patient to reconstructive failure.
- A multidisciplinary approach is critical for an effective and thorough preoperative workup.

P. K. Dekker · K. G. Kim · K. L. Fan
Department of Plastic and Reconstructive Surgery, MedStar Georgetown University Hospital, Washington, DC, USA
e-mail: pkd15@georgetown.edu; kgk31@rwjms.rutgers.edu; Kenneth.L.Fan@medstar.net

K. K. Evans (✉)
Department of Plastic and Reconstructive Surgery, MedStar Georgetown University Hospital, Washington, DC, USA

Department of Plastic and Reconstructive Surgery, Center for Wound Healing and Hyperbaric Medicine, Washington, DC, USA
e-mail: karen.k.evans@medstar.net; Karen.K.Evans@gunet.georgetown.edu

7.1 Introduction

Thorough preoperative workup plays a key role in avoiding perioperative complications and optimizing wound healing and ambulation after reconstructive surgery. Several modalities such as vascular studies, thermograms, and transcutaneous oximetry measurements provide objective data that can guide perioperative management as well as surgical planning. This chapter provides an overview of these available modalities and their utility in planning a successful diabetic foot reconstruction.

7.2 Relevance to Surgical Outcome

Each step of the preoperative evaluation plays an important role in optimizing reconstructive success. Patients and their family members should be counseled early and often regarding the importance of strict adherence to instructions for postoperative weight-bearing and ambulation. A patient who is too aggressive with his or her return to ambulation risks compromised flap perfusion and subsequent flap failure. In patients with diabetes, failure to achieve adequate blood sugar control prior to surgery is associated with an increased risk of dehiscence and reoperation [1]. Proactive identification of arterial and venous

J. P. Hong, H. Suh (eds.), *Diabetic Foot Reconstruction*,
https://doi.org/10.1007/978-981-16-9816-3_7

pathologies is also of critical importance: endovascular procedures done prior to reconstructive surgery coupled with adequate consideration of vascular pathologies in the surgical plan can help ensure adequate reperfusion of ischemic areas and prevent flap congestion and/or thrombosis [2–4]. A thorough assessment for hereditary and/or acquired thrombophilias prior to surgery can help optimize a patient's perioperative anticoagulation regimen, thereby minimizing the risk of flap thrombosis and subsequent flap failure with a high risk of nonsalvageability [3, 5–8]. Patients should also undergo a comprehensive biomechanical exam: addressing gait abnormalities is an important step in preventing wound recurrence.

7.3 Preoperative Evaluation and Special Considerations

Our management algorithm (Fig. 7.1) utilizes multidisciplinary collaboration to identify and proactively manage risks for flap failure, optimize comorbidities prior to surgery, and develop a personalized surgical plan. In addition to an early and aggressive focus on comorbidity optimization, the first layer of surgical preparation includes vascular studies to optimize donor and recipient vessel selection, hypercoagulability studies to minimize perioperative clotting risk, and a biomechanical exam to address mechanical factors that may compromise lower extremity

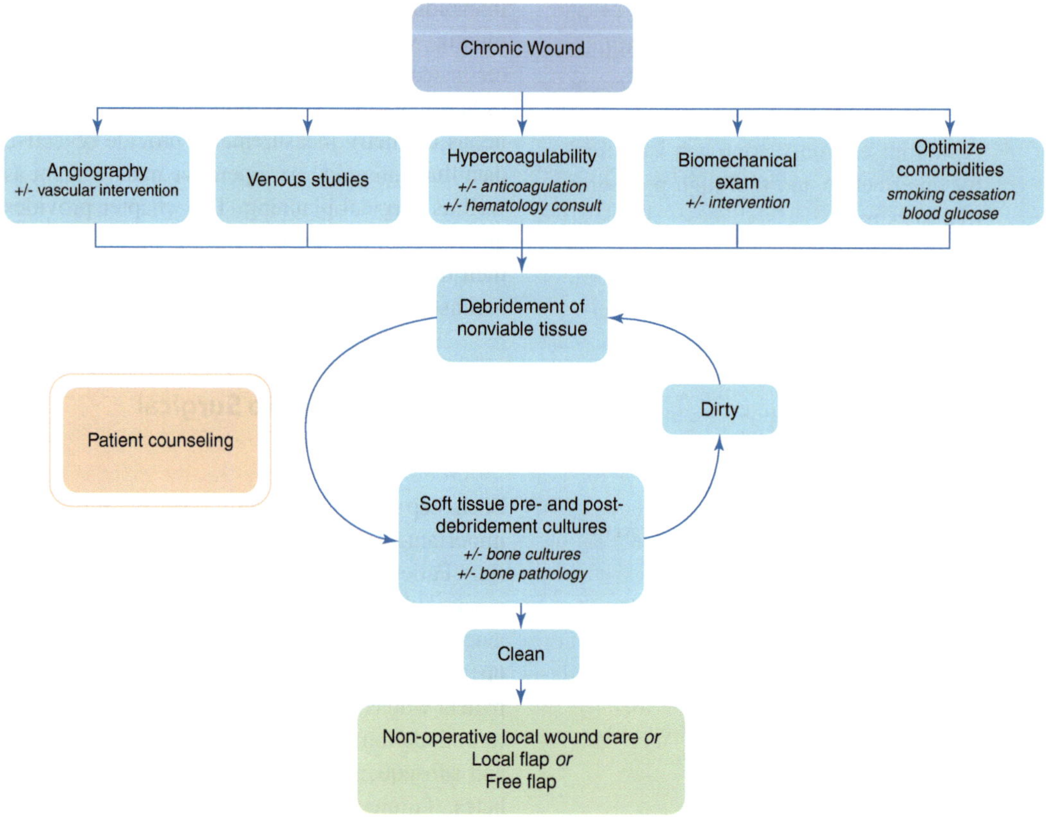

Fig. 7.1 Management algorithm

wound healing. The next phase of preparation involves serial surgical debridement to prepare a culture-negative wound bed before pursuing further wound management with reconstruction.

Counseling the patient and family should occur frequently throughout the preoperative process, with an emphasis on postoperative ambulation and expectations for the patient's weight-bearing status as he or she rehabilitates postoperatively. Strict compliance with ambulation instructions is critical for reconstructive success.

7.3.1 Comorbidity Optimization

Comorbid conditions increase surgical complications and should thus be evaluated with thorough history taking and optimized appropriately before surgery [9]. In patients with diabetes, adequate blood sugar control is critical: blood glucose levels above 200 mg/dl and HbA1c above 6.5% increases risk of dehiscence and reoperation by over three and four times, respectively [1]. All patients who smoke should be encouraged to quit or otherwise abstain for a minimum of 4–8 weeks prior to surgery [10]. Postoperatively, patients are in a hypermetabolic state and should undergo preoperative nutritional screening. Malnutrition can be managed with nutritional prehabilitation and exercise therapy [11] and tracked via albumin and prealbumin levels, although utility of these tests as markers of nutrition has recently come into question [12]. In a retrospective review of patients undergoing lower extremity free tissue transfer (FTT) at our institution, albumin levels lower than 2.7 g/dL preoperatively were associated with significantly increased healing times and decreased flap healing rates. Conversely, low prealbumin levels (traditionally defined as lower than 20 mg/dL) were not associated with increased time to flap healing or flap healing rates [13].

7.3.2 Vascular Examination

Flap success is highly dependent on adequate perfusion of the transferred tissue; therefore, a thorough vascular exam is critical to optimizing flap survival. By focusing this exam on the vascular supply defining the 6 foot and ankle angiosomes, a surgeon can (1) predict the viability of a given tissue for harvest, (2) plan for optimal surgical incision placement, and (3) coordinate with a vascular surgeon for preemptive revascularization to ensure adequate reperfusion to areas of ischemic ulceration [2, 3].

7.3.3 Arterial Examination

There are several options for arterial examination, including palpating for pulses, ankle-brachial indices, handheld Doppler examination, computed tomographic (CT) angiography, and catheter arteriography [14]. The contrast dye load required for conventional arteriography is significantly less than that required for lower extremity CT angiography; therefore, arteriography is more renal protective and thus may be preferred in the diabetic patient population, in which many patients have renal insufficiency [14]. In our practice, routine preoperative arteriography identified arterial pathology in 67.8% of patients undergoing FTT for chronic lower extremity wounds [14]. Furthermore, diabetes was associated with the presence of stenosis or occlusion on angiography as well as the need for endovascular intervention [14]. This imaging modality is thus particularly helpful in the preoperative workup of this population.

7.3.4 Venous Examination

Insufficient venous outflow leading to congestion and delayed venous thrombosis is a leading cause of flap loss [15]. Venous studies with lower extremity duplex ultrasound can identify venous anomalies and venous insufficiency that results in high venous pressure and may predispose a patient to congestive complications in the deep or superficial venous system. Preoperative venous studies are therefore useful when selecting recipient veins for FTT and help guide whether the superficial or deep venous system should be used. At our institution, venous duplex ultrasonography detected venous insufficiency (defined as <0.5 seconds of reflux) in 39% of patients undergoing FTT for lower extremity wounds [4]. Deep vein thrombosis requiring anticoagulation was identified in 6.78% of patients [4].

7.3.5 Thrombophilia Assessment

While the literature demonstrates that FTT can be performed with a high success rate in hypercoagulable patients [5], patients with hereditary or acquired factors for thrombophilia are at increased risk of microvascular thrombosis and subsequent flap failure with high rates of nonsalvageability [6–8]. Preoperative workup should include a thorough thrombophilia screening to assess propensity for perioperative flap thrombosis, optimize individual anticoagulation protocol, and subsequently obtain hematology consultation, if necessary, prior to surgery [3, 5, 6].

In our practice, all patients are screened for potential thrombophilia via thorough history taking and a preoperative thrombophilia panel [8]. Patients should be asked about any personal or familial history of blood clots, use of blood thinners, previous miscarriage, as well as any diagnoses of clotting disorders, autoimmune disease, and/or purpura fulminans [8]. In addition to complete blood count (CBC), prothrombin time (PT), and partial thromboplastin time (PTT), a comprehensive laboratory workup includes testing for antiphospholipid antibodies; activity levels for antithrombin III, protein C, and protein S; homocysteine and factor VIII levels; genotypes for factor V Leiden *G1691A* and prothrombin *G20210A*; testing for MTHFR polymorphisms (*A1298C* and *C677T*); and testing for the 4G/5G polymorphism of the plasminogen activator inhibitor-1 (PAI-1) gene [8]. Implementation of this preoperative assessment in our practice revealed that 61% of patients undergoing FTT for lower extremity salvage had at least one thrombophilic trait; 20% of patients were found to have three or more separate diagnoses.

Patients with either known or newly detected thrombophilia should receive a hematology consult to assist with preoperative risk stratification and anticoagulation regimen optimization. Implementation of a risk-stratified anticoagulation algorithm in our practice resulted in lower rates of total (3.0 vs. 19.0%) and partial (10.0 vs. 37.0%) flap loss in the risk-stratified group when compared to non-stratified controls. Successful limb salvage in the setting of postoperative thrombosis was 0% in both groups, reiterating the risk of nonsalvageability in thrombophilic patients who develop thrombosis postoperatively and reinforcing the potential benefits of a risk-stratified anticoagulation protocol [6].

7.3.6 Biomechanical Exam

All patients should undergo biomechanical examination to identify any mechanical issues contributing to wound formation and persistence. If left unaddressed, such issues may lead to wound recurrence. A thorough biomechanical exam is of critical importance in patients with diabetic peripheral neuropathy, as these patients often have altered plantar pressure and stance times [16]. In our practice, we routinely address equinus gait with Achilles tendon lengthening.

7.3.7 Transcutaneous Oximetry

Transcutaneous oximetry (TcPO2) is a noninvasive method that can be used as an adjunctive clinical tool to guide the selection between local wound management and surgical reconstruction. It functions by measuring capillary oxygen content through electrodes placed on the skin. TcPO2 is a valuable tool in determining the likelihood of wound healing in diabetic foot ulcers, with a substantial diagnostic odds ratio (DOR) of 15.8, compared to 1.0 for ankle-brachial index (ABI) [17]. Furthermore, ABI is inaccurate in the presence of arterial calcinosis and toe-brachial index is inappropriate in the presence of an existing ulcer or amputation, making TcPO2 particularly helpful in these cases [17]. A TcPO2 value ≥25 mmHg generally indicates adequate perfusion and significantly improves odds of wound healing [18, 19]. In one study, all wounds with

TcPO2 ≥ 40 mmHg achieved healing, while those with measurements < 10 mmHg failed to heal [19]. In addition to compromised healing, low (< 25 mmHg) TcPO2 measures have also been shown to more than double one's risk of mortality at 1 year [20]. TcPO2 is also significantly correlated with ulcer size and Wagner ulcer grade [21].

The utility of TcPO2 in predicting amputation is less clear, with a DOR of 4.4 compared to 2.9 for ABI [17]. A large prospective cohort by Boyko et al. found that TcPO2 did not significantly correlate with overall amputation rates [22]. Although the risk of amputation based on TcPO2 is inconclusive, it can be used to guide selection of amputation site and should read ≥ 20 mmHg, which confers an 80% chance of wound healing [23, 24].

7.3.8 Thermograms

Thermoanalysis has emerged as an adjunctive method in the early prediction of diabetic foot complications and can thus guide appropriate interventions. Amputations in the diabetic patient are often due to ulcers on the plantar foot, which is prone to ischemic and neuropathic pathophysiology [25]. Infrared thermoanalysis is a fast and noninvasive method used to visualize temperature distribution of the plantar foot without subjecting the patient to radiation [26, 27]. Healthy patients exhibit mirrored symmetry of temperature distribution across both feet, with temperature hottest at the medial longitudinal arch and decreasing distally along the plantar foot [28]. Multiple methods of thermogram analysis exist. Asymmetric temperature analysis is the most common method and assesses for mirrored symmetry of temperature distribution in both feet, with asymmetry suggesting disease [27]. A colder foot on exam may suggest compromised local autonomic control, placing that tissue at risk of ischemic ulceration and warranting further investigation with vascular ultrasound [25, 28]. Contrarily, hot spots may signify areas of inflammation; however, many diabetics will show increased plantar temperatures bilaterally [25]. Temperature distribution analysis is less common and assesses plantar temperature within each individual foot. However, distribution patterns between diabetic patients may be irregular [27]. Nonetheless, evaluation may reveal decreased temperature under the first metatarsal head, fifth metatarsal head, the heel, or the big toe [26]. Thermograms are limited by subjective analysis and susceptibility to the external environment and are most useful for clinical correlation [27].

7.3.9 Considerations for Transplant Patients

Existing evidence demonstrates that free tissue transfer can be successfully performed in patients who have undergone solid organ transplantation and require lifelong immunosuppression [29, 30]. This is particularly important in the diabetic population, as many of these patients may develop chronic kidney disease and eventually require kidney transplantation. Despite demonstrated success of microvascular FTT in this patient population, chronic immunosuppression may put these patients at increased risk of complications such as flap thrombosis, infection, and delayed wound healing [29, 30]. Many immunosuppressive agents can also cause hypertension and thrombocytopenia, which may increase the risk of hematoma formation [30]. Immunosuppressive agents may also exacerbate the atherosclerotic-predisposing effects of diabetes, hypertension, and hyperlipidemia [31], highlighting the importance of aggressive optimization of these comorbidities and preoperative vascular studies in this patient population. Multidisciplinary collaboration between the reconstructive surgeon and the surgical transplant team is essential in ensuring that both the transplanted organ and transferred tissue have adequate monitoring postoperatively [30].

7.3.10 Infection Control

Prior to proceeding with reconstructive surgery, the wound bed must be clear of infection. Serial debridement procedures performed in conjunction with culture-driven antibiotic therapy should continue until negative cultures are obtained. A detailed description of infection control is described in Chaps. 4 and 5 ("Understanding Infection" and "Understanding Wound Bed Preparation," respectively) of this textbook.

7.4 Conclusion

Comprehensive surgical preparation is key in achieving successful diabetic limb reconstruction. Aggressive management of comorbidities, particularly perioperative blood glucose levels in the patient with diabetes, is essential for reducing the risk of dehiscence and necessity for reoperation. Ancillary clinical testing such as vascular studies, hypercoagulable screening, thermoanalysis, transcutaneous oximetry, and a biomechanical exam can all add vital information necessary for planning and executing the most optimal reconstruction for the presenting patient.

7.5 Case

A 43-year-old male with a past medical history significant for type I diabetes mellitus initially presented with a fissure on the left heel (Fig. 7.2). Over the course of the next 3 weeks, the wound developed erythema, swelling, warmth, and sanguineous drainage (Fig. 7.3). The patient also reported severe constant, deep pain of the left lower extremity which he rated as 9+/10 in severity and limited his ability to ambulate. When he presented to the emergency room 3 weeks after initial presentation, the patient was complaining of subjective fever, chills, malaise, and worsening pain and redness of the area. On exam, the patient was afebrile (36.2) but was hypotensive (97/64). Exam of the left heel ulcer revealed fluctuant eschar and purulent drainage (Fig. 7.3b). The area was warm, swollen, and tender to palpation, and erythema was noted, extending distally to the dorsal foot and proximally up the posterior calf. X-ray and CT of the limb were negative for osteomyelitis and subcutaneous emphysema, but

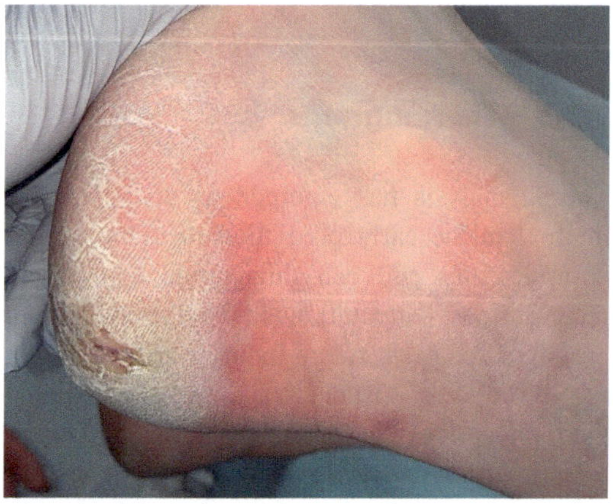

Fig. 7.2 Initial presentation of small fissure on left heel

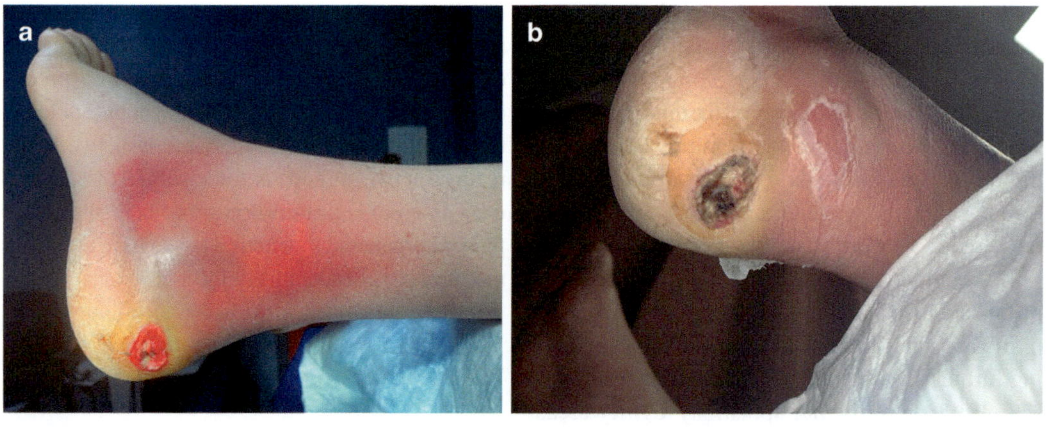

Fig. 7.3 (**a**) Left heel wound, 3 weeks after initial presentation. (**b**) Left heel wound with wet gangrene necessitating admission

the patient was admitted for emergent surgical exploration and debridement due to concern for necrotizing fasciitis.

In the operating room (OR), excision of the ulcer down to fascia was performed, as well as complete excision of the area over the peroneal tendons (Fig. 7.4). The patient returned to the OR on postoperative day one (POD1) for repeat debridement to ensure complete removal of infected tissue. This procedure included partial excision of the lateral wall of the calcaneus bone. The resulting open defect was substantial, and it was determined that definitive closure with FTT may be required (Fig. 7.5). We then proceeded with our management algorithm as outlined above in preparation for free flap reconstruction.

- *Two additional debridement procedures* were performed until cultures were negative and a clean wound bed was achieved. Figure 7.6 depicts the clean wound prior to FTT.
- Vascular surgery was consulted for *arteriogram*, which was performed 1 week prior to FTT. Findings were significant for an approximately 8–10 cm segment of high-grade subsegmental stenoses of the posterior tibial artery. This finding in conjunction with the location of the patient's wound necessitated revascularization of the posterior tibial artery with percutaneous transluminal angioplasty.
- Vascular surgery was also consulted for *venous studies*. Venous duplex was performed 5 days prior to FTT, and findings were significant for reflux in the external iliac vein and a non-occlusive thrombus in the small saphenous vein at the distal calf.
- *Hypercoagulability studies* revealed that the patient had neither the Factor V Leiden *G1691A* mutation nor the prothrombin *G20210A* mutation nor the MTHFR polymorphisms (*A1298C* or *C677T*). Screening for antiphospholipid antibodies and lupus anticoagulants was also negative. His protein S activity was slightly low (62, normal 65–140), as was his protein C activity (63, normal 70–130). His antithrombin III activity was also slightly low (76, normal 80–125). Homocysteine was within normal limits (6.1, normal 3.2–10.7). The patient's hypercoagulability studies did not necessitate further workup or specialized intraoperative management.

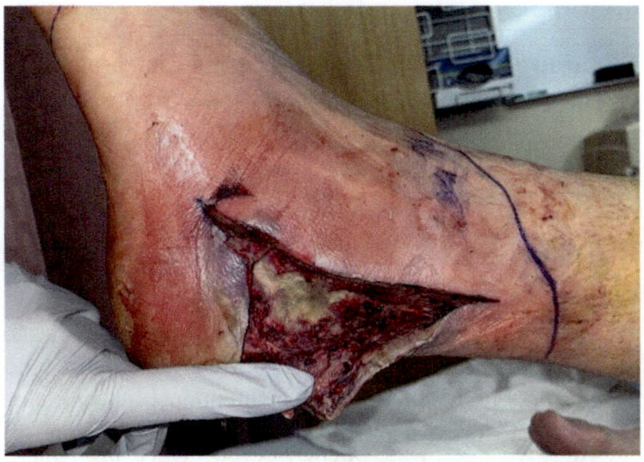

Fig. 7.4 Left heel wound after initial exploration and debridement

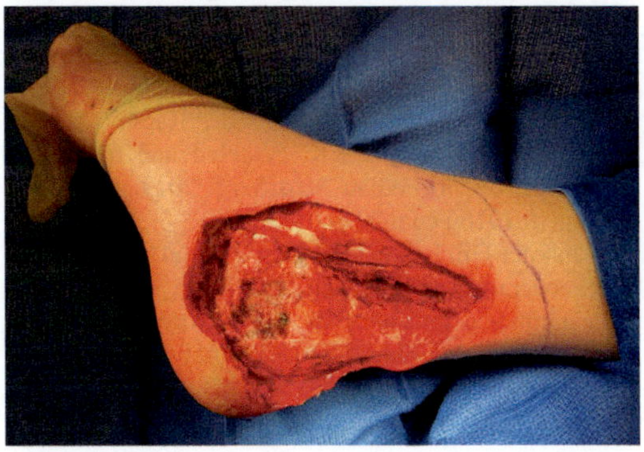

Fig. 7.5 Left heel wound after second debridement and partial excision of calcaneus bone

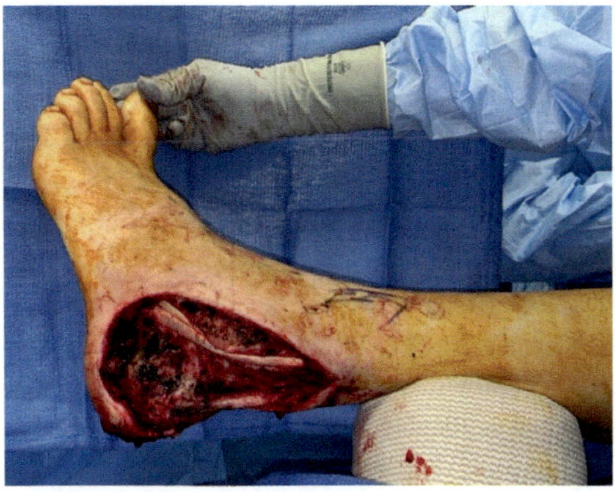

Fig. 7.6 Preoperative image of wound with exposed calcaneus bone and peroneal tendon prior to FTT

- Internal medicine was consulted for *optimization of blood glucose levels*. On admission, the patient's hemoglobin A1c was 10.7% and he had glucometer readings as high as 326 mg/dL several days prior to FTT. The patient was a nonsmoker.

At the time of FTT, the defect requiring coverage measured 13 × 9 cm (Fig. 7.6). Closure was performed with an anterolateral thigh (ALT) perforator fasciocutaneous flap (Fig. 7.7) with end-to-side anastomosis to the anterior tibial artery and two venous anastomoses (Fig. 7.8). He was discharged 11 days after FTT. His flap donor and recipient sites are now well healed (Fig. 7.9a, b), and the patient is able to ambulate.

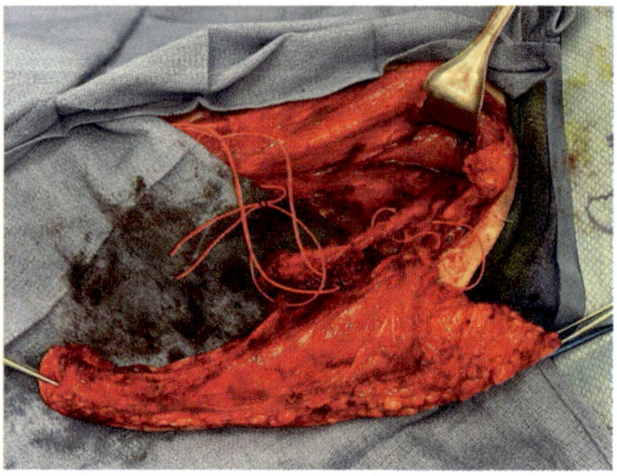

Fig. 7.7 Two perforator ALT flap

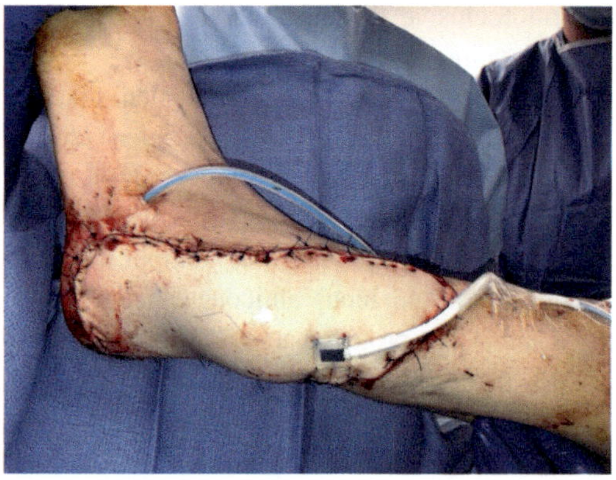

Fig. 7.8 Postoperative image of ALT flap covering defect on the left lateral ankle and leg

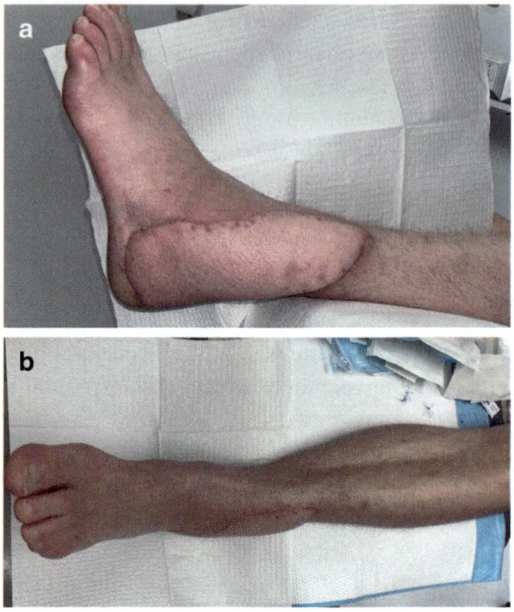

Fig. 7.9 (**a, b**) Four months after FTT

Disclosure Statement There are no financial disclosures, commercial associations, or any other conditions posing a conflict of interest to report for any of the above authors.

References

1. Endara M, Masden D, Goldstein J, Gondek S, Steinberg J, Attinger C. The role of chronic and perioperative glucose management in high-risk surgical closures: a case for tighter glycemic control. Plast Reconstr Surg. 2013;132:996–1004. https://doi.org/10.1097/PRS.0b013e31829fe119.
2. Attinger CE, Evans KK, Bulan E, Blume P, Cooper P. Angiosomes of the foot and ankle and clinical implications for limb salvage: reconstruction, incisions, and revascularization. Plast Reconstr Surg. 2006;117(7 SUPPL):261–93. https://doi.org/10.1097/01.prs.0000222582.84385.54.
3. Black CK, Kotha VS, Fan KL, Ragothaman K, Attinger CE, Evans KK. Pedicled and free tissue transfers. Clin Podiatr Med Surg. 2019; https://doi.org/10.1016/j.cpm.2019.03.002.
4. Janhofer DE, Lakhiani C, Kim PJ, et al. The utility of preoperative venous testing for lower extremity flap planning in patients with lower extremity wounds. Plast Reconstr Surg. 2020;145(1):164e–71e. https://doi.org/10.1097/PRS.0000000000006384.

5. Kotamarti VS, Shiah E, Rezak KM, Patel A, Ricci JA. Does anticoagulation improve flap outcomes in hypercoagulable patients? A systematic review. J Reconstr Microsurg. 2020; https://doi.org/10.1055/s-0039-3400531.
6. DeFazio M, Economides J, Anghel E, Tefera E, Evans K. Lower extremity free tissue transfer in the setting of thrombophilia: analysis of perioperative anticoagulation protocols and predictors of flap failure. J Reconstr Microsurg. 2019;35(04):270–86. https://doi.org/10.1055/s-0038-1675145.
7. Wang TY, Serletti JM, Cuker A, et al. Free tissue transfer in the hypercoagulable patient: a review of 58 flaps. Plast Reconstr Surg. 2012;129(2):443–53. https://doi.org/10.1097/PRS.0b013e31823aec4d.
8. Defazio MV, Hung RWY, Han KD, Bunting HA, Evans KK. Lower extremity flap salvage in thrombophilic patients: managing expectations in the setting of microvascular thrombosis. J Reconstr Microsurg. 2016; https://doi.org/10.1055/s-0035-1571249.
9. Levy N, Dhatariya K. Pre-operative optimisation of the surgical patient with diagnosed and undiagnosed diabetes: a practical review. Anaesthesia. 2019;74:58–66. https://doi.org/10.1111/anae.14510.
10. Lumb AB. Pre-operative respiratory optimisation: an expert review. Anaesthesia. 2019;74:43–8. https://doi.org/10.1111/anae.14508.
11. Gillis C, Wischmeyer PE. Pre-operative nutrition and the elective surgical patient: why, how and what? Anaesthesia. 2019;74:27–35. https://doi.org/10.1111/anae.14506.
12. Lee JL, Oh ES, Lee RW, Finucane TE. Serum albumin and Prealbumin in calorically restricted, non-diseased individuals: a systematic review. Am J Med. 2015;128(9):1023.e1–1023.e22. https://doi.org/10.1016/j.amjmed.2015.03.032.
13. Kim KG, Mishu M, Zolper EG, Bhardwaj P, Rogers A, Dekker PK, Fan KL, Evans KK. Nutritional markers for predicting lower extremity free tissue transfer outcomes in the chronic wound population. Microsurgery. 2021 Aug 6. https://doi.org/10.1002/micr.30794. Epub ahead of print. PMID: 34357655.
14. Janhofer DE, Lakhiani C, Kim PJ, et al. The utility of preoperative arteriography for free flap planning in patients with chronic lower extremity wounds. Plast Reconstr Surg. 2019;143(2):604–13. https://doi.org/10.1097/PRS.0000000000005265.
15. Fischer JP, Wink JD, Nelson JA, et al. A retrospective review of outcomes and flap selection in free tissue transfers for complex lower extremity reconstruction. J Reconstr Microsurg. 2013; https://doi.org/10.1055/s-0033-1343952.
16. Fernando M, Crowther R, Lazzarini P, et al. Biomechanical characteristics of peripheral diabetic neuropathy: a systematic review and meta-analysis of findings from the gait cycle, muscle activity and dynamic barefoot plantar pressure. Clin Biomech. 2013;28(8):831–45. https://doi.org/10.1016/j.clinbiomech.2013.08.004.
17. Wang Z, Hasan R, Firwana B, et al. A systematic review and meta-analysis of tests to predict wound healing in diabetic foot. J Vasc Surg. 2016;63(2):29S–36S.e2. https://doi.org/10.1016/j.jvs.2015.10.004.
18. Brownrigg JRW, Hinchliffe RJ, Apelqvist J, et al. Performance of prognostic markers in the prediction of wound healing or amputation among patients with foot ulcers in diabetes: a systematic review. Diabetes Metab Res Rev. 2016;32:128–35. https://doi.org/10.1002/dmrr.2704.
19. Yang C, Weng H, Chen L, et al. Transcutaneous oxygen pressure measurement in diabetic foot ulcers mean values and cut-point for wound healing. J Wound Ostomy Cont Nurs. 2013;40(6):585–9. https://doi.org/10.1097/WON.0b013e3182a9a7bf.
20. Fagher K, Katzman P, Löndahl M. Transcutaneous oxygen pressure as a predictor for short-term survival in patients with type 2 diabetes and foot ulcers: a comparison with ankle–brachial index and toe blood pressure. Acta Diabetol. 2018;55(8):781–8. https://doi.org/10.1007/s00592-018-1145-8.
21. Zubair M, Ahmad J. Transcutaneous oxygen pressure (TcPO 2) and ulcer outcome in diabetic patients: is there any correlation? Diabetes Metab Syndr Clin Res Rev. 2019;13(2):953–8. https://doi.org/10.1016/j.dsx.2018.12.008.
22. Boyko EJ, Seelig AD, Ahroni JH. Limb- and person-level risk factors for lower-limb amputation in the prospective Seattle diabetic foot study. Diabetes Care. 2018;41(4):891–8. https://doi.org/10.2337/dc17-2210.
23. Ladurner R, Küper M, Königsrainer I, et al. Predictive value of routine transcutaneous tissue oxygen tension (tcpo2) measurement for the risk of non-healing and amputation in diabetic foot ulcer patients with non-palpable pedal pulses. Med Sci Monit. 2010;16(6):273–7.
24. Wütschert R, Bounameaux H. Determination of amputation level in ischemic limbs: reappraisal of the measurement of TcPO2. Diabetes Care. 1997;20(8):1315–8. https://doi.org/10.2337/diacare.20.8.1315.
25. Renero-C F-J. The abrupt temperature changes in the plantar skin thermogram of the diabetic patient: looking in to prevent the insidious ulcers. Diabet Foot Ankle. 2018;9(1):1430950. https://doi.org/10.1080/2000625X.2018.1430950.
26. Astasio-Picado Á, Martínez EE, Gómez-Martín B. Comparison of thermal foot maps between diabetic patients with neuropathic, vascular, neurovascular, and no complications. Curr Diabetes Rev. 2019;15(6):503–9. https://doi.org/10.2174/1573399815666190206160711.

27. Adam M, Ng EYK, Tan JH, Heng ML, Tong JWK, Acharya UR. Computer aided diagnosis of diabetic foot using infrared thermography: a review. Comput Biol Med. 2017;91:326–36. https://doi.org/10.1016/j.compbiomed.2017.10.030.
28. Renero-C F-J. The thermoregulation of healthy individuals, overweight–obese, and diabetic from the plantar skin thermogram: a clue to predict the diabetic foot. Diabet Foot Ankle. 2017;8(1):1361298. https://doi.org/10.1080/2000625X.2017.1361298.
29. Sbitany H, Xu X, Hansen SL, Young DM, Hoffman WY. The effects of immunosuppressive medications on outcomes in microvascular free tissue transfer. Plast Reconstr Surg. 2014; https://doi.org/10.1097/PRS.0000000000000012.
30. Lee AB, Dupin CL, Colen L, Jones NF, May JW, Chiu ES. Microvascular free tissue transfer in organ transplantation patients: is it safe? Plast Reconstr Surg. 2008; https://doi.org/10.1097/PRS.0b013e31817123b0.
31. Craig-Schapiro R, Nejim B, Arhuidese I, Malas MB. Aggressive infrainguinal revascularization in renal transplant patients is justifiable. Am J Transplant. 2018; https://doi.org/10.1111/ajt.14636.

When and How to Perform Local Flap

8

S. Raja Sabapathy and Madhu Periasamy

Key Points

- Local flaps are useful for the reconstruction of small defects in a vascular foot.
- Cutaneous flaps and muscle flaps are possible in the foot.
- Cutaneous flaps are preferred for reconstruction of the weight-bearing surfaces.
- Muscle flaps are preferred for coverage of defects in non-weight-bearing areas of the feet and to fill small bony cavities.
- Local flaps when done for plantar trophic ulcers need to be followed by surgical offloading procedures to prevent ulcer recurrence.

Supplementary Information The online version contains supplementary material available at [https://doi.org/10.1007/978-981-16-9816-3_8].

S. R. Sabapathy (✉) · M. Periasamy
Department of Plastic, Hand and Reconstructive Microsurgery, Ganga Hospital, Coimbatore, Tamil Nadu, India

Department of Plastic, Hand and Reconstructive Microsurgery, Ganga Medical Centre and Hospital, Coimbatore, Tamil Nadu, India

8.1 Introduction

Locoregional flaps for reconstruction of the Diabetic foot ulcers have been in use for a long time. A local flap is a three-dimensional unit of tissue that is harvested from the area adjacent or interpolated to the tissue defect. Most flaps follow a geometrical basis during the transfer. Local flaps were initially raised as random pattern flaps. Attinger defined the angiosomes of the foot and ankle [1], which led to the local flaps being preferentially designed by including named vessels or perforators in the base. This has made the survival of local flaps more predictable. Cutaneous local flaps have the advantage of providing skin cover with tissue of a similar nature.

8.2 General Principles

1. Size: Local flaps in the diabetic foot are indicated to cover small defects with the wound size of about 3 × 6 cm with exposed critical structures in the base [2, 3]. Local flaps for defects larger than this would result in a donor site defect in the weight-bearing plantar surface of the foot, causing considerable morbidity.
2. Vascularity of the foot: Local flaps are indicated in a vascular foot, with palpable pulses of either the dorsalis pedis or posterior tibial arteries. When raised from the bed, all local flaps endure a reduction in tissue perfusion.

J. P. Hong, H. Suh (eds.), *Diabetic Foot Reconstruction*,
https://doi.org/10.1007/978-981-16-9816-3_8

Hence the chances of full or partial necrosis of flaps is high in a dysvascular foot. An ulcer in a dysvascular foot will have a poorly vascularized wound bed which is prone for infection. Local flaps need to be placed on a good bed for optimal healing. A poorly vascular bed leads to infection and dehiscence of flap margins. Raising a big local flap in a poorly vascular foot may cut off collaterals to the part of foot distal to the flap resulting in secondary distal gangrene. We prefer to have at least one palpable foot pulse before choosing local flaps for reconstruction.

3. Neuropathy: Diabetic neuropathy is not a contraindication for local flaps. Most of the patients with neuropathy have good palpable pulses and local flaps are a viable option in such patients. While performing cutaneous flaps pose no specific problem in a neuropathic foot, may need to exercise caution in choosing muscle flaps in such feet. The volume of intrinsic muscles of the foot is approximately reduced by 50% in patients with diabetic neuropathy [4]. Planning and raising adequate flaps to cover defects can be tricky, and the final volume of the muscle flap may be inadequate to complete the reconstruction.
4. Infection: The wound bed must be free of infection and slough before performing the local flap. Radical debridement prior to flap cover is the key to success. Sub-flap collection and infection lead to flap necrosis or dehiscence of wound margins. Muscle flaps are relatively better in tolerating infection. In the presence of infection, we would do a radical debridement, wait for a few days for the inflammation to settle down and then do the local flap. In situations with a compelling need for flap cover, radical debridement is done and irrespective of the size of the wound, a microsurgical free flap option must be entertained, which would also bring in fresh blood supply.
5. Need for future access: Ulcer healing is not the end goal of management of a diabetic ulcer. It also includes the prevention of the recurrence. In most cases, the cause of the ulcer is due to the derangement of the biomechanics of the foot and that would need correction after ulcer healing. Any flap that is done must facilitate future access for surgical procedures, which may also include implant placement. If local flaps would not suffice, a larger regional flap or a free flap would be a better option.

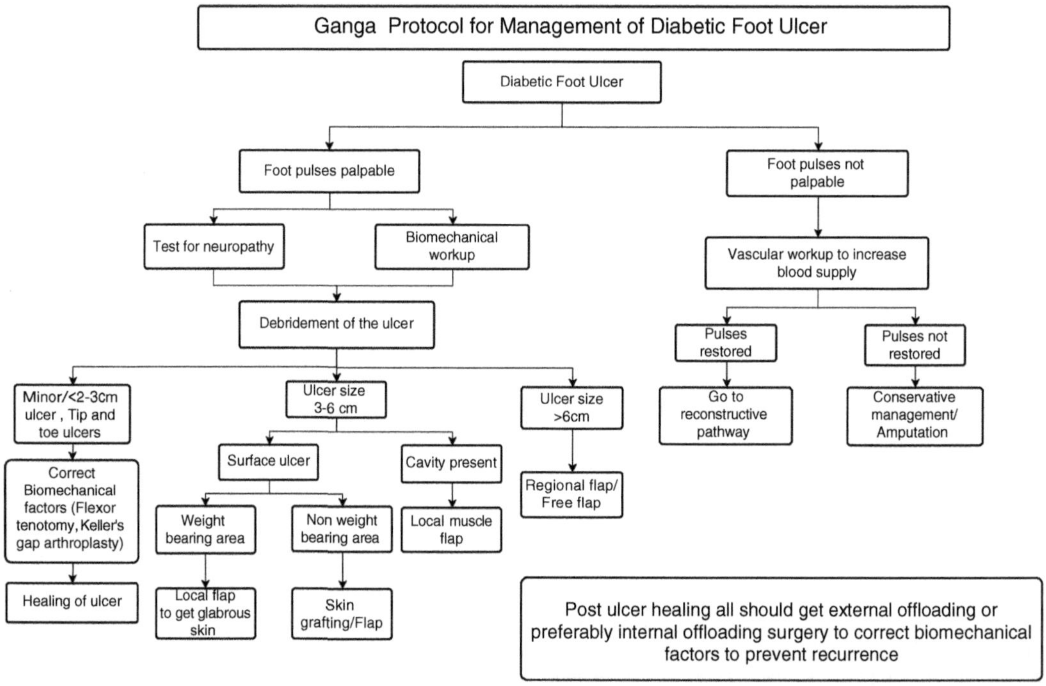

8.2.1 Choice of Flap: How Do We Choose Which Flap?

Local Flaps are chosen primarily based on the location of the defect and the purpose of the flap for which it is intended. A plantar ulcer exposing a critical structure would require a glabrous skin flap to preserve the durable load bearing and shear resistant properties of the sole. Such flaps necessitate the movement of adjacent skin with similar properties into the defect by using one of the numerous plastic surgical techniques of movement of flaps. When choosing local skin flaps to cover the metatarsal heads, one should avoid ending up placing skin grafts on the forefoot. It would lead to recurrence of the ulcer during weight bearing. Sommerlad and McGrouther showed that after reconstruction of the plantar surface of the foot, patients preferentially bear weight on the non-reconstructed part of the foot [5]. Since it is not possible for the patient to avoid forefoot loading during gait, skin grafts are poorly tolerated on the forefoot.

Intrinsic muscle flaps are used to fill cavities in addition to providing cover. Based on the location of the wound and reach of the adjacent muscle appropriate muscle flap is chosen. Nearly all the intrinsic muscle flaps of the foot belong to Type II of the Mathes and Nahai classification and can survive on a single dominant pedicle [6]. An intrinsic muscle flap with a skin graft is also chosen for coverage of plantar defects with a deficiency of overlying or adjacent skin. Such flaps do not have the resilience of the glabrous skin flaps and must be followed up with good skin graft care and offloading methods. The skin graft on the muscle flaps often undergoes a hypertrophic change in response to axial and shear pressures of the underlying bony prominences. Even when these areas are excised and re-grafted, these hypertrophic skin changes adamantly recur until the underlying cause of the excessive stress is corrected.

8.2.1.1 Timing of Local Flap Cover

Local flaps in a diabetic foot are done once the wound bed is devoid of any slough and clinical evidence of active invasive infection has subsided. We do not wait for a negative bacteriological swab result before flap cover. However, if there has been significant infection, we do a post debridement tissue culture to know the presence of the organisms and the antibiotic sensitivity for the choice of antibiotics in the postoperative period. We prefer to allow local inflammation and infection to settle with appropriate rest and antibiotic therapy before flap cover. Local skin flaps are relatively hypo-vascular once they are raised from their bed and hence are not very resistant to sub-flap infection, which can lead to partial or complete flap loss. Hence it is important to rule out infections of the bed and, also to prevent any postoperative sub-flap collection by placing large, drains.

8.3 Preoperative Evaluation of the Patient

Tissue loss in a diabetic foot ulcer is often secondary to a spreading and necrotizing infection. Diabetes is often poorly controlled in such patients, as reflected by the HbA1c levels. The mean HbA1c of 100 consecutive patients presenting with diabetic foot ulcer in our institution was 7.4 with a range of 5.2–14.7. Poor glycemic control predisposes the patient to associated complications like nephropathy, atherosclerosis, and ischemic heart disease [7]. Optimization of the patient's general condition for surgery includes control of chronic comorbid conditions and, also the immediate effects of wound sepsis. Radical debridement helps to optimize the patient's general condition much faster. With popularization of peripheral nerve blocks, debridement could be done without risking the systemic stress associated with spinal or general anaesthesia. Debridement should be done as early as possible, and the timing of flap cover would depend upon the status of the bed after debridement.

We prefer to wait to assess the blood counts and blood C Reactive Protein (CRP) levels to reflect a reducing trend to plan a definitive flap cover. Serial measurement of inflammatory markers like CRP, IL6 help to assess the level of general inflammation [8] and indirectly also reflect the inflammation in the peri-wound areas. We do not wait for complete normalization of values but go ahead with flap cover once we see a consistently declining trend of inflammatory markers coupled with clinical assessment of the wound and the patient. Clinical assessment includes the absence of a foul smell, necrotic tissue in the bed, and resolution of peri-wound edema and erythema. We also clinically examine tendon tracts to check for extension of infection along the long and short tendons.

It is ideal to wait for a culture-negative wound before attempting a flap cover as it has been shown that flaps performed in the setting of a culture-positive post debridement wound have a higher risk of flap failure necessitating further complex surgery [9]. If, however, the exposure of critical structures warrants early cover, then we prefer to do a more radical debridement and go ahead with flap cover. If the wound size becomes bigger, we switch to a microvascular free tissue transfer. The flap donor site is also preoperatively assessed by the same parameters that are applied to the peri-wound area. Raising a flap in an inflamed donor area poses inherent risks of excessive bleeding and flap necrosis from the demand-supply gap in tissue requirement of oxygen and its availability [10]. Further, inflammation obliterates tissue planes and makes it difficult to identify pedicles (even when done under tourniquet) with increased risk of pedicle injury. The inflammatory edema and capillary ooze also make it difficult to graft the donor site if necessary.

8.4 Surgical Procedures

Local flaps can be either cutaneous flaps or muscle flaps.

8.4.1 Cutaneous Flaps

Cutaneous flaps are designed based on the available local tissue and the possible arc of movement. The most commonly used flaps are the rotation (Fig. 8.1), the transposition, and advancement flaps (Fig. 8.2). The skin flaps can be reliably raised based on the knowledge of angiosomes of the foot. The skin flaps can also be raised on a single perforator as an islanded propeller flap (Fig. 8.3). Transposition flaps leave behind a defect that needs to be grafted while rotation flaps leave no secondary defect (Fig. 8.4). We prefer the modified rotation flap [11]—an extrapolation of the transposition flap geometry, to, the standard rotation flap design (Fig. 8.5). Another flap that torques into place is the “Hatchet flap” which is a triangular flap with a small retained cutaneous pedicle and a non-circumferential scar [12] (Fig. 8.6). Circular defects can be closed by raising double opposing hatchet or VY flaps (Fig. 8.7). Advancement flaps are mostly V-Y flaps (Video 8.1). Any of the above adipocutaneous flaps can also be raised as an islanded flap based on a perforator from the underlying medial plantar or lateral plantar source vessel and can be moved or propelled into place as required.

Cutaneous flaps can also be raised along with the underlying fascia based on named vessels. These flaps will be elaborated later in relation to each angiosome they are based upon.

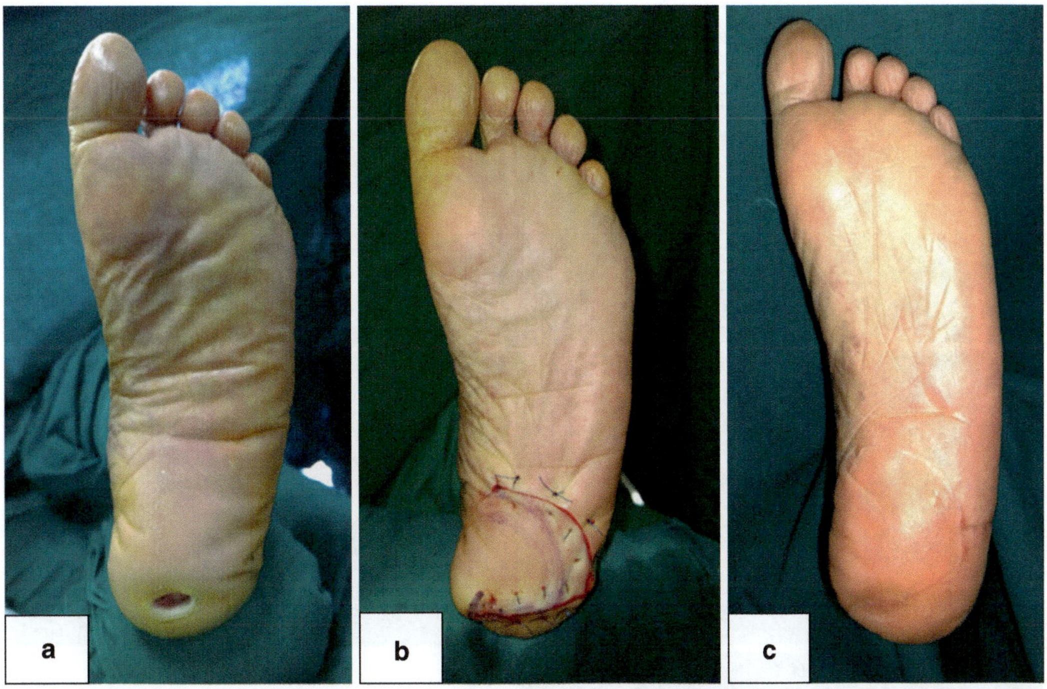

Fig. 8.1 Classic rotation flap: (**a**) A case of chronic nonhealing ulcer over the left heel region (**b**) Rotation flap used to cover the defect. (**c**) 8 month follow up picture showing the settled flap

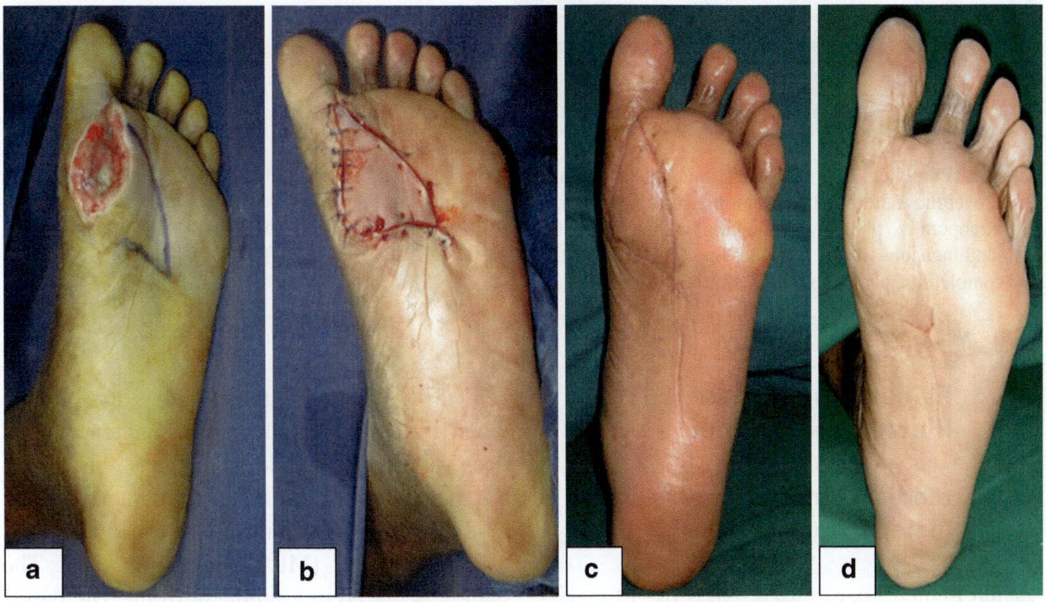

Fig. 8.2 VY advancement flap: (**a**) Post infective raw area over the first metatarsal head region of the right foot with the marking of the V-Y advancement flap (**b**) Flap raised and advanced into the defect. (**c** and **d**) 3 months and 1.5 years follow up pictures showing the settled flap

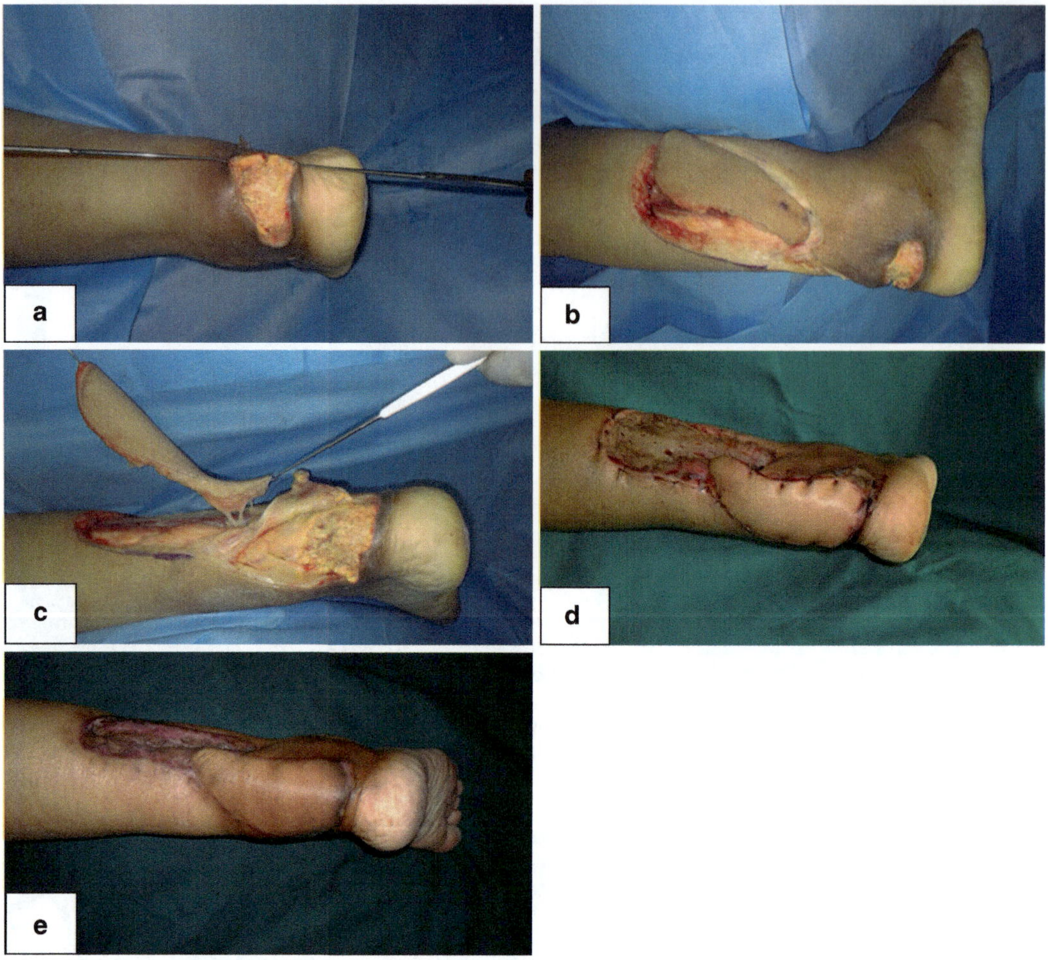

Fig. 8.3 Propeller flap: (**a**) A chronic post-traumatic defect over the Achilles tendon region in a diabetic patient (**b**) Intraoperative photograph showing the marked perforator and incisions for the propeller flap (**c**) The propeller flap completely islanded on the perforator (**d**) Immediate follow up picture showing the propeller flap cover for the defect and the donor raw area covered with split skin graft (**e**) 4 months follow up photograph showing the settled propeller flap and skin graft

8.5 Flaps from the Medial Plantar Angiosome

8.5.1 Medial Plantar Artery Instep Flap (Video 8.2)

Medial Plantar artery instep flap is used for coverage of heel defects. It is based on perforators arising from the medial plantar artery in between the bellies of the flexor digitorum brevis laterally and the abductor hallucis muscle medially. The medial plantar artery runs on a deeper plane adjacent to the flexor digitorum brevis muscle and when traced proximally passes underneath the deep surface of the abductor hallucis muscle into the medial division of the tarsal tunnel. A hand-held doppler is used to identify the medial plantar artery perforator (MPAP) [13] (Fig. 8.8). The patient is placed in a supine position. The flap is raised in the sub plantar fascial plane, and the perforators to the abductor hallucis are identified medially and divided. The skin perforator is identified, and the dissection is carried over to the lateral side. The flap is then islanded on the

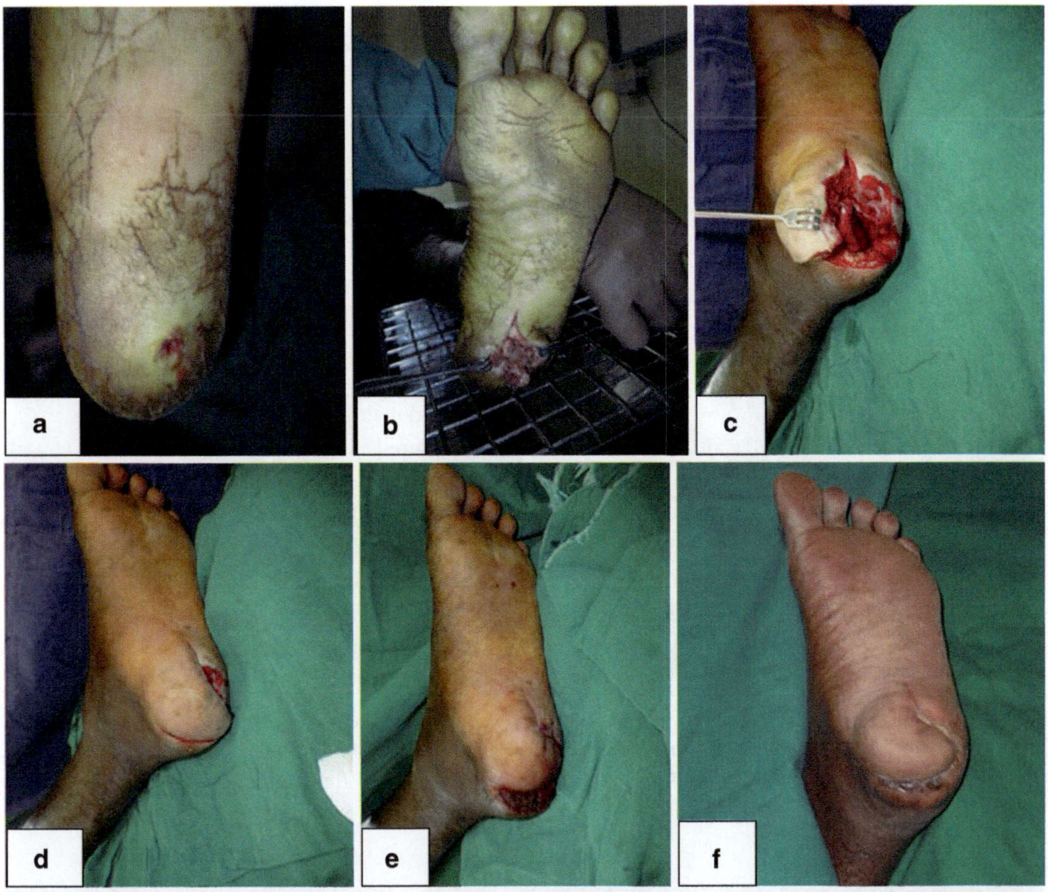

Fig. 8.4 Transposition Flap: (**a**) A case of chronic heel ulcer with calcaneal osteomyelitis (**b**) Intraoperative photograph showing the extent of the disease process (**c**) The post debridement picture showing the defect in the weight-bearing region of the heel (**d**) The. transposition flap has been marked and incised (**e**) The transposed flap has been inset and the donor area of the flap has been covered with split skin graft (**f**) 5 months follow-up photograph showing the reconstructed heel and settled scars

MPAP. One needs to be careful when islanding the flap as the veins are prone to get damaged, leading to venous congestion. The flap can also be raised as a distally based flap for the cover of forefoot defects, albeit with a higher likelihood of complications [14].

8.5.2 Abductor Hallucis Muscle Flap

The muscle originates from the calcaneum and inserts on to the medial sesamoid, the medial capsule of the first MTP joint, and ultimately into the base of the proximal phalanx of the hallux. The dominant vessel is found at its proximal end, which originates from the medial plantar artery. The flap is approached by an incision over the medial border of the foot. The muscle is in the first layer of the sole and becomes tendinous just distal to the midfoot. The flap is raised after dividing the tendon and dissecting the muscle off the deeper flexor hallucis brevis. The flap can be used to cover defects of the ankle, hindfoot, and midfoot on its medial border (Fig. 8.9).

If raised on a skeletonized pedicle its reach can be extended [15]. It can also be raised as a distally based flap [16, 17], however, it is not recommended in feet with ischemia.

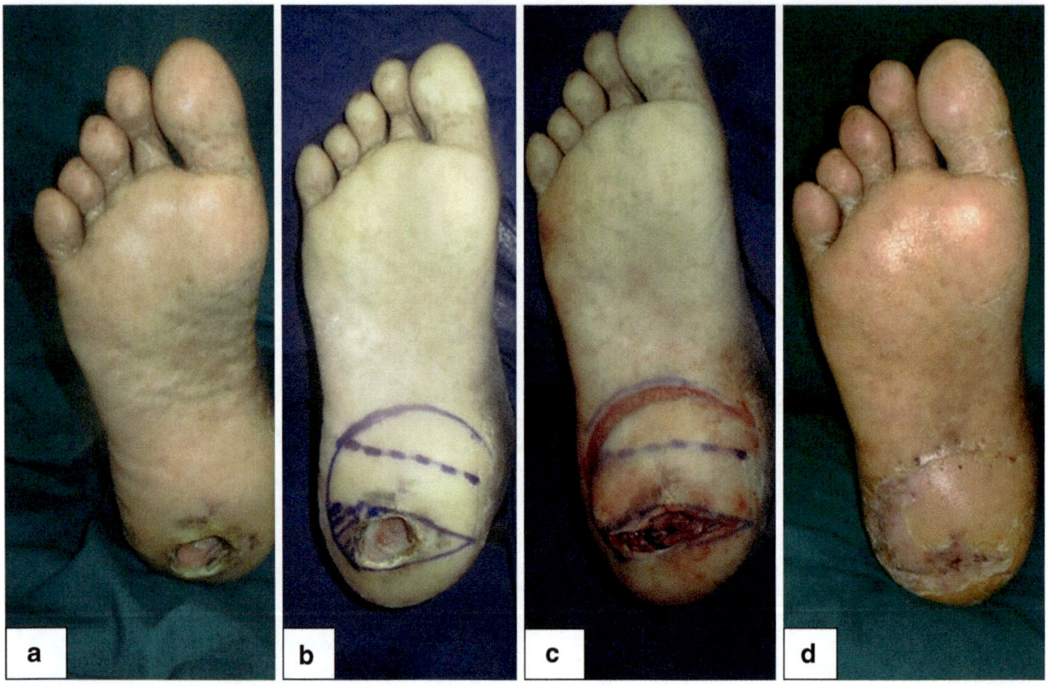

Fig. 8.5 Modified rotation flap: (**a**) A case of nonhealing ulcer over the right heel region (**b**) The marking of the planned rotation flap extended from the marking of the transposition flap. Shaded triangular region will be excised before the inset of the flap (**c**) Rotation flap used to cover the defect. (**d**) 6 month follow up picture showing settled flap

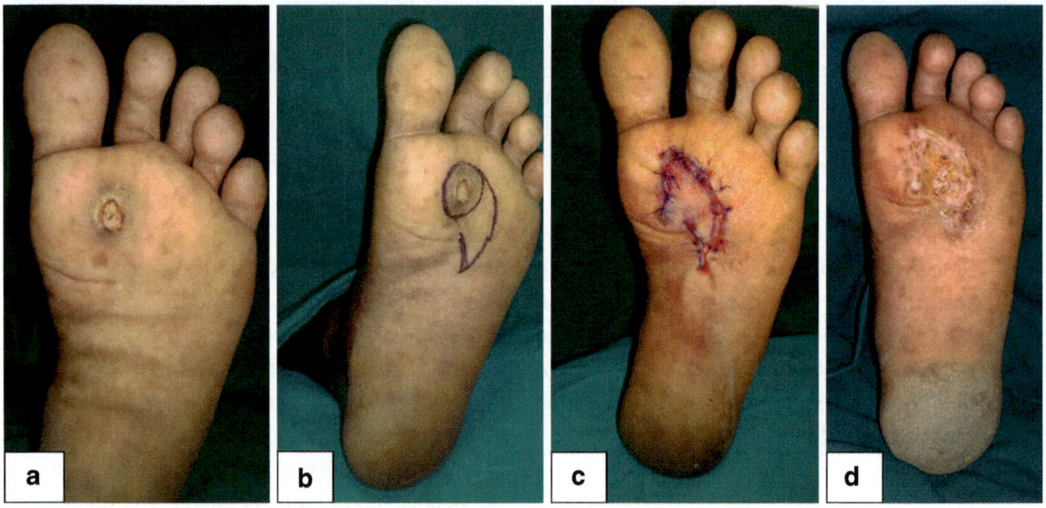

Fig. 8.6 Hatchet flap: (**a**) A case of forefoot ulcerated corn planned for excision (**b**) Hatchet flap and the corn to be excised are marked (**c**) Immediate postoperative photograph showing the suture line of the flap. (**d**) 3 month follow up photograph showing the settled flaps and supple scar

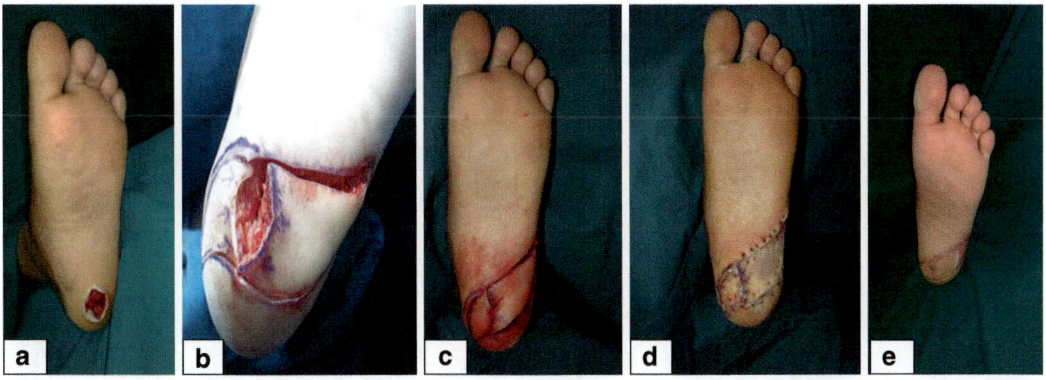

Fig. 8.7 Double opposing V-Y advancement flap: (**a**) A case of heel ulcer after debridement showing the skin and soft tissue loss. (**b**) The double opposing V-Y advancement flap marked and incised (**c**) Both the V-Y flaps advanced to cover the defect (**d**) Immediate postoperative photograph showing the suture line of the flap. (**e**) 4 months follow up photograph showing the settled flaps

8.6 Flaps from the Lateral Plantar Angiosome

8.6.1 Flexor Digitorum Brevis Flap (Video 8.3)

This is a muscle flap that is raised by a midline plantar incision extending from the heel to just proximal to the metatarsal heads. It is ideally used as a turnover flap to fill in cavities of the distal calcaneum and heel. The patient is placed in a supine position and an incision made on the midline extending from the defect distally. The plantar fascia is incised and raised along with the skin flaps. Below the plantar fascia, one can visualize the flexor digitorum brevis (FDB) muscle originating from the calcaneum and its four tendinous slips to the lateral four toes inserting into the respective middle phalanx bases. The tendon slips to the toes are divided at the forefoot, and the flap is raised from distal to proximal. The main pedicle from the lateral plantar artery can be seen entering the muscle at its proximal third on its lateral border. Minor pedicles from the medial plantar artery also supply the muscle at its proximal third. The flap is mostly used to cover heel defects. The raw area over the muscle is grafted or if adequate skin is available, it is loosely closed over the muscle (Fig. 8.10).

8.6.2 Abductor Digiti Minimi Flap

The Abductor digiti minimi flap was found to be the most commonly used flap amongst all intrinsic muscle flaps of the foot in a systematic review by Ramanujam [16, 17]. The muscle arises from the calcaneum and inserts into the lateral aspect of the base of the proximal phalanx of the little toe. The blood supply is mainly from branches of the lateral plantar artery, which if skeletonized, increases the reach of the flap [18]. The flap can be used for coverage of the heel and lateral ankle defects. The patient is positioned with the lateral side of the involved foot up. A curvilinear incision connects the wound and extends along the lateral border of the foot to the forefoot (Fig. 8.11). The distal tendinous part is divided, and the flap is raised from distal to proximal, taking care to preserve the branches from the lateral plantar artery, which enter it near the base of the fifth metatarsal.

8.7 Flaps from the Posterior Tibial Angiosome

The Posterior tibial artery supplies the area of the lower leg starting from the medial border of the tibia to the posterior midline of the leg overlying

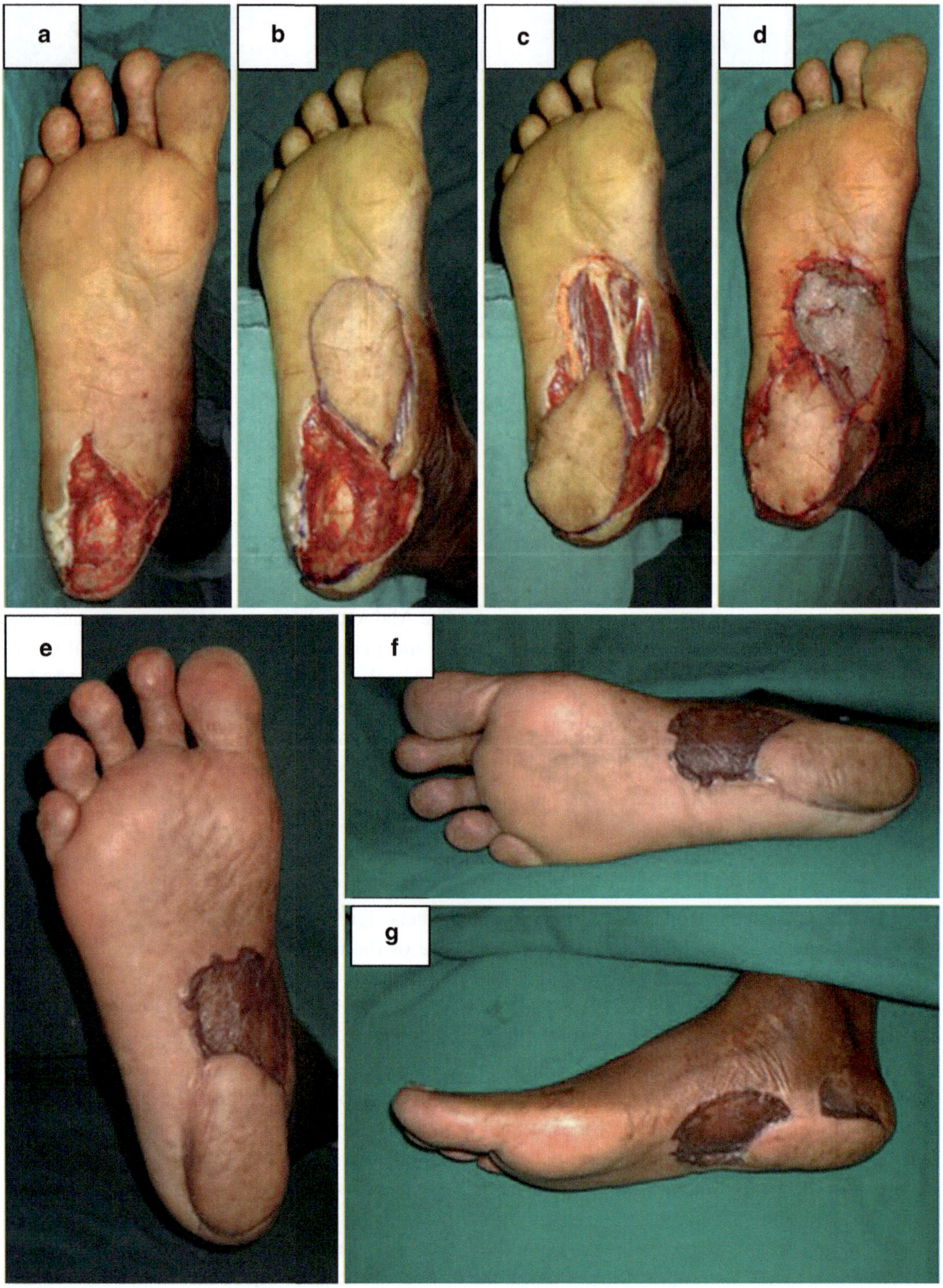

Fig. 8.8 Medial plantar artery perforator flap: (**a**) A case of hind foot infected ulcer after debridement showing near total loss of heel region (**b**) Medial plantar artery perforator flap marked in the instep region (**c**) Medial plantar artery perforator flap islanded on the MPAP and propelled into the defect (**d**) Donor area of the flap and the non-critical raw areas were covered with split skin graft (**e–g**) 7 months follow up picture showing well settled flap and split skin grafts

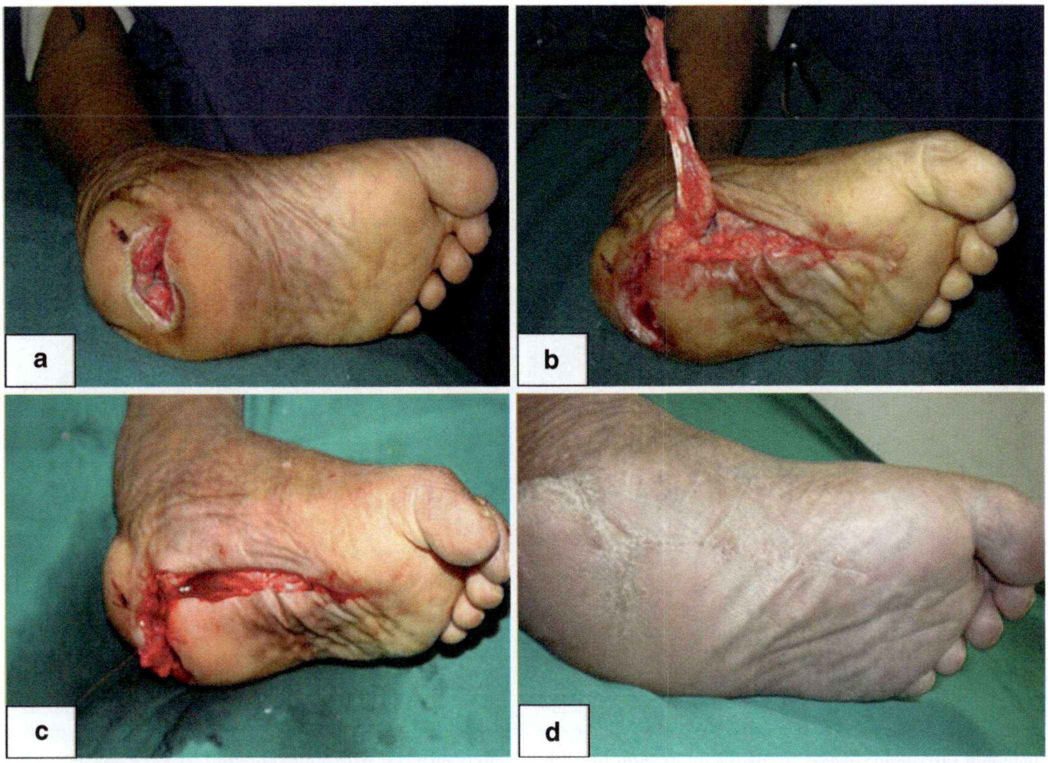

Fig. 8.9 Abductor hallucis flap: (**a**) Skin and soft tissue defect over the left heel region (**b**) Abductor hallucis muscle flap raised based on the proximal pedicle (**c**) Flap inset into the defect (**d**) Long term follow up picture showing the well-settled scar

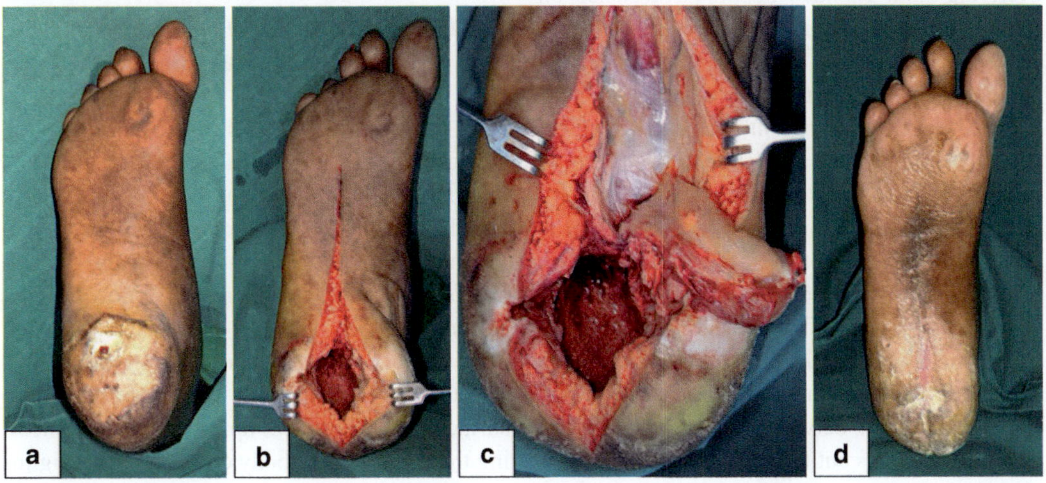

Fig. 8.10 Flexor digitorum brevis flap: (**a**) Chronic ulcer over the right heel region with underlying osteomyelitis of calcaneum (**b**) Post debridement picture showing the skin, soft tissue and the bony defect. (**c**) Flexor digitorum brevis muscle flap elevated on the branches from lateral plantar artery (**d**) 2 year follow-up picture showing a well-settled flap

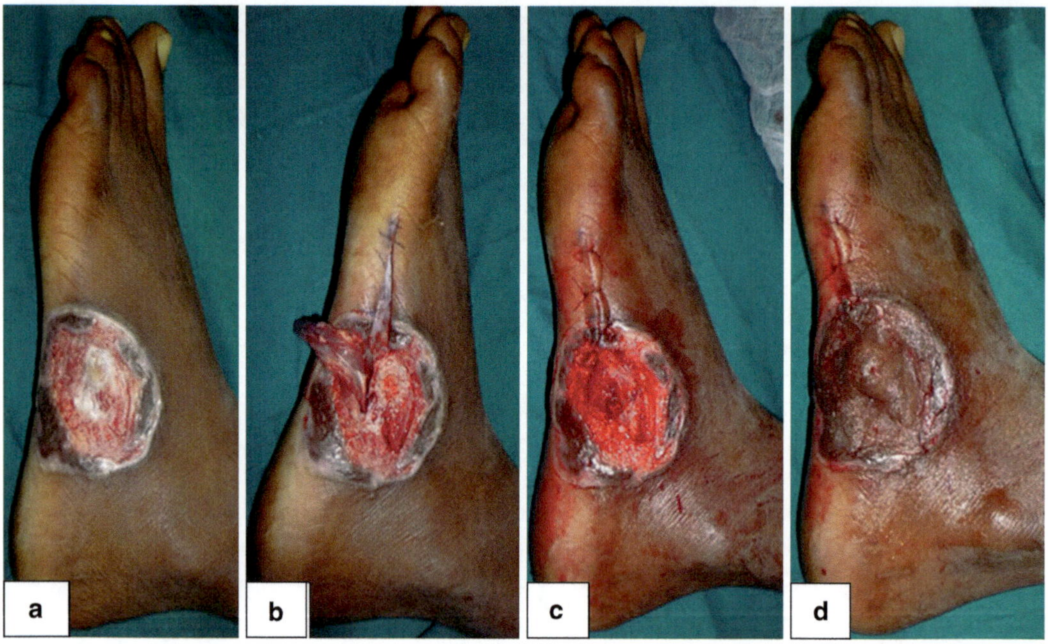

Fig. 8.11 Abductor digiti minimi flap: (**a**) A case of chronic ulcer over left fifth metatarsal base post a failed attempt at split skin graft cover. (**b**) Status post debridement and proximally based Abductor digiti minimi muscle flap elevated on branches from the lateral plantar artery, which enter the muscle near the base of the fifth metatarsal. (**c**) Flap inset into the defect. (**d**) The muscle flap resurfaced with split skin graft

the Achilles tendon. It gives a series of septocutaneous and musculocutaneous perforators to the overlying skin. Islanded flaps can be raised on these perforators and used to cover defects over the distal tibia, ankle, and heel. The perforators are identified preoperatively by a hand-held doppler and the flap planned in reverse. An exploratory incision is made along the anterior edge of the flap and the previously marked perforators are visualized and their suitability for transfer is assessed. If a series of perforators are isolated, then the most prominent pedicle closest to the defect is chosen. The flap is then planned on the axis of the chosen pedicle and the skin incision completed to island the flap. The fascia is then cut and the septum between the deep and superficial compartments cut to raise the flap. The pedicle is isolated by careful dissection taking care to divide all fibrous attachments, which can impede free rotation of the pedicle (Fig. 8.3). The flap is then inset loosely to allow for postoperative edema. The donor site is grafted.

8.8 Flap from the Anterior Tibial Angiosome

8.8.1 The Extensor Digitorum Brevis (EDB) Flap

EDB flap like many other intrinsic muscles of the foot originates from the calcaneum. The muscle flap can be raised from the dorsum of the foot based on the lateral tarsal communicating branch. It can have a forward flow from the anterior tibial/dorsalis pedis system or reverse flow through communicating branches from the peroneal artery. The patient is positioned supine with a slight tilt to the opposite side so that the lateral surface of the foot faces up. An incision connecting the wound to the body of the extensor digitorum brevis muscle is made and skin flaps laid open. The tendon slips to the lateral four toes are cut and bunched and the flap is raised from distal to proximal. The lateral tarsal artery and the main pedicle can be seen entering the muscle on its deep surface. One needs to be careful with branches taking off from the lateral tarsal artery to the underlying tarsal bones to avoid damage to the main vessel [19]. The origin from the calcaneum is dissected to mobilize the muscle fully and it can be used to cover defects around the ankle joint (Fig. 8.12).

8.9 Reverse First Dorsal Metatarsal Artery (FDMA) Perforator Flap

Reverse First Dorsal Metatarsal Artery perforator flap is a cutaneous flap that can be reliably raised from the dorsum of the foot for coverage of the distal toes. It is a reverse flap based on the communications between the distal first dorsal metatarsal artery and the plantar lateral plantar arterial system [20]. The perforator is marked with a hand-held doppler and the flap designed on the dorsum of the foot. The flap is then raised in the subfascial plane in a proximal to distal fashion. The dissection is then carried out by identifying the FDMA which lies in between the interossei. The vessel is included in the flap as it is raised from proximal to distal upto the point of the perforator, which has been previously identified. The flap can either be completely islanded or the base left intact for future division (Fig. 8.13).

8.10 Flaps from the Peroneal Angiosome

Both muscle flaps and cutaneous flaps can be raised on the distal branches of the peroneal artery. The muscle flap that can be raised based on the distal branches of the peroneal artery is the distally based peroneus brevis muscle flap. The peroneus brevis muscle is exposed through a longitudinal incision just behind and parallel to the fibula. Retraction of the peroneus longus exposes the underlying peroneus brevis muscle. The main pedicle to the muscle from the peroneal artery enters the proximal end of the muscle along with its motor nerve branch and travels down the muscle

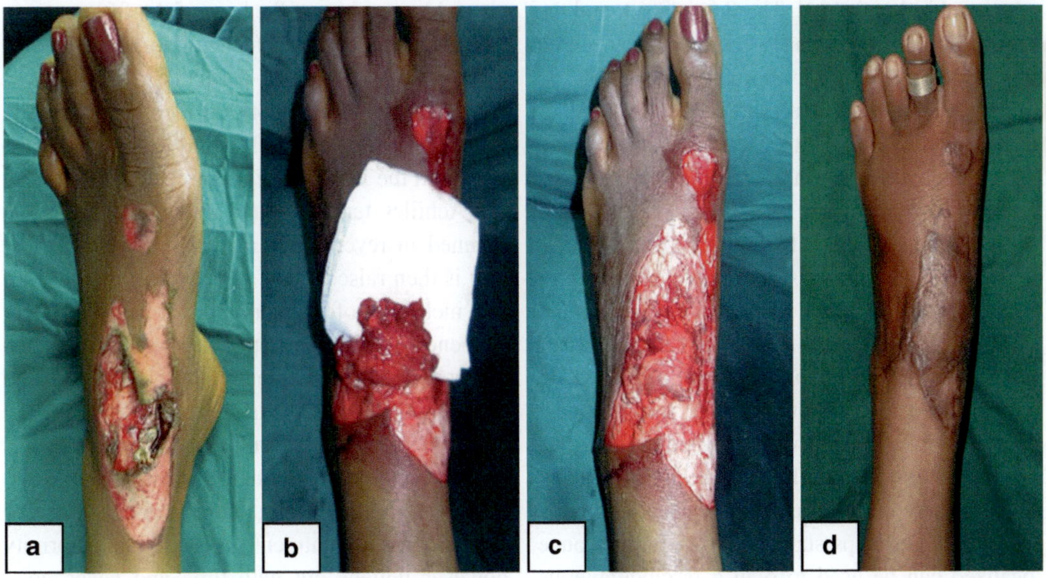

Fig. 8.12 Extensor digitorum brevis flap: (**a**) Post-traumatic defect over the right ankle region exposing the tibia and head of talus in a diabetic women (**b**) Picture showing the defect post debridement and Extensor digitorum brevis muscle elevated. The main pedicle enters the flap in the deeper surface (**c**) Flap covering the defect. The muscle flap was resurfaced with split skin graft. (**d**) Long-term follow-up picture showing well-settled flap with split skin graft

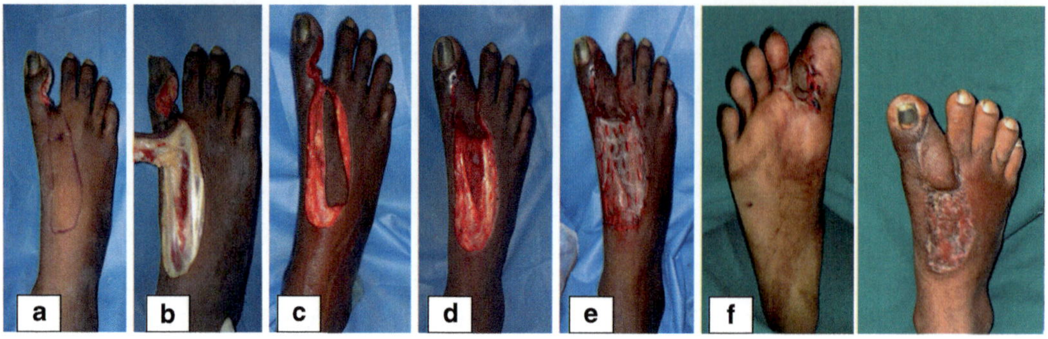

Fig. 8.13 Reverse FDMA flap: (**a**) Infected raw area over the medial aspect of right great toe requiring flap cover. The perforator location of the FDMA flap has been marked by handheld doppler and the outline of the required flap is indicated. (**b** and **c**) The reverse FDMA flap elevated. (**d** and **e**) The flap inset into the defect and the donor area covered with split skin graft (**f**) 1 year follow up showing the well-settled flap and skin graft

as an axial vessel [21, 22]. The neurovascular pedicle is divided, and the muscle is raised off its origin from the fibula and the anterolateral septum. Arterial branches from the anterior tibial vessels and the peroneal vessels are divided as the muscle is raised. The distal-most pedicle is from the peroneal vessel and is about 4–5 cm from the lateral malleolus [23] and hence it is prudent to limit the distal dissection above this level. The flap has been shown to survive even when used in limbs with peripheral ischemia [22]. The flap is inset, and the donor site closed primarily taking care to avoid any pressure at the site of flap turndown. The flap can be covered with skin graft either primarily or secondarily. We prefer to use this flap for small defects around the lateral malleolus and the distal fibular areas.

The cutaneous flaps from the peroneal angiosome include the lateral supramalleolar perforator flap, the terminal lateral calcaneal artery flap and the interpolated reverse sural artery flap. The lateral supramalleolar flap can be raised based on septocutaneous perforators from the peroneal artery that lie about midway between the Achilles tendon and the fibula. They travel along the deep posterior septum between the peroneal compartment and the triceps surae. The perforators once localized can be used to plan a fasciocutaneous propeller flap that can be used to cover the Achilles tendon, lateral malleolar region, and lateral heel.

8.10.1 The Lateral Calcaneal Artery Flap

The Lateral Calcaneal artery flap is a cutaneous flap based on the lateral calcaneal artery a terminal branch of the peroneal artery coursing along the lateral side of the heel. The flap can be designed to include the skin of the lateral heel from the posterior lateral part of the lateral malleolus and can be curved forward up to the base of the fifth metatarsal if necessary as an extended flap. Small defects of the posterior heel, particularly around the Achilles tendon insertion are ideally covered by this flap. The patient is placed in semi lateral position with the involved leg lower and tilted so that the Achilles tendon points upwards. The flap is planned in reverse and markings are made. The flap is then raised as an adipocutaneous flap with the inclusion of the sural nerve and the short saphenous vein in the flap. The plane of dissection is just above the periosteum of the calcaneum and the secondary raw area is grafted (Fig. 8.14). The resultant contour deformity at the donor site is obvious, and this cosmetic deformity must be discussed with the patient preoperatively to avoid potential disappointment. The contour deformity however flattens out with time and needs good postoperative graft care to prevent hypertrophic changes.

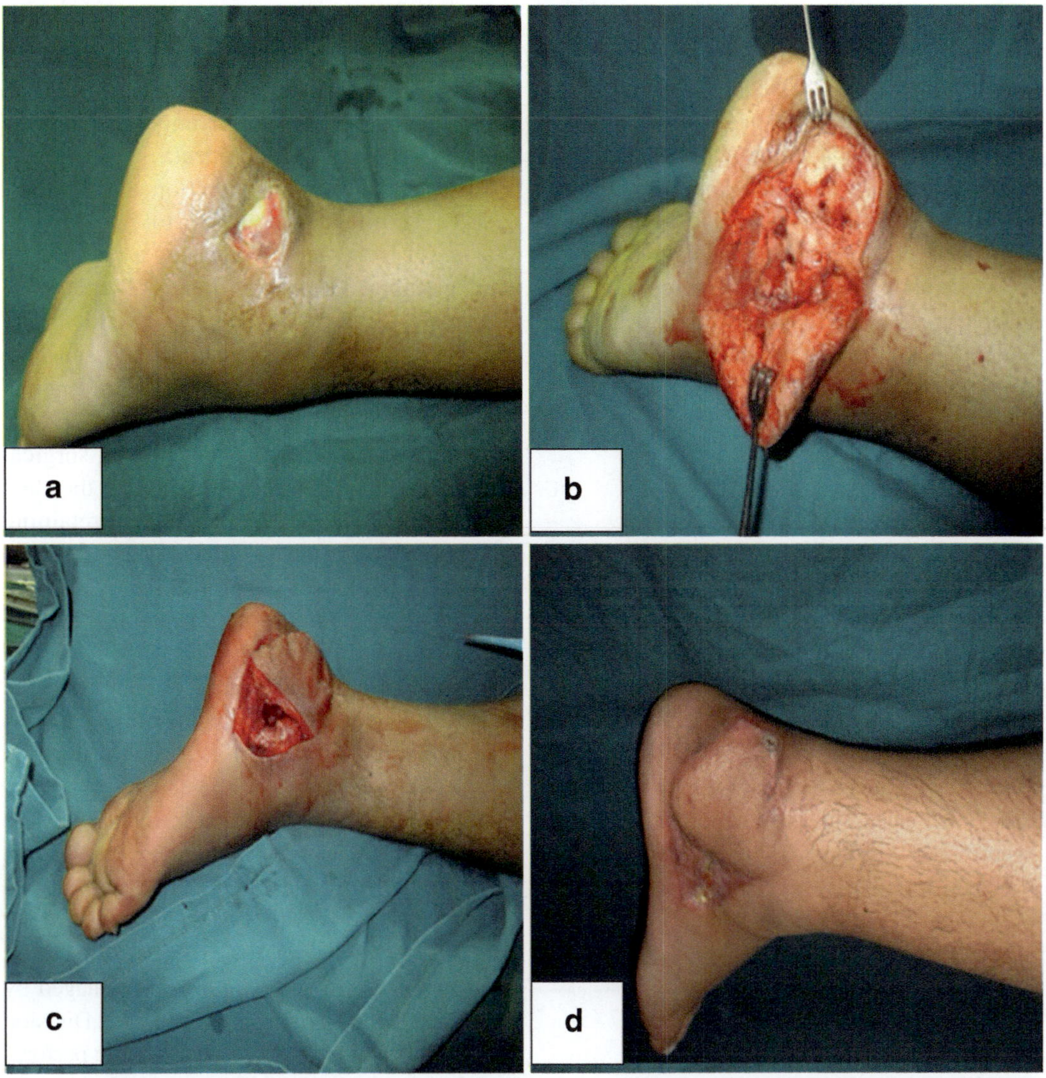

Fig. 8.14 Lateral calcaneal artery flap: (**a**) Infected ulcer over the Achilles tendon region of the right foot. (**b**) Lateral calcaneal artery flap elevated based on the lateral calcaneal artery, which is one of the terminal branches of the peroneal artery (**c**) Flap transposed to cover the defect. Donor region of the flap was resurfaced with split skin graft. (**d**) 6 month follow up showing well-settled flap and split skin graft

8.11 Postoperative Care and Expected Outcome

8.11.1 Immediate Postoperative Care

We prefer to immobilize the operated limb is a plaster of Paris slab that is contoured suitably to avoid pressure on the flap but accommodate the swelling of the flap in the postoperative period. The patient is continued on culture-specific antibiotics. The flap is dressed at least once in 48 h to watch for any sub-flap collection or discharge. The patient is kept in bed for a week and then allowed non-weight-bearing mobilization. We prefer to keep sutures for about 3 weeks for flaps raised on glabrous skin.

8.11.2 Late Postoperative Care

Once the flap has settled well and the wound closure has been achieved the patient is allowed full weight-bearing mobilization with adequate protective orthoses. A removable knee-high offloading device or in those who do not tolerate a knee-high device, an ankle-high orthotic device or prescription footwear is prescribed [24]. Suitable prescription footwear is provided for the opposite foot to prevent new ulcers and to correct any mismatch in height for patients using a cast or orthotic boot for the affected foot.

8.11.3 Follow-Up Care and Surveillance

The patient is initially followed up monthly and the review period is gradually increased to once every 3 months. During each review, the flap is assessed for any evidence of breakdown. The patient is then offered correction of the altered biomechanics, which was the predisposing factor for the occurrence of the ulcer. This is an important step in the completion of treatment, as ulcers invariably recur if the patient is not very compliant with external offloading methods.

8.12 Management of Complications

Complications include bleeding in the immediate postoperative period. Many of the patients are on antiplatelet drugs for comorbid conditions, and it is advisable to stop potent drugs like clopidogrel and ticagrelor. They may be substituted with aspirin or low molecular weight heparin at least 4 days before the planned procedure. These drugs can be skipped on the day of the procedure and continued postoperatively.

Venous congestion may complicate an island flap due to pedicle damage or obstruction of venous outflow due to pedicle compression or sub-flap hematoma. When identified early, the flap can be re-explored and any fibrous band released or hematomas evacuated. If identified late, then an approach of decompression by releasing a few sutures and observation with regular dressings to await demarcation and judge the extent of flap survival is prudent.

If there is sub-flap infection and the discharge is minor, we prefer to immediately decompress the flap by releasing a few sutures and washing out any purulent collection frequently (at least twice daily) with dressings. A culture of the discharge and antibiotic sensitivity is done and change of antibiotics made if necessary. If the infection does not resolve with these measures, we proceed to surgical debridement of the bed after raising the flap. The flap is then hitched with a few retaining sutures to prevent retraction and frequent dressings continued. Once the sub-flap infection settles, a formal re-inset of the flap is done if necessary.

Flap necrosis may be partial or complete. One might incur flap necrosis despite all precautions and interventions to avoid it. If such a situation arises, we prefer to wait for demarcation and separation unless flap removal and a redo procedure is emergent. Many a time, the deep layer of the flap survives by the crane principle and the surgeon can get away with SSG once the superficial areas sloughs out. Partial flap necrosis in a pedicled flap like a rotation flap can be managed by re-advancing the flap to cover the defect. Division of the source artery may be attempted in perforator flaps to further mobilize them.. However, if the residual flap is inadequate then the procedure of choice would be either a free microsurgical flap or a cross leg flap rather than attempt a second local flap from the same foot, which has already lost a considerable amount of tissue.

8.13 Case Demonstrations

Case 1 V-Y flap cover for heel defect (Video 8.1)

Case 2 Medial plantar artery flap cover for heel defect (Video 8.2)

Case 3 Flexor Digitorum Brevis flap for heel defect (Video 8.3)

8.14 Discussion

Local flaps should be viewed as a solution for small defects exposing critical structures which if left untreated could progress to further tissue loss. They have a high chance of success when done in foot with good vascularity. Adequate muscle bulk must be ascertained when attempting muscle flaps. Local flaps do not tolerate infection well, and hence it is important to debride the wound well and ensure a good bed for flap cover.

Local flaps must preferably be raised from an adjacent uninvolved angiosome. Glabrous skin flaps are preferable for small defects of the weight-bearing areas considering their durable nature. Intrinsic muscle flaps are useful for non-weight-bearing areas over the medial and lateral borders of the foot and to fill bony cavities. Intrinsic muscle flaps are limited by their size and hence can only be used to fill cavities of a small to moderate size. Large cavities would be better served by a free muscle flap. Defects that are too large for a flap from adjacent tissue require a distant pedicled flap or a free flap.

Our preference of flaps for specified defects is summarized below.

- Plantar Forefoot—Local V-Y advancement/Rotation flap/Hatchet Flap/bilateral V-Y Flaps/Perforator flap
- Plantar Midfoot—Local Transposition/Perforator with propeller/Abductor Hallucis/Abductor digiti minimi.
- Plantar Heel ulcers—Rotation/Instep Flap/Flexor Digitorum Brevis flap/Reverse Sural/Posterior tibial artery perforator flap
- Ankle and Achilles Tendon—Propeller flaps/Reverse Sural Flap/Distally based Peroneus Brevis/Lateral Calcaneal artery flap
- Dorsum and Toes—Fillet flap/Cross Toe flap/Reverse First Dorsal Metatarsal artery perforator flap

8.15 Conclusion

Local flaps are very useful for coverage of defects less than 3 cm × 6 cm in a vascular foot. Radical debridement of the bed prior to flap cover, attention to detail in performing the flaps, and good after care will ensure success. Follow-up procedures like off-loading surgeries for the correction of predisposing factors will prevent ulcer recurrence.

Disclosure Statement The authors have nothing to disclose.

References

1. Attinger C, Cooper P, Blume P. Vascular anatomy of the foot and ankle. Oper Tech Plast Reconstr Surg. 1997;4(4):183–98.
2. Ducic I, Attinger CE. Foot and ankle reconstruction: pedicled muscle flaps versus free flaps and the role of diabetes. Plast Reconstr Surg. 2011;128(1):173–80.
3. Black CK, Kotha VS, Fan KL, Ragothaman K, Attinger CE, Evans KK. Pedicled and free tissue transfers. Clin Podiatr Med Surg. 2019; 36 [cited 2021 Jan 2]. p. 441–55. Available from http://www.podiatric.theclinics.com/article/S0891842219300266/fulltext
4. Andersen H, Gjerstad MD, Jakobsen J. Atrophy of foot muscles: a measure of diabetic neuropathy. Diabetes Care. 2004;27(10):2382–5. https://doi.org/10.2337/diacare.27.10.2382.
5. Sommerlad BC, McGrouther DA. Resufracing the sole: long-term follow-up and comparison of techniques. Br J Plastic Surg. 1978;31(2):107–16. Available from https://pubmed.ncbi.nlm.nih.gov/638300/
6. Clemens MW, Attinger CE. Functional reconstruction of the diabetic foot. Semin Plast Surg. 2010;24(1):43–56.
7. Bain SC, Bekker Hansen B, Hunt B, Chubb B, Valentine WJ. Evaluating the burden of poor glycemic control associated with therapeutic inertia in patients with type 2 diabetes in the UK. J Med Econ. 2020 [cited 2021 Jan 2];23(1):98–105. Available from https://pubmed.ncbi.nlm.nih.gov/31311364/
8. Weigelt C, Rose B, Poschen U, Ziegler DAN, Friese G, Kempf K, et al. Immune mediators in patients with acute diabetic foot syndrome. Diabetes Care. 2009;32(8):1491–6. Available from: http://creativecommons

9. Shuck J, Nolan J, Kanuri A, et al. The effect of positive post-debridement cultures on local muscle flap reconstruction of the lower extremity. 2015. journals.lww.com. Available from https://journals.lww.com/plasreconsurg/fulltext/2015/10001/The_Effect_of_Positive_Post_Debridement_Cultures.16.aspx
10. Feng LJ, Price DC, Mathes SJ, Hohn D. Dynamic properties of blood flow and leukocyte mobilization in infected flaps. World J Surg. 1990 Nov [cited 2021 Jan 2];14(6):796–803. Available from https://link.springer.com/article/10.1007/BF01670526
11. Ahuja RB. Mechanics of movement for rotation flaps and a local flap template. Plastic Reconstruct Surg. 1989;83(4):733–7. Available from http://journals.lww.com/00006534-198904000-00024
12. Emmett AJJ. The closure of defects by using adjacent triangular flaps with subcutaneous pedicles. Plastic Reconstruct Surgery. 1977;59(1) Available from https://journals.lww.com/plasreconsurg/Fulltext/1977/01000/THE_CLOSURE_OF_DEFECTS_BY_USING_ADJACENT.8.aspx
13. Scaglioni MF, Rittirsch D, Giovanoli P. Reconstruction of the heel, middle foot sole, and plantar forefoot with the medial plantar artery perforator flap: clinical experience with 28 cases. Plast Reconstr Surg. 2018;141(1):200–8.
14. Guillier D, Cherubino M, Oranges CM, Giordano S, Raffoul W, di Summa PG. Systematic reappraisal of the reverse-flow medial plantar flap: from vascular anatomical concepts to surgical applications. J Plastic Reconstruct Aesthetic Surg. 2020;73:421–33.
15. Michlits W, Gruber S, Windhofer C, MacHeiner P, Walsh M, Papp C. Reconstruction of soft tissue defects overlying the achilles tendon using the super extended abductor hallucis muscle flap. J Trauma. 2008;65(6):1459–62.
16. Schwabegger AH, Shafighi M, Harpf C, Gardetto A, Gurunluoglu R. Distally based abductor Hallucis muscle flap: anatomic basis and clinical application. Ann Plast Surg. 2003;51(5):505–8.
17. Lee S, Kim MB, Lee YH, Baek JK, Baek GH. Distally based abductor hallucis adipomuscular flap for forefoot plantar reconstruction. Ann Plast Surg. 2015;75(3):319–22.
18. Elfeki B, Eun S. Lateral malleolar defect coverage using abductor Digiti Minimi muscle flap. Ann Plast Surg. 2019;83(6):e50–4.
19. del Piñal F, Herrero F. Extensor digitorum brevis free flap: anatomic study and further clinical applications. Plastic Reconstruct Surg. 2000;105(4):1347–56. Available from https://pubmed.ncbi.nlm.nih.gov/10744224/
20. Hallock GG. The first dorsal metatarsal artery perforator propeller flap. Ann Plastic Surg. 2016 [cited 2021 Jan 2];76(6):684–7. Available from https://pubmed.ncbi.nlm.nih.gov/25003433/
21. Bajantri B, Bharathi R, Ramkumar S, Latheef L, Dhane S, Sabapathy SR. Experience with peroneus brevis muscle flaps for reconstruction of distal leg and ankle defects. Indian J Plastic Surg. 2013;46(1):48–54. Available from: /pmc/articles/PMC3745121/?report=abstract
22. Nguyen T, Rodriguez-Collazo ER. Healing heel ulcers in high-risk patients: distally based peroneus brevis muscle flap case series. J Foot Ankle Surg. 2019;58(2):341–6.
23. Masadeh S, Bibbo C. Distally based peroneus brevis flap: a reliable and versatile flap to cover the lateral foot and ankle. Curr Orthop Pract. 2016;27:499–507.
24. Bus SA, Armstrong DG, Gooday C, Jarl G, Caravaggi C, Viswanathan V, et al. Guidelines on offloading foot ulcers in persons with diabetes (IWGDF 2019 update). Diabetes Metab Res Rev. 2020;36(S1) Available from https://onlinelibrary.wiley.com/doi/abs/10.1002/dmrr.3274

9 When and How to Perform Free Flaps

Joon Pio Hong and Hyunsuk Peter Suh

9.1 Introduction

The treatment of diabetic foot ulceration is complex with multiple considerations involving the multidisciplinary team. Despite the efforts of the team, the aggravation of the wound often leads to limb amputation. Throughout this book, important concepts such as multidisciplinary approach, understanding the overall systemic condition, improving vasculopathy, treating infection, and wound bed preparation all leads to enhance the outcome for reconstructive surgery. Thus understanding what value the multidisciplinary team brings to the overall treatment is crucial for reconstructive surgeons. An example would be evaluating the patient's nutrition status and correcting accordingly prior to surgery. Prealbumin with a half-life of 2–3 days is a good indicator for acute nutritional status. Low prealbumin values have been reported to be a risk factor for poor healing and postoperative infection [1]. Another example would be to properly control blood sugar level prior and after surgery as poor glycemic control is related with significantly higher complications after surgery [2]. Most of all, understanding the vascularity of the limb is crucial when planning the reconstructive surgery as flap success is determined by the vascular status and supply. Building from the foundation of previous chapters, this chapter will focus on the reconstructive aspect of using free flaps to salvage the diabetic limb. The reconstructive surgeon brings on the capability to achieve healing by soft tissue manipulation. The surgeon may follow a reconstruction algorithm to manage and salvage diabetic foot ulcers. Having the reconstructive option in the treatment spectrum may enhance the healing process and increase the chances for salvage. Figure 9.1 shows the spectrum of care for diabetic foot. Understanding the spectrum of care and the role of each discipline will increase the chance for healing. While the systemic condition of the patient is being optimized wound specialists or surgeons can direct attention to the foot ulcer. Depending upon general condition, peripheral vascular status, bone pathology, wound depth, location, duration, involvement of chronic osteomyelitis, and patient motivation, wounds can be treated with debridement and other related surgical procedures [3].

Traditionally patients with diabetic foot have been regarded as relative contraindication for microsurgical free tissue transfer as it was felt that diabetic patients have arteriolar occlusive disease, which can cause vascular compromise to the flap and complication during the postoperative course [4]. But studies have failed to

J. P. Hong (✉) · H. P. Suh
Department of Plastic Surgery, Asan Medical Center
University of Ulsan, Seoul, Korea
e-mail: joonphong@amc.seoul.kr;
hyunsuk.suh@amc.seoul.kr

J. P. Hong, H. Suh (eds.), *Diabetic Foot Reconstruction*,
https://doi.org/10.1007/978-981-16-9816-3_9

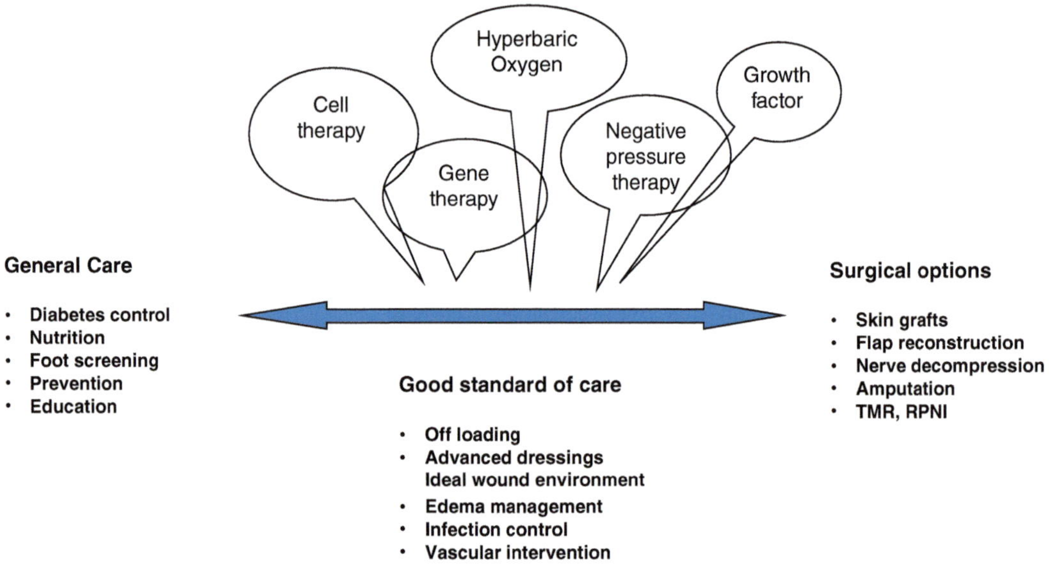

Fig. 9.1 The treatment spectrum of diabetic foot. Note the surgical options are listed on the right as the options for complex and complicated diabetic foot wounds

demonstrate significant increase of arteriolar occlusive disease or endothelial proliferation in diabetic foot [5–8]. A thickening of the capillary basement membrane has been documented, but capillary narrowing or occlusion has not [8]. The same study showed that diabetics often have atherosclerotic occlusion of the tibial arteries, but the occlusive disease occurs mainly in the leg so that the arterial system in the foot is less involved. Colen stated that diabetic neuropathy rather than microvascular disease is the primary cause of foot lesions in the presence of normal or near-normal arterial systems and advocated reconstruction [9]. However, the diabetic foot with complex conditions and often leading to amputations are the ischemic types. In clinical reality, the diabetic foot cases are often mixed with neuropathic as well as ischemic types complicating the reconstructive process. Thus reconstruction should be dependent upon the patient's overall condition rather than types of diabetic foot. Understanding the relative risk factors for failure and managing to reduce these risks can be the right strategy for successful reconstruction. The multidisciplinary approach as mentioned above is the critical step toward reducing these risks.

Today, the microvascular free flaps to reconstruct diabetic foot have been reported as comparable to nondiabetic patients [3, 9–23]. A meta-analysis of a systematic review of free tissue transfer in 528 diabetes patients in 18 studies showed that flap survival was 92% and limb salvage rate of 83.4% over a 28 months average follow-up period [24]. Furthermore, the impact of limb salvage by reconstructive microsurgery against 5-year survival rate has shown to reach 86.8% compared to the amputation group, which the 5-year mortality rate can range from 39% to as high as 80% [21, 25, 26].

This chapter will explore the aspect of microsurgical approach, indication, preoperative evaluation, intraoperative techniques, and postoperative care for diabetic foot reconstruction using free flaps.

9.2 Reconstruction Algorithm

While the medical care for the patient with diabetic foot ulceration begins with control of blood sugar, maintaining adequate nutrition and stabilization of the patient, the surgical care begins with debridement and control of infection. After the patient and the wound are stabilized, further evaluation of the wound is made. Unless immediately indicated for major amputation, the reconstructive algorithm may guide you through the necessary steps, as shown in Fig. 9.2. If simple with minimal or no vital structures exposed, conservative care with various treatments can be considered. If the wound is large that may take a long time to heal and healthy granulations are noted after wound preparation, skin graft or a small local flap can be performed [27]. Well-granulating wounds are an indication for good vascularity. The use of NPWT often enhances granulation formation and can be used to prepare the wound for reconstruction. However, if healing is stalling, then further evaluation using transcutaneous oxygen pressure measurement (TcPO2) or angiograms may be warranted to evaluate the arterial flow and prepare for vascular intervention. The same evaluation and approach to ensure vascularity is needed for complex wounds waiting for reconstructive procedure.

The philosophy to reconstruct diabetic foot follows the principle of reconstructive elevator and orthoplastic approach. Although reconstructive ladder still valued and widely taught, the reconstructive ladder comes from the concept of wound closure ladder dating back beyond the era of modern reconstructive surgery [28]. In the era of modern reconstructive surgery, one must consider not only adequate closures but form and function. A skin graft after plantar defects will provide coverage, but a skin or muscle flap with good padding and thicker skin will provide superior functional results in addition to coverage. A simpler reconstructive option may not necessarily produce optimal results. This is especially true for diabetic foot reconstruction, where consequences of inadequate coverage will lead to complications such as additional soft tissue loss, osteomyelitis, functional loss, increased medical cost and even amputation. Furthermore, one should understand the orthoplastic approach to assure adequate biomechanics of the foot is achieved to have optimal function after reconstruction [29]. Often requiring to have secondary or tertiary procedures of the bone, adequate coverage is essential. Correct skeletal correction is also essential to minimize post-reconstruction

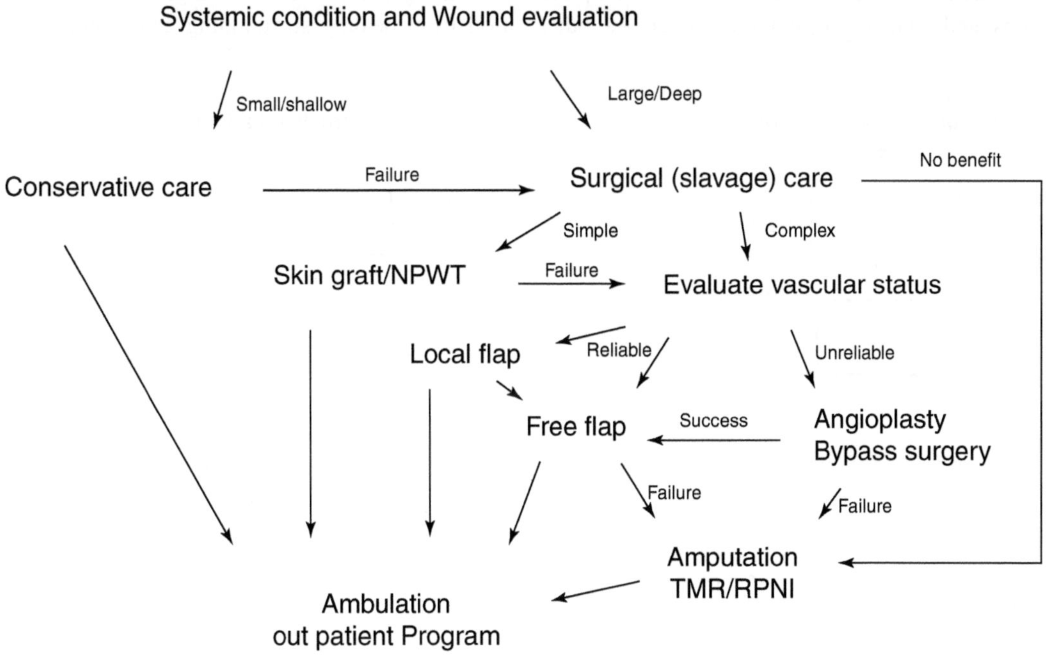

Fig. 9.2 The reconstruction algorithm

complications. Often missed is to correct tight Achilles tendon. If the Achilles is not lengthened, then the forefoot will have increased pressure during the gait and will likely cause additional ulceration due to the increased pressure. Thus to provide optimal form and function, we jump up and down the rungs of the ladder to correct the not only the soft tissue but the skeletal and tendon deformities as well. This paradigm of thought does not eliminate the concept of reconstructive ladder but replaces it as a ladder of wound closure and makes its mark in the field where variety of advanced reconstructive procedures and techniques are not readily available (Fig. 9.3). Based on the reconstructive elevator and orthoplastic approach, method of reconstruction of soft tissue and bone should be chosen based on procedures that results in optimal function as well as appearance [30].

9.3 Debridement and Infection Control

The first step of treatment for diabetic foot wound is to evaluate, debride, and treat infection [31]. Missing timely management will lead to amputations and longer hospital days [32]. As other chapters has covered these topics, this chapter will focus on the reconstruction perspectives. Optimal management of diabetic foot infection can potentially reduce incidence of major limb amputations and other related morbidities. All nonviable and infected soft tissue and bone should be excised during debridement. Milking along the proximal tendon can be helpful to identify and limit ascending infection. Tissue culture should be sent prior to debridement and after debridement. Post-debridement antibiotics selection should be based on the post-debridement culture. Sufficient irrigation should follow after debridement to reduce bacterial count [33]. Recent advance in technology introduced a hydrosurgery system that allows debride while preserving viable tissues and irrigating simultaneously allowing reduced surgical time [34, 35].

The understanding of vascular distribution of the foot, angiosome, helps to plan not only reconstruction but debridement [36]. When planning for reconstruction, one can avoid violating the angiosome territory while designing a local flap that may lead to flap breakdown [37]. Also by performing debridement according to the angiosome territory, one may enhance flap survival by increasing the chance for marginal vascularization from healthy surrounding angiosome terri-

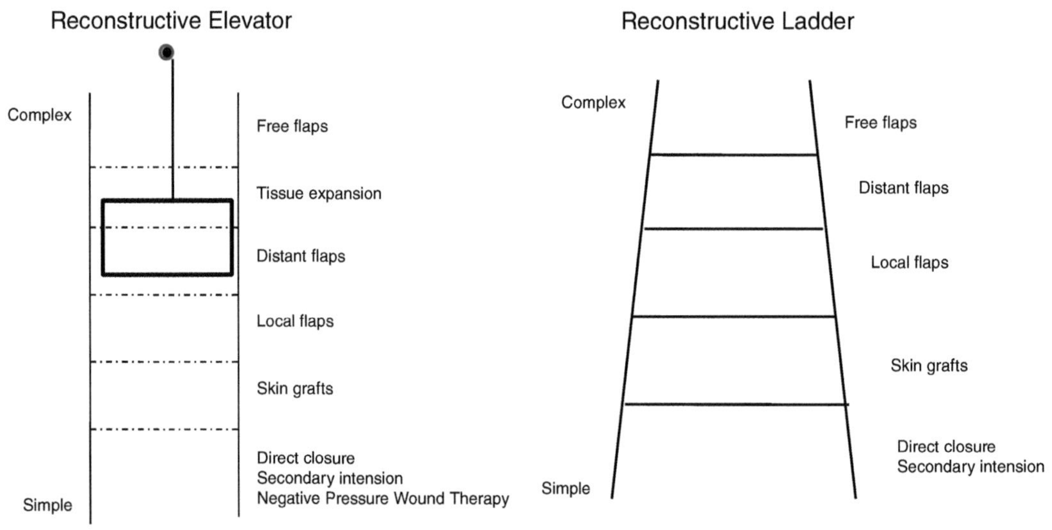

Fig. 9.3 The reconstructive elevator versus the ladder. Note that the reconstructive elevator finds the ideal option based on the reconstructive needs rather than climbing up each rung of options from simple to complex

tory [23]. This approach of using angiosome based debridement can be critical to allow inosculation from well-vascularized tissue, especially when reconstructing ischemic diabetic foot [23, 36]. The transcutaneous oxygen measurement (TcPO2) also plays a role in our protocol. Measurement over 30 mmHg in normobaric oxygen is a relative predictive factor for successful healing whereas pressure less than that of 30 mmHg is likely to follow an unfavorable course [38, 39]. If peri-wound $TcPO_2$ measurements were over 30 mmHg, then further treatment, including reconstructive procedures, were planned otherwise, amputations at according levels were performed.

Repetitive debridement should be performed as part of wound preparation for reconstruction while monitoring c-reactive protein for possible hidden infections and using it as an index for possible infection after reconstruction. In between the debridements, the use of NPWT can increase the rate of granulation and prevent the communication of external and internal bacteria from entering and escaping from the wound.

If the obvious wound and infection do not improve or subside even after the proper surgical debridement and antibiotics, surgeons should question the current treatment and seek the cause behind the uncontrolled infection. Monitoring the C-reactive protein (CRP) can be a good indicator to monitor inflammatory states in regard to infection [40]. When the infection focus is in question, the use of magnetic resonance imaging can help find hidden pockets of infection.

9.4 Evaluating and Enhancing the Vascular Status

As mentioned in the reconstruction algorithm, all patients considered for reconstruction using flaps should be evaluated for the vascular status. Although there are multiple evaluation tools, direct visualization of the vessels is preferred when considering reconstruction. The Ankle Brachial Index (ABI) is not used as it is not reliable in diabetic patients due to the high incidence of calcified vessels causing falsely elevate values [41]. Typically, the neuropathic type will have a patent vessels but often is accompanied by an ischemic component. Often the distinction between ischemic and neuropathic type is not clear and the foot and the extremity can be a mixed neuroischemic type showing early signs of calcification even in neuropathic types. Thus it will be prudent to perform angiograms for patients undergoing any reconstruction with flaps. The CT angiogram provides information regarding general vascular anatomy of the lower extremity, shows atherosclerotic change of vessels, which is useful information when choosing recipient's vessels and allows to select the flap donor site on the leg. This overview of the vascularity of the entire limb is important as collateral vessels may be the main supply to the distal limb, and the wrong selection of donor flaps can end in catastrophic complication (Fig. 9.4). After the examination, if vascular status is in doubt, then revascularization by angioplasty or bypass surgery is required. Although preoperative angiograms may indicate intact anatomy of the artery to the foot, actual findings upon surgery can be different. In order to confirm the distal vascular flow, we use ultrasound duplex scans to obtain physiologic information regarding the quality of the flow [3, 23, 42]. Our recent experience shows that peak blood flow velocity over 15–20 cm/s on the recipient vessels allows the flap to survive [23, 42]. Thus, one of the aims for intervention in regard to flap reconstruction is to reach this minimal flow velocity that allows free flap reconstruction.

In our center, the first approach for vascular intervention is endovascular approach using balloon angioplasty and stents. It is preferred due to the simplicity and minimal invasiveness of the approach. In diabetic patients, the atherosclerosis most significant occlusions occur in the crural arteries often sparing the arteries of the foot [8]. Bypass to dorsalis pedis or posterior tibial artery of the foot or angioplasty with or without stent placement procedures result in high success to restore perfusion pressure to the distal circulation of the foot reestablishing palpable pulse.

The role of vascular intervention may also extend to the postoperative period. Re-stenosis after

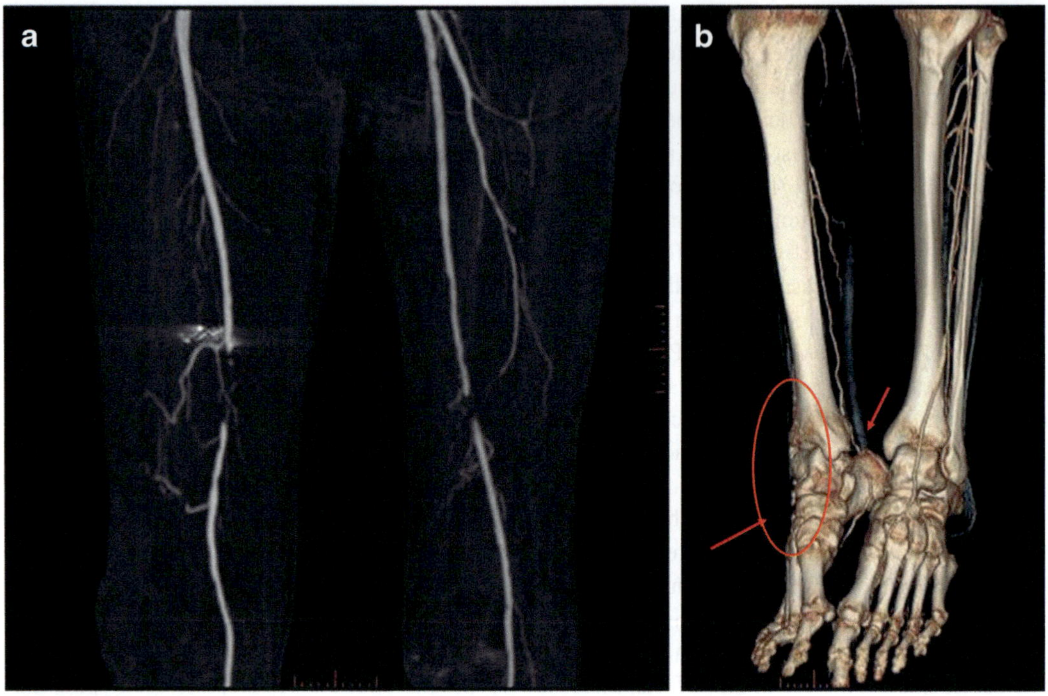

Fig. 9.4 CT angiogram of the flap donor site. Note that the femoral artery is totally obstructed and the flow distal to the leg is mainly supplied by the descending branch of the lateral femoral circumflex artery bypassing the obstruction (**a**). The 3D reconstruction of the CT angiogram shows the calcified and the calcification spared segment of the major arteries (**b**)

endovascular intervention can be as high as 50–60% within the first 6–12 months, and this can happen as early as the first or second week after surgery [43, 44]. In these cases, the flap can be salvaged by emergency angiogram to identify the obstruction leading to angioplasty reestablishing the flow to the flap. It is prudent to keep a keen observation for any early ischemic changes of the flap.

Reperfusion is most essential prior to any reconstruction using graft, local flaps and microsurgical reconstruction. If vascular intervention fails and wound progresses, amputation is warranted.

Skin grafts and local flaps have been discussed in other chapters.

9.5 Indications for Free Flap

1. Stagnant healing despite good wound care.
2. Wounds that are complex and/or exposed vital structures needing timely coverage.
3. No significant systemic illness likely to be exacerbated by multiple operations and prolong rehabilitation.
4. Previously ambulatory with the aim to restore a functional limb.
5. Reasonably patent crural vascular status with minimal recipient artery flow velocity of 15–20 cm/s.

An inclusion criteria from a meta-analysis of free tissue transfer in 528 diabetes patients in 18 studies suggests: (1) Lower limb defect which has not displayed any signs of granulation or healing despite adequate debridement or necrotic tissue and conservative treatment; (2) No significant renal function impairment; (3) No significant systemic illness likely to be exacerbated by multiple operations and prolong rehabilitation; (4) Previously ambulatory with the aim to restore a functional limb; (5) Likely to engage with the significant physiotherapy required for return to normal living; and (6) Peak flow velocity of >40 cm/s in recipient artery [24]. We generally agree with the suggested inclusion criteria except for the significant renal disease. In our experience, we have not found an increased risk for failure despite the fact that uremia may causes a decrease in cell-mediated immunity and impair wound healing [45, 46]. However, patients after kidney transplantation who received immunosuppression had an odds ratio of 4.857 of having flap failure ($p = 0.041$). I would rather prefer to present the contraindication rather than the indications for flap reconstruction as microsurgery technique evolves using small recipient vessels rather than a major vessels for reconstruction [47]. The most important factor may be the perfusion of the recipient vessel. If any small vessel is seen with good pulsatile flow, it would be indicated for microsurgery. As mentioned above, our experience shows that recipient vessels with minimal flow velocity of 15–20 cm/s will be adequate. Thus an absolute contraindication would be no flow to the foot without any sign of perfusion from any distal small vessels.

9.6 Timing for Reconstruction

As shown in the indication, when the systemic condition of the patient can tolerate the surgery, vascular supply is reasonable, wound bed prepared, and infection controlled, reconstruction can take place. However, the timing for reconstruction can be challenging when vascular status is compromised.

The timing of when to perform reconstruction after vascular intervention is not clear. Reports have shown successful free flap transfer with simultaneous vascular reconstruction to salvage the limb [48]. But early bypass failures within 30 days are reported to be high [18, 49]. In our experience, partial flap loss or total loss was suddenly noted after 2–3 weeks in the cases combined with simultaneous or reconstruction following few days after vascular interventions. This may suggest that there should be a sufficient stabilization period after vascular bypass surgery. However, for endovascular angioplasties, we usually perform microsurgery as soon as possible. Knowing that re-stenosis after endovascular intervention can be as high as 50–60% within the first 6–12 months, early reconstruction will increase the chance of flap survival during the window period of the patent flow [43, 44].

9.7 Choosing the Recipient Vessel and Microanastomosis

1. Preoperative diagnostic tools should be used to map out the ideal recipient artery in terms of anatomy, physiology, and pathology.
2. When selecting a major artery, end-to-side approach will maintain adequate distal flow.
3. If the target artery is calcified, search for a calcification free segment (end-to-side) or a branch from the major artery (end-to-end).
4. Perforator or small arteries can be used as a recipient vessel when the flow velocity is at least 15–20 cm/s.
5. Understand the angioplasty technique and if possible avoid the segment of the artery that underwent angioplasty.

The biggest challenge in reconstructive microsurgery for diabetic foot is finding an adequate recipient vessel, especially in ischemic diabetic foot. Biphasic pulsatile signal or acoustic wave from handheld Doppler does not guarantee a good recipient vessel for anastomosis. The sensitivity of handheld Doppler is very high and can trace a vessel less than 0.2–0.3 mm diameter and even severely calcified vessels often misleading the surgeon to think that it can be a reliable recipient source. The surgeon should select the recipient vessel based on anatomical knowledge, preoperative angiograms, ultrasound findings, and intraoperative visual inspection. When the major vessels are calcified, it may be very difficult to select the recipient vessel. Careful examination of CT angiograms may provide clues on how to find a reliable recipient vessel [50]. Even with a visual pulsation to the artery of the foot, atherosclerosis of the artery can make anastomosis very difficult. The separation of intima and adventitia layers of the artery caused by calcification makes intima to intima contact difficult and may increase the risk for thrombosis. Thus calcification spared segments of the major artery can be used to anastomose the flap in an end-to-side manner, or you can find a branch from the major artery and use it to anastomose end-to-end (Fig. 9.5) [3, 20, 22]. In our experience, using the branch from the major artery as a recipient may be a better choice. It is not common to see branches from posterior tibial and dorsalis pedis arteries to be calcified and by using these branches, one can easily anastomose to a supple and soft artery without diminishing distal flow. An alternative anastomosis may be the T-style anastomosis, where bypassing artery segment with a branch to the flap is inter-anastomosed between the proximal and distal recipient artery. If a T-style anastomosis is not possible, using a vein graft in between the calcified artery, then anastomosing the flap pedicle as an end-to-side fashion on the vein graft can be an alternative. We try to avoid using major artery as an end-to-end fashion as using the major vessel in this manner will decrease the distal flow to the foot and will have a negative impact on the overall circulation of the foot [3, 23].

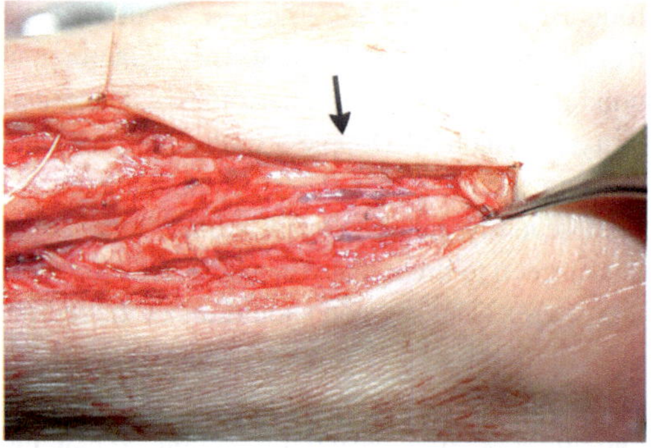

Fig. 9.5 Calcification of the dorsalis pedis artery is shown. Note that there is a calcification spared segment that allows for side of the dorsalis pedis artery to be used as a recipient to the end of the flap donor artery. Also note that the branches from the dorsalis pedis are spared from calcification being a potential source for recipient artery in an end-to-end fashion

When approaching arteries that underwent angioplasties, one must be aware how the angioplasty was performed. After angioplasties, frequently damage to the intimal layers can occur, and this will increase the burden to an already challenging anastomosis. Avoiding the segment that underwent angioplasty will make the anastomosis but easier. Sometimes, angioplasty can be performed between the intima and adventitia as the lumen of the artery is collapsed, making angioplasty impossible. In these cases, the microsurgery will become very difficult not to mention the increased risk for thrombosis. Thus knowing how the angioplasty was performed may guide the microsurgeon in selecting the right recipient for microsurgery.

However, what if there are no major vessels available? Is microsurgery possible? One can often see even when limbs have no sufficient major vessels, most of the skin of the ischemic limb is still intact with good bleeding. This is most likely due to the slow occlusion of the major artery leading to persistent formation of collateral vessels supplying the distal limb and subdermal plexus of the skin [50]. Often, the territory of ischemia and necrosis coincides with the angiosome territory, and the surrounding angiosome is spared from necrotic change [23, 31, 36, 37]. Thus, a terminal perforator artery or a small vessel within the healthy angiosome adjacent to the necrotic lesion can be used as a recipient vessel. These small perforators can be traced using a handheld Doppler or Duplex ultrasound to confirm an adequate velocity of the arterial flow. In our experience, a small artery can be used when the flow velocity was over 15–20 cm/s [23, 42]. As most of the perforator flaps have a flow velocity over 20 cm/s for the perforating artery, these small recipient perforators can be an ideal recipient source. However, one must visually confirm the adequacy of the recipient vessel prior to anastomosis. The use of these small perforators or vessels require a supermicrosurgery technique and usually perform end-to-end as perforator-to-perforator (Fig. 9.6) [23]. The overall success rate for supermicrosurgery approach can be high as 90.5% [22, 23]. This it is comparable but slightly lower to any nondiabetic foot

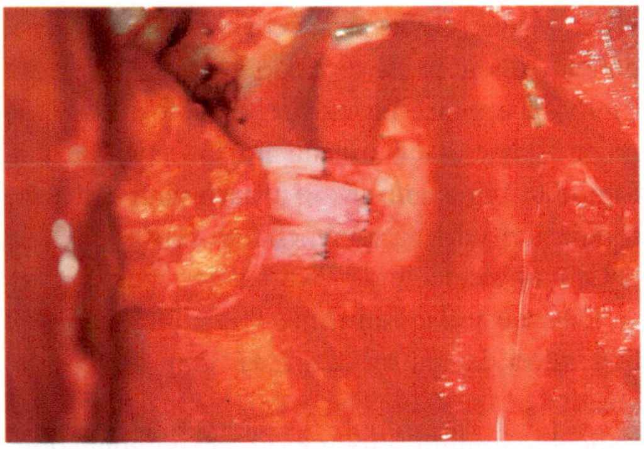

Fig. 9.6 Perforator-to-perforator anastomosis is shown. The recipient and the donor vessels needs to be sufficiently enlarged by using a vessel dilator prior to microanastomosis

reconstruction as well as diabetic foot reconstruction using the classical approach.

The selection for veins is relatively easier compared to the artery. Usually, the veins are spared from developing any pathology. Superficial veins can be used reliably. However, when the diabetic foot undergoes ischemic change, the soft tissue may be fibrosed, and perivascular scarring can make the dissection difficult.

As the recipient's vessel, despite the preoperative evaluation, can be different when actually dissected. The recipient's vessels need to be isolated and visually confirmed first prior to flap elevation. This will allow for better planning to select the right flap. The surgeons should always have a flexible mind and adjust accordingly when challenges are met.

9.8 Free Flaps

The flap for reconstruction of diabetic foot should provide a well-vascularized tissue to control infection, adequate contour for footwear, durability, and solid anchorage to resist shearing forces. Controversy still remains which flap, whether muscle flaps with skin grafts, fasciocutaneous flaps and recently added perforator flaps, offers the optimal solution to reconstruct the foot, especially the weight-bearing surface. But as long as the large defect is covered with any well-vascularized tissue, it will provide an independent and well-nourished vascular supply to eradicate infection, increase local oxygen tension, enhancing antibiotics activity, and neovascularization to the adjacent ischemic tissue [51, 52]. In our clinical experience, we are shifting toward using perforator flaps such as anterolateral thigh (ALT) perforator flap, gluteal artery perforator (GAP) flap, superficial circumflex iliac perforator (SCIP) flap and medial plantar perforator flap as it provides, a thin flap to minimize shearing, can take only the superficial fat to imitate the fibrous septa of the sole to adhere tightly, enhance neovascularization of the subdermal plexus with adjacent tissue, and provide adequate blood supply to fight infection. In this section, we will focus on the perforator flaps.

Our experience shows that microsurgical approach to reconstruct diabetic foot may have flap survival rate of 91.7% and limb salvage rate of 84.9%, which are similar with other reports [21, 24]. Although significant increase of failure was noted in patient with poor arteries requiring multiple angioplasties, with peripheral arterial disease and taking immunosuppressive agents after kidney transplantation, the overall success rate and the limb salvage rate justifies the use of reconstructive microsurgery [21]. What was more interesting was that the impact on free flap reconstruction and limb salvage may have not only on the improving quality but on patient survival. The death rate after 5 years for a major amputation can be as high as 78% [53–55]. In our previous reported series, according to the Kaplan-Meier survival estimate curve, the 5-year survival rate for reconstructed patients against patients amputated above the ankle showed 86.8% and 41.4%, respectively [21]. Although the average age and ASA (American Society of Anesthesiologists) physical status classification of the major amputated patients was relatively higher (63 against 54.6 years, 2.7 against 2.3) than the reconstructed patients in that series, it was not statistically significant. This strongly suggests that reconstruction rather than amputating above the ankle will increase 5-year-survival rate.

As mentioned briefly above, the introduction of supermicrosurgery concept allows exploring more options for the recipient vessels. Based on the idea that surrounding angiosomes around the ischemic defects are healthier, one can find a very small artery or a perforator which is an end vessel going into the skin and use it as a recipient vessel [22, 23]. The overall success rate for supermicrosurgery approach in diabetic foot is 90.5%. This it is comparable but slightly lower to any nondiabetic foot reconstruction as well as diabetic foot reconstruction using the classical approach [23]. The reconstruction by perforator flap using supermicrosurgery approach provides well-vascularized tissue that covers diabetic foot defect without being dependent on major vessels. This concept may provide solution to even to the more progressed ischemic diabetic foot. Figure 9.7 illustrates an approach with using the supermicrosurgery approach to reconstruct a diabetic foot ulcer.

One must also remember to correct any bone or tendon deformity that may alter the biomechanics of the foot. The orthoplastic approach is critical to minimize long-term flap complications such as re-ulcerations of the flap.

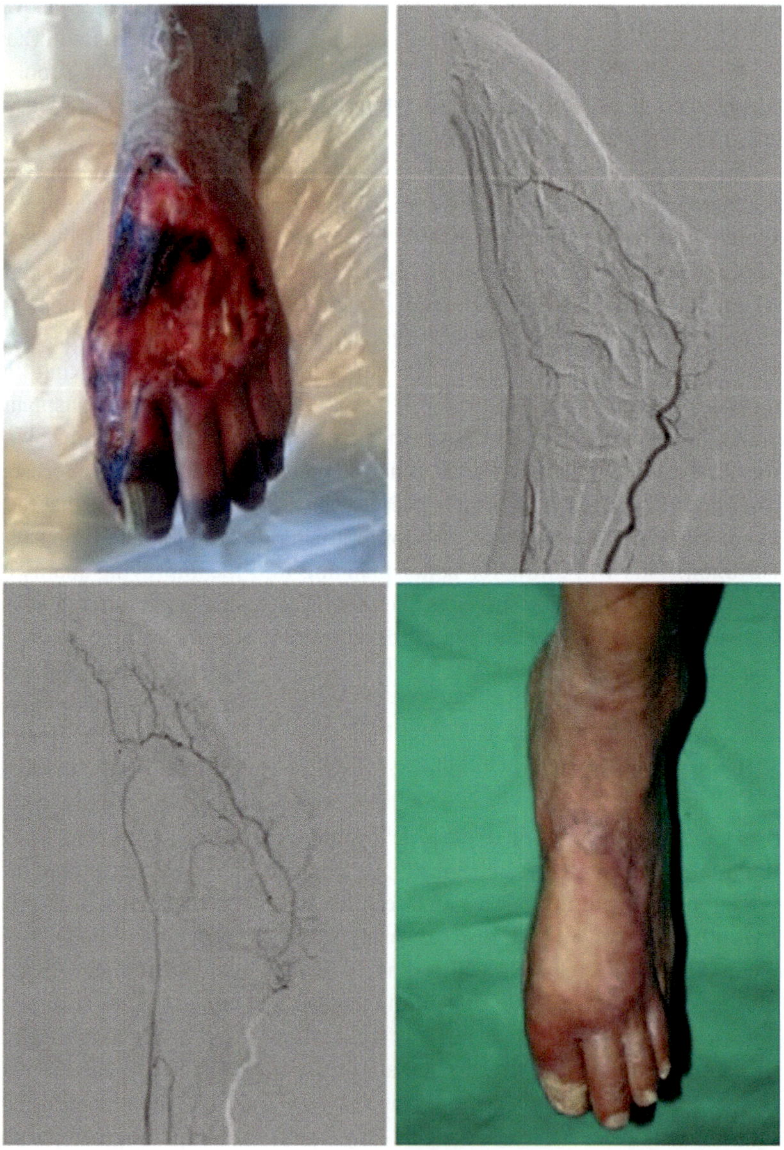

Fig. 9.7 Demonstrating the supermicrosurgery approach. After angioplasty and increasing the flow, small collaterals are seen more vividly. One of the collateral near the defect after debridement was used as the recipient artery for the SCIP free flap

9.8.1 Flap Selection Algorithm for Perforator Flaps

When we consider to select a flap for reconstruction, these are the factors to consider; (1) patient position, (2) flap size, (3) Thickness of the flap, (4) flap composition and (5) pedicle length required [56]. We believe this approach helps to optimize form and function, decrease operative time, while minimizing donor site morbidity and secondary procedures. Although this algorithm was evaluated based on our experience with perforator flaps, this can be applied to muscle flaps as well.

We prefer to select a flap based on the patient's position following defect preparation. Avoidance of an intraoperative position change helps to minimize operative time and avoids potential anesthetic complications such as inadvertent extubation, peripheral nerve compression or intravascular line malposition [57, 58]. Flaps can be selected without changing the patient position to harvest the flap. Defect sizes dictate which flap to select and although not all flaps can be designed large, most flaps can be designed small. Understanding the limit of the flap is important when selecting the flap. The thickness of the flap is an important issue as the thicker the flap, the more shearing can occur, leading to future complications of ulceration [20]. For optimal footwear and to minimize shearing achieving the right thickness is essential. However, if the thickness cannot be controlled, secondary debulking will allow to achieve the right thickness. The SCIP flap can be one of the thinnest flap possible to elevate, and when other perforator flaps are used, elevation on a superficial plane may help to harvest the perforator flap with the right thickness [59–61]. The flap composition required is determined by the defect dimensions and missing components. Many flaps, such as the ALT or the SCIP flap, can be used as combined/chimeric flap. Understanding what component each flap can add will allow to have a better reconstruction addressing the missing components of the defect. Regarding the pedicle length, any flap can be harvested with a short pedicle. However, there are flaps with a short maximum pedicle length, limiting their universal use. Thus one should consider the pedicle length required in flap selection, despite other ideal characteristics it may have for coverage. This is especially important in ischemic diabetic foot, where the source of recipient vessels can be limited. In our experience, we often reside in using the anterior tibial artery and vein for heel defects as defects in this region frequently occur from having a poor peroneal and posterior tibial arterial supply requiring a flap with a long pedicle [62]. Fig. 9.8 shows the algorithm for perforator flap selection.

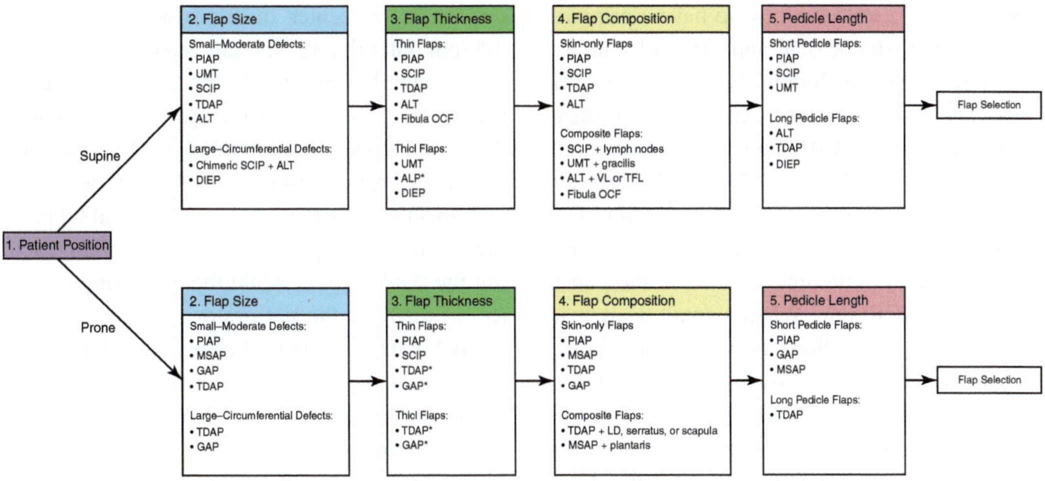

Fig. 9.8 The algorithm for perforator flap selection is shown

9.8.2 Perforator Flaps: Technical Aspects

9.8.2.1 SCIP (Superficial Circumflex Iliac Artery Perforator) Flap

The SCIP flap is an evolution from groin flap. The groin flap, supplied by the superficial circumflex iliac artery (SCIA), is one of the first free flaps successful in reconstruction. This flap was first described as a pedicle flap by McGregor and Jackson and then introduced as a free flap by Daniel and Taylor [63, 64]. Koshima et al. modified it as a skin flap elevated above the deep fascia based on the SCIA perforator overcoming some disadvantages such as bulkiness and variable arterial anatomy [65–67]. But even with these evolved technique and concept, the SCIP flap was still challenging to use due to the short pedicle, small vessel caliber, relative bulkiness, especially in obese patients, and donor site morbidity such as lymphorrhea. Further modifications were made where Hong et al. harvested the flap on the superficial fascia making the flap thinner (superthin flaps) while avoiding injuries to the lymphatic system which is located on the deep fat below the superficial fascia, thus minimizing lymphorrhea [47, 60, 68–71].

The advantages of using the SCIP flap is; (1) to obtain a thin flap, (2) to have reliable perforator anatomy (medial and lateral branches) and superficial vein, (3) to have the capability to either elevate a small or a large flap (from 4 × 3 cm to 12 × 35 cm), (4) to have a primarily closed hidden donor scar, and (5) to elevate as a composite flap (including lymph nodes, iliac bone, and part of Sartorius muscle). The disadvantages of using SCIP flap is; (1) to have a relatively short pedicle, and (2) small perforator artery diameter (Table 9.1). The use of skin flaps for chronic osteomyelitis has been shown to have no difference in outcome, and the same can be said for the SCIP flap. When a small dead space is noted, part of the flap can be de-epithelialized to obliterate the dead space [72]. The main contraindications for the SCIP flap would defects that needs a long pedicle to reach the recipient vessels. A relative contraindication would be defects that exceed the coverage potential of the SCIP flap and unable to close primarily. Although one can perform skin grafts for the donor defect, it would less ideal to utilize the advantages of the flap. The authors also recommend to avoid harvesting the SCIP flap on the side that underwent percutaneous angiograms or angioplasty prior to surgery. When hematoma is collected, it makes identifying the perforators very difficult.

Table 9.1 Advantages and disadvantages of the SCIP flap

Pros	Cons
Well concealed donor site	Smaller vessel lumen
Thin and pliable skin flap – allows single stage resurfacing	Short pedicle
Septocutaneous pedicle (medial branch)	Learning curve to elevate as thin flap
Expedient harvest	Supermicrosurgery technique required for certain defects
Composite with lymph node and bone	
Medium to large skin dimension	

Preoperative ultrasound Doppler or a handheld Doppler is used to mark the potential perforators of the SCIP flap. There are two major perforators to base the SCIP flap on. In 95% of the SCIP flaps, of the medial (superficial) perforator of the SCIA penetrates the deep fascia within an oval of 4.2 × 2 (vertical × horizontal) cm, with the center of the oval point located 4.5 cm lateral and 1.5 cm superior from the superolateral corner of the pelvic tubercle (Fig. 9.9) [73]. The medial perforating branch then can be divided into two distinctive patterns; The axial pattern (44%) shows the perforator runs in an axial pattern on the superficial fat passing the anterior superior iliac spine (ASIS) reaching the flank region, while the anchoring pattern (56%) displays the perforator reaching the subdermal plexus without further branching [73]. This anatomy becomes relevant, especially when longer SCIP flaps need to be harvested, which the axial pattern would be safer to use. The lateral (deep) branch can be detected on the lateral region of the axis drawn from the pubic tubercle to the ASIS. It usually traveling laterally beneath the deep fascia and often with an intramuscular pathway perforating the deep fascia on the lateral aspect (deep branch) near the ASIS. The CT angiogram allows to visualize the medial (deep) and lateral (superficial) branches with accuracy, allowing safer design, especially in respect to size of the flap [73]. Recently, the use of ultrasound has helped to define the not only the exact location but the pathway of the perforator and the superficial vein as well with high accuracy. One should remember that the SCIP flap can be designed based on the either the medial and lateral perforators or take both when needed (Fig. 9.10). Table 9.2 shows the points to consider when selecting either the medial or lateral branch of the SCIA of the SCIP flap. The venous drainage of the flap often can be based on the superficial vein. When the superficial vein is not available or is not included in the flap, accompanying vein can be used as well but will have a very small vessel diameter to work with. The most common presentation of the venous drainage is the accompanying vein draining into the superficial venous system [60].

Elevation of the flap should first keep in mind which perforator will be the main pedicle. The medial branch is always a direct cutaneous perforator having an easy dissection, while the lateral branch travels underneath the deep fascia, often

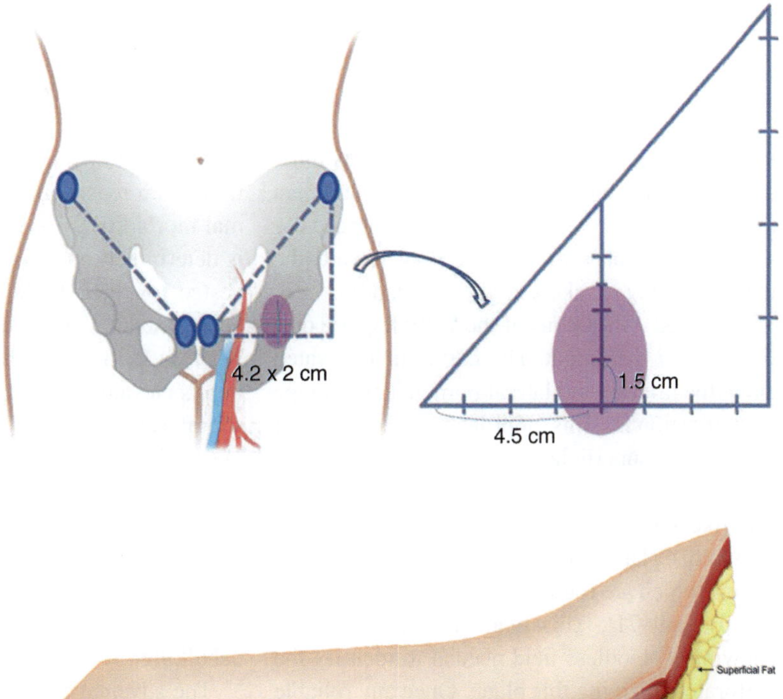

Fig. 9.9 The medial perforators of the SCIA penetrate the deep fascia within an oval of 4.2 × 2 (vertical × horizontal) cm with the center of the oval point located 4.5 cm lateral and 1.5 cm superior from the superolateral corner of the pelvic tubercle

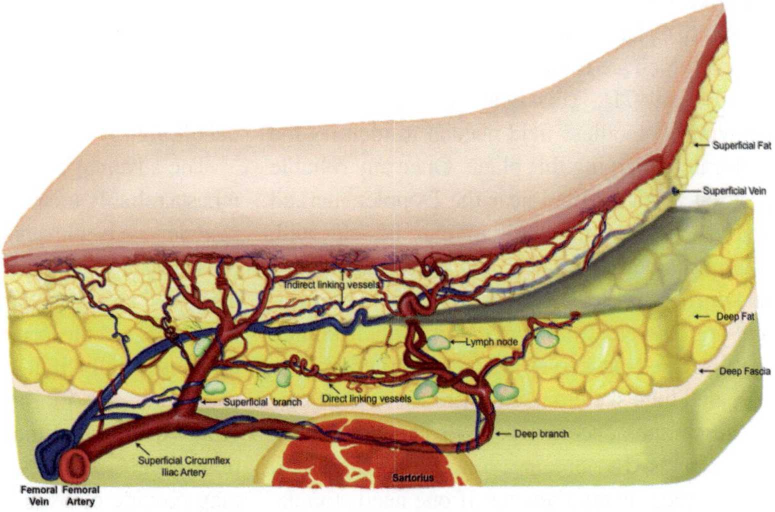

Fig. 9.10 There are two major perforators of the SCIP flap. The medial (superficial) branch is a direct cutaneous branch with and easy and quick dissection while the lateral (deep) branch travels laterally beneath the deep fascia and often with an intramuscular pathway perforating the deep fascia on the lateral aspect near the ASIS

Table 9.2 Comparison between the flaps based on medial versus lateral branches of the superficial circumflex iliac artery. Note that flaps can be based on both medial and lateral branch as well

Medial (superficial) branch	Lateral (deep) branch
Septocutaneous perforator	Muscular path included
Short pedicle	Relatively longer pedicle
Topographically constant perforator	Non-constant perforator
Two distinct type of perforator – Axial pattern – Anchoring pattern	Mostly axial pattern perforator
Medium size skin paddle (anchoring type) Large size skin paddle (axial pattern)	Large size skin paddle
Expedient harvest	Slower harvest
Composite with lymph node	Composite with bone and muscle

needing dissection near or in the Sartorius muscle making the dissection more complicated than the medial branch. The lateral branch is usually an axial pattern perforator traveling toward the flank, allowing to take a larger skin paddle.

Required dimensions of the SCIP flap are outlined as per the defect. The flap is first elevated along the inferior and lateral borders under loupe magnification as this approach allows to best identify the superficial fascia lying between the superficial and deep fat. This is a distinct white film-like layer, and elevation of the flap on or above this plane avoids injury to the lymphatic system which are found in the deeper adipose tissue [60, 69–71]. This plane is also avascular, allowing a bloodless field needed to identify the perforators piercing this plane. Once any reliable perforator is identified near the Doppler marked region, the rest of the flap can be elevated. Multiple other perforators can be further identified during the elevation. When multiple perforators are dissected, one can decide which branch (perforator) best serves the reconstructive purpose and then skeletonize toward the source vessel passing the deep fascia [60]. The deep fascia can be incised to obtain a longer pedicle length and a larger vessel diameter. If one needs to take part of the iliac bone, a branch toward the crest from the lateral (deep) branch can be identified and elevated together [74–76]. A superficial vein running from the ASIS toward the pubis is normally identified and is preserved. The accompanying vein of the medial branch often drains into the superficial vein thus need to harvest only one vein. In cases where there is a small or absent superficial vein, the accompanying vein of the perforator is usually of a larger caliber. Whenever the donor vessels are small, dissection is should be performed under the microscope. Figure 9.11 shows the overall sequence of elevation.

9.8.2.2 Anterolateral Thigh (ALT) Free Flap

One of the most used workhorse flaps among the perforator flaps is the anterolateral thigh perforator flaps. First described by Baek and Song and with refinements from Wei et al., it has become one of the ideal flaps for reconstruction providing reliable anatomy, long pedicles, thin flaps, sensation and a reasonable donor site scar with minimal morbidity [77–79]. The method of elevation is determined on whether the deep fascia is harvested together. If the flap is elevated with the deep fascia, it is called a subfascial elevation, whereas if the deep fascia is left intact and the flap is elevated above the deep fascia, it is called suprafascial elevation [79]. In either case, the flap may still be bulky in some cases and additional debulking may be required to achieve the right thickness after elevation. Thus the superficial fascia located between the deep and the superficial fat can be used as a plane of elevation (superthin flap), minimizing the need for immediate or late debulking [59, 80].

The advantages of using the ALT flap are that it has a reliably located perforator, provides a long pedicle, can be elevated as a thin flap on the superficial fascia plane, can be innervated, and can be harvested as a large flap. The major disadvantages can be the tedious process of dissecting the perforator especially if it has an intramuscular path, and donor site morbidity, especially when harvested in a large dimension. Preoperative evaluation using CT angiograms or Duplex ultrasound may provide clues in selecting the ideal pathway

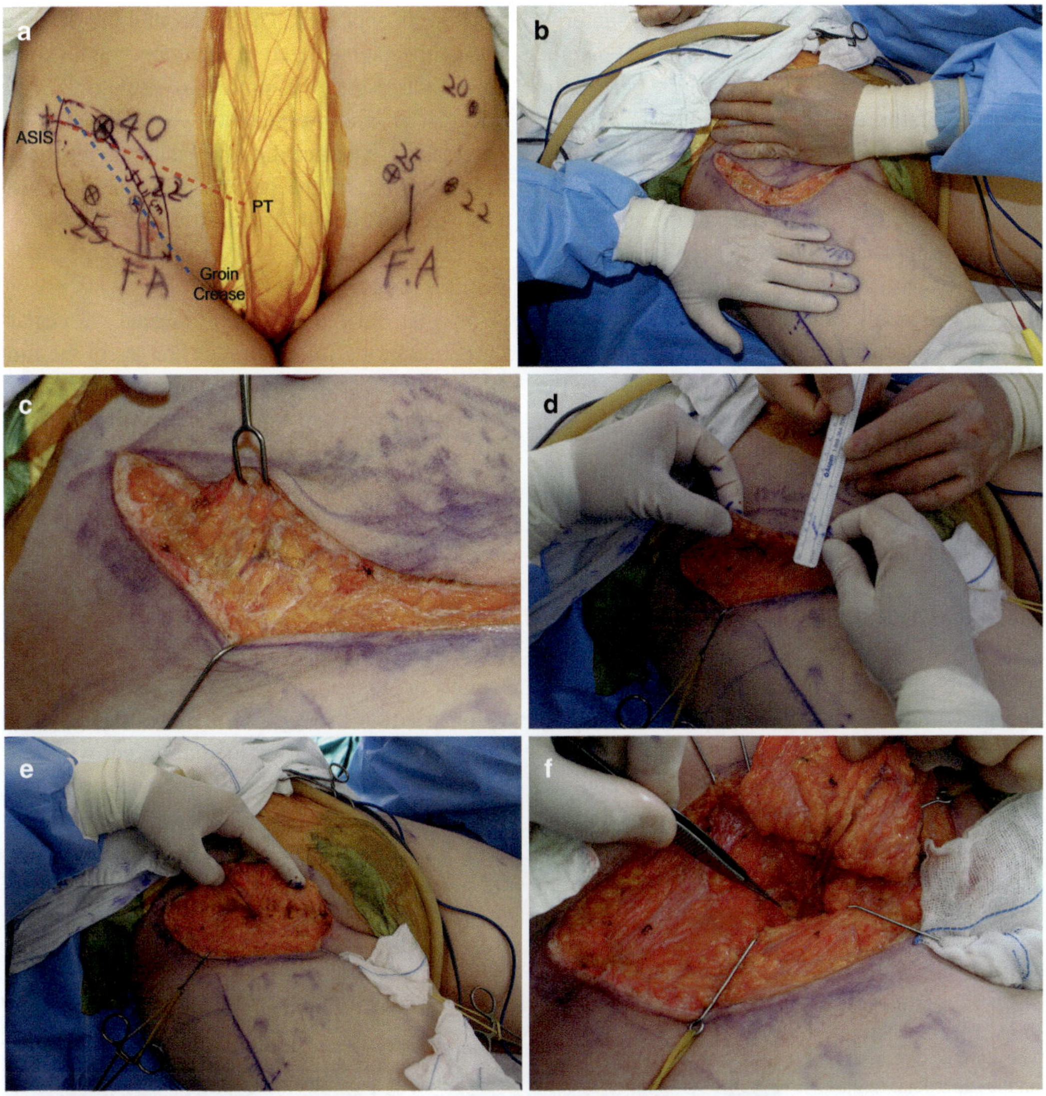

Fig. 9.11 The sequence of the elevation of the SCIP flap is shown. The SCIP flap design should be made along the axis between the groin crease and the ASIS (anterior superior iliac spine) where the SCIA usually travels. Using the handheld Doppler, the medial and lateral perforators can be identified and marked (**a**). The elevation begins from the lateral inferior margin with traction as the superficial fascia will be most evident (**b**). Once the superficial fascia plane is found, the elevation proceeds from lateral to medial and caudal to cephalic until the perforators are seen (**c**). Note that the superficial vein is included in the flap (**d**). The lateral branches are identified first followed by the medial branch (**e**). After dissecting both medial and lateral branches, one can determine which perforator to use or can use both (**f**)

of the pedicle as well as the most dominant perforator [42, 81, 82]. Another advantage of using preoperative CT angiogram is that it can provide information about the status of the flap pedicle. The descending branch can often be affected with calcification, and one should consider to use the side with less calcification to minimize complication. One should also remember that the descending branch can be the major collateral when the femoral artery is totally obstructed.

The elevation begins after identifying the perforators with handheld Doppler or Duplex ultrasound tracing along the axis between the anterior superior iliac spine (ASIS) and the lateral patella, the skin flap is designed to include the perforator. Once perforators are marked, the elevation begins from either margins of the flap, but the authors prefer approaching the lateral border of the flap first. The incision is made deep to the superficial fascia dividing superficial and deep fat. It is easy to identify based on the characteristics of the fat lobule. The small lobules suddenly become bigger as it passes a very thin fascia-like structure. It is easier to identify this fascia while retracting the skin from both sides of the incision (Fig. 9.12). After locating the fascia, then elevation is made on this plane until reaching the axis between ASIS and the lateral patella. Dissection under loupe magnification allows to see the small perforators and minimizes the risk of trauma. The same approach is performed from the medial side. When elevating far outside where the perforators are suspected (hot zone), one can quickly elevate without worrying about perforator injury (cold zone). One must keep this plane of dissection clean as possible, performing meticulous coagulation as bleeding can cause identifying the perforator difficult. After locating multiple perforators, the favorable one or multiple perforators are traced through the deep fat and deep fascia in a freestyle approach. The fat around the perforator can be skeletonized or maintained with some surrounding fat. We prefer to skeletonize the deep fat around the pedicle. Once traced to the deep fascia, a vertical linear incision on the fascia allows to dissect the pedicle proximally to harvest adequate length for anastomosis [59, 80].

9.8.2.3 Case

A 55-year-old female patient is seen with bilateral ulcerations and ischemic changes of the foot (Fig. 9.13). The right foot shows ischemic first and second toes and exposed tendons on the dorsum of the foot, while the left foot shows chronic wound that led to rupture and contracture of the Achilles tendon with an open wound (Fig. 9.13a, b). After angioplasty and minor surgery of both foot, the foot showed improved circulation with marginal epithelization and granulation. Repetitive angioplasty was performed as the wound no longer improved. On the day of the reconstruction the right foot shows the first two toes amputated with the medial defect with tendon exposure, and the right foot shows reconstructed Achilles tendon with skin defect (Fig. 9.13c, d). The SCIP flap was harvested from the left groin to reconstruct the right dorsum of the foot and the ALT was harvested to reconstruct

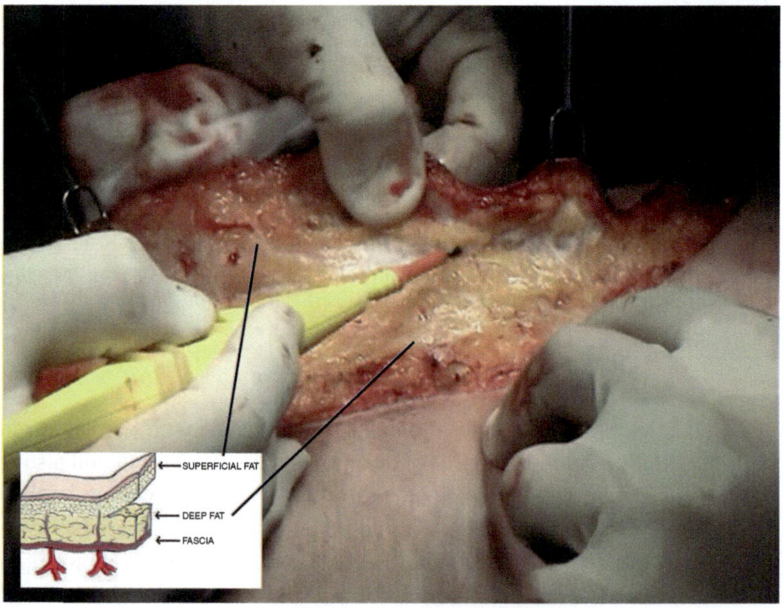

Fig. 9.12 Elevation of the ALT flap is shown. The plane of elevation is on the superficial fascia plane (superthin) between the superficial and the deep fat

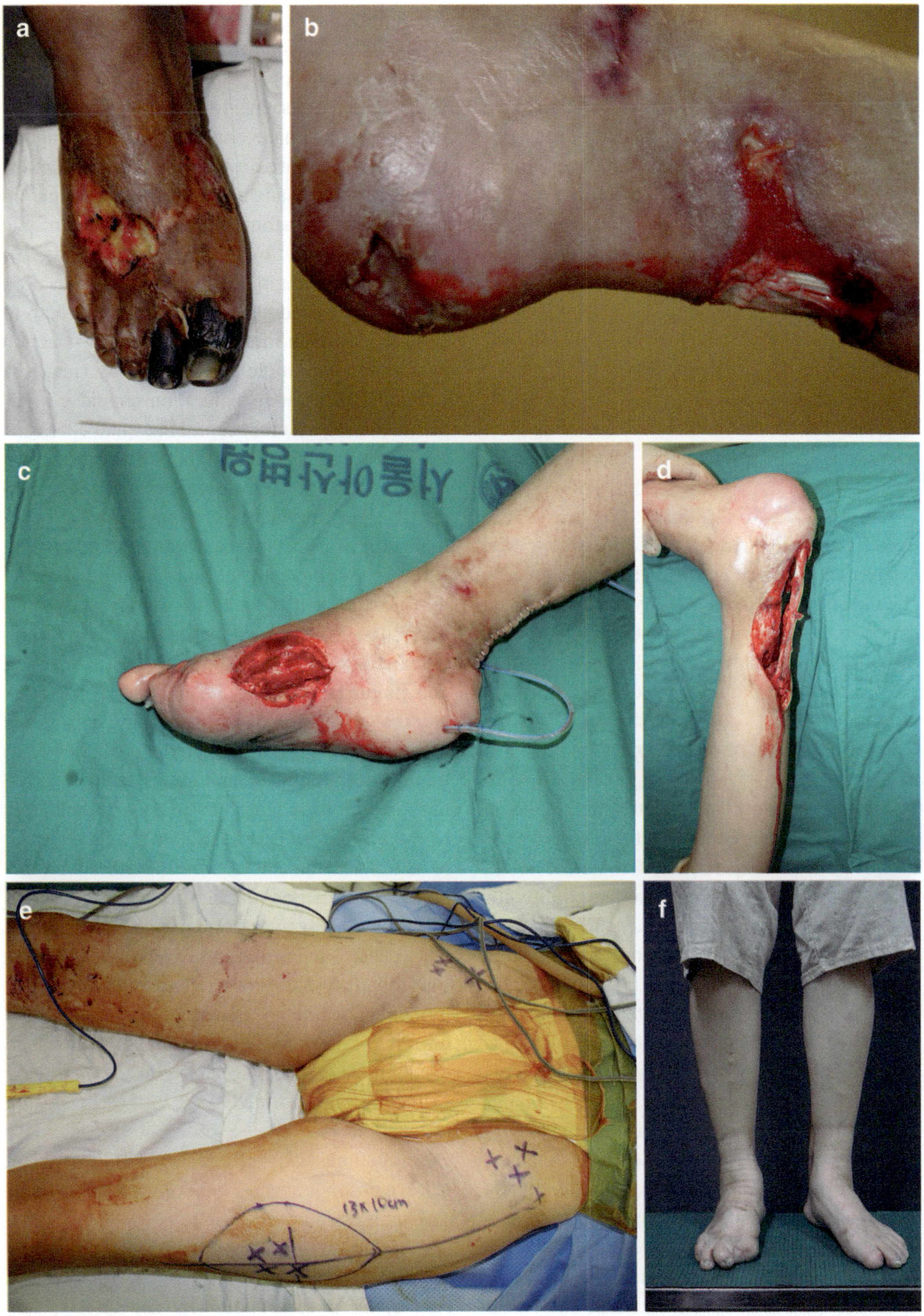

Fig. 9.13 Case presentation using both SCIP and the superthin ALT to reconstruction bilateral diabetic foot wounds. (**a**) Ischemic ulcer of the right foot. (**b**) Chronic ulceration leading to Achilles tendon ruture and surrounding granulation. (**c**) After debridment and toe anputations of the right foot. (**d**) After debridement and Achilles tendon repair. (**e**) Desing for elevation using ALT free flap on the left thigh and scip flap from the left groin. (**f**, **g**) Postoperative view after 2 years

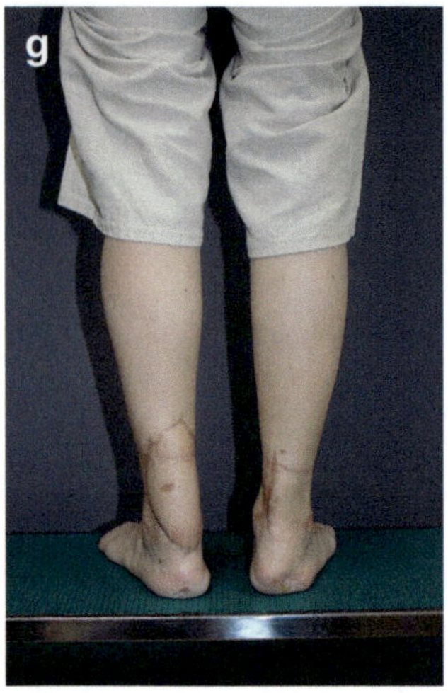

Fig. 9.13 (continued)

the left heel (Fig. 9.13e). In both reconstructions, anterior tibial artery was used as it was the only patent artery available. At 3 years after reconstruction the patient shows good function and contour of both sides (Fig. 9.13f, g).

9.9 Postoperative Care

Monitoring during the postoperative period should not only be focused on the flap but on the overall systemic condition of the patient as diabetic patients may have increased morbidity. It is especially important to monitor hemodynamic and blood sugar level. Input and output of fluid should be monitored closely as distal perfusion is primarily affected by hypotensive episodes. Patients who have chronic renal failures and require the assistance of dialysis often remove large volumes which can make fluid maintenance difficult. Limiting the range of motion may be needed for flaps covering the joints as extension or flexion may increase the tension of the pedicle. Monitoring flaps, especially free flaps in the first 24 h is essential due to the majority of thrombosis occurring at this time. According to Chen et al., up to 85% of the compromised flaps can be salvaged when the first sign of vascular compromise is clinically noted during the first 3 days after microsurgery [83]. There is no ideal method of flap monitoring but recent techniques such as tissue oxygen measurement, implantable Doppler device, laser Doppler flowmetry, Duplex ultrasound and fluorescent dye injections may assist the judgment made from clinical evaluation which remains as the golden standard of monitoring. One thing that the surgeons should keep in mind is the possibility of re-occlusion of the artery proximal to the anastomosis, as re-occlusion after angioplasty can be as high as 60% in 6 months. Emergency angiogram can help to actually pin point the location of the obstruction and determine whether angioplasty may be needed. Emergent reexploration should be performed once pedicle compromise is noted.

Although there are no clinical reviews that conclusively show any agents that increase flap survival rate, about 96% among surveyed 106 microsurgeons use some form of prophylactic antithrombotic treatment such as heparin, dextran, and aspirin or in combinations with other agents [84–86]. The routine use of dextran should be carefully approached due to allergic reaction and pulmonary edema, but aspirin, heparin, or low molecular weight heparin can be considered on theoretical basis and related studies from different disciplines. Thrombolytics such as urokinase can be used when flow is not immediately re-established after pedicle rearrangement or revision anastomosis [86]. But no agent can replace the meticulous surgical technique and early diagnosis of flap compromise.

Leeches have a role in the postoperative care for jeopardized flap. In cases of venous congestion, by injecting a salivary component called hirudin which inhibits platelet aggregation and coagulation cascade, leeches can decongest by extracting blood directly and further by oozing after it detaches. The use of leeches for 5–7 days can sometimes help salvage the flap that does not resolve despite reexploration of the venous flow.

Compression of the flap after the flap is taken and stabilized may help to reduce edema and allow the patient to engage in early ambulation [87]. If the patient underwent angioplasty, then compression needs to wait until the flap is fully incorporated with the surrounding skin. If the patient has stable vascular flow, then early compression can be performed on day 4 or 5 with about 30–40 mmHg using compression bandages. The bandages are maintained for 6 months until swelling is no longer seen during weight bearing. If the reconstruction was performed on the plantar aspect, the patient is asked to maintain the compression for longer duration and especially during the gait.

After discharge, constant education on how the patient monitors the flap is essential. Measuring the temperature of the flap as well as visual inspection can be critical in detecting early complications as the patient frequently will have peripheral neuropathy.

9.10 Conclusion

Plastic surgeons are an important component in any multidisciplinary approach for the treatment of diabetic foot wounds. When technically feasible, the trend of management has shifted from major amputation to limb salvage [88]. Using free flaps with an elevator approach can be a critical component in salvaging the limb with diabetic foot.

References

1. Steed DL, Attinger C, Colaizzi T, Crossland M, Franz M, Harkless L, et al. Guidelines for the treatment of diabetic ulcers. Wound Repair Regen. 2006;14(6):680–92.
2. Endara M, Masden D, Goldstein J, Gondek S, Steinberg J, Attinger C. The role of chronic and perioperative glucose management in high-risk surgical closures: a case for tighter glycemic control. Plast Reconstr Surg. 2013;132(4):996–1004.
3. Hong JP, Oh TS. An algorithm for limb salvage for diabetic foot ulcers. Clin Plast Surg. 2012;39(3):341–52.
4. Goldenberg S, Alex M, Joshi RA, Blumenthal HT. Nonatheromatous peripheral vascular disease of the lower extremity in diabetes mellitus. Diabetes. 1959;8(4):261–73.
5. Barner HB, Kaiser GC, Willman VL. Blood flow in the diabetic leg. Circulation. 1971;43(3):391–4.
6. Conrad MC. Large and small artery occlusion in diabetics and nondiabetics with severe vascular disease. Circulation. 1967;36(1):83–91.
7. LoGerfo FW, Coffman JD. Current concepts. Vascular and microvascular disease of the foot in diabetes. Implications for foot care. N Engl J Med. 1984;311(25):1615–9.
8. Strandness DE Jr, Priest RE, Gibbons GE. Combined clinical and pathologic study of diabetic and nondiabetic peripheral arterial disease. Diabetes. 1964;13:366–72.
9. Colen LB, Reus WF, Kalus R. Posterior hindfoot reconstruction. J Reconstr Microsurg. 1990;6(2):143–9.
10. Colen LB. Limb salvage in the patient with severe peripheral vascular disease: the role of microsurgical free-tissue transfer. Plast Reconstr Surg. 1987;79(3):389–95.
11. Dabb RW, Davis RM. Latissimus dorsi free flaps in the elderly: an alternative to below-knee amputation. Plast Reconstr Surg. 1984;73(4):633–40.
12. Godina M. Early microsurgical reconstruction of complex trauma of the extremities. Plast Reconstr Surg. 1986;78(3):285–92.
13. Irons GB, Wood MB, Schmitt EH. Experience with one hundred consecutive free flaps. Ann Plast Surg. 1987;18(1):17–23.
14. Khouri RK, Shaw WW. Reconstruction of the lower extremity with microvascular free flaps: a 10-year experience with 304 consecutive cases. J Trauma. 1989;29(8):1086–94.
15. May JW, Halls MJ, Simon SR. Free microvascular muscle flaps with skin graft reconstruction of extensive defects of the foot: a clinical and gait analysis study. Plast Reconstr Surg. 1985;75(5):627–41.
16. Oishi SN, Levin LS, Pederson WC. Microsurgical management of extremity wounds in diabetics with peripheral vascular disease. Plast Reconstr Surg. 1993;92(3):485–92.
17. Searles JM, Colen LB. Foot reconstruction in diabetes mellitus and peripheral vascular insufficiency. Clin Plast Surg. 1991;18(3):467–83.
18. Shenaq SM, Dinh TA. Foot salvage in arteriolosclerotic and diabetic patients by free flaps after vascular bypass: report of two cases. Microsurgery. 1989;10(4):310–4.
19. Ducic I, Attinger CE. Foot and ankle reconstruction: pedicled muscle flaps versus free flaps and the role of diabetes. Plast Reconstr Surg. 2011;128(1):173–80.
20. Hong JP. Reconstruction of the diabetic foot using the anterolateral thigh perforator flap. Plast Reconstr Surg. 2006;117(5):1599–608.
21. Oh TS, Lee HS, Hong JP. Diabetic foot reconstruction using free flaps increases 5-year-survival rate. J Plast Reconstr Aesthet Surg. 2013;66(2):243–50.
22. Suh HS, Oh TS, Hong JP. Innovations in diabetic foot reconstruction using supermicrosurgery. Diabetes Metab Res Rev. 2016;32(Suppl 1):275–80.
23. Suh HS, Oh TS, Lee HS, Lee SH, Cho YP, Park JR, et al. A new approach for reconstruction of diabetic foot wounds using the Angiosome and Supermicrosurgery concept. Plast Reconstr Surg. 2016;138(4):702e–9e.
24. Fitzgerald O'Connor EJ, Vesely M, Holt PJ, Jones KG, Thompson MM, Hinchliffe RJ. A systematic review of free tissue transfer in the manage-

ment of non-traumatic lower extremity wounds in patients with diabetes. Eur J Vasc endovasc Surg. 2011;41(3):391–9.
25. Moulik PK, Mtonga R, Gill GV. Amputation and mortality in new-onset diabetic foot ulcers stratified by etiology. Diabetes Care. 2003;26(2):491–4.
26. Reiber GE. The epidemiology of diabetic foot problems. Diabet Med. 1996;13(Suppl 1):S6–11.
27. Knox KR, Datiashvili RO, Granick MS. Surgical wound bed preparation of chronic and acute wounds. Clin Plast Surg. 2007;34(4):633–41.
28. Gottlieb LJ, Krieger LM. From the reconstructive ladder to the reconstructive elevator. Plast Reconstr Surg. 1994;93(7):1503–4.
29. Azoury SC, Stranix JT, Kovach SJ, Levin LS. Principles of orthoplastic surgery for lower extremity reconstruction: why is this important? J Reconstr Microsurg. 2019;37(1):42–50.
30. Hong JP. Reconstructive surgery: lower extremity coverage. In: Neligan P, editor. Plastic surgery. 4th ed. London: Elsevier; 2018. p. 127–50.
31. Attinger CE, Bulan EJ. Debridement. The key initial first step in wound healing. Foot Ankle Clin. 2001;6(4):627–60.
32. Reiber GE, Vileikyte L, Boyko EJ, del Aguila M, Smith DG, Lavery LA, et al. Causal pathways for incident lower-extremity ulcers in patients with diabetes from two settings. Diabetes Care. 1999;22(1):157–62.
33. Badia JM, Torres JM, Tur C, Sitges-Serra A. Saline wound irrigation reduces the postoperative infection rate in guinea pigs. J Surg Res. 1996;63(2):457–9.
34. Granick M, Boykin J, Gamelli R, Schultz G, Tenenhaus M. Toward a common language: surgical wound bed preparation and debridement. Wound Repair Regen. 2006;14(Suppl 1):S1–10.
35. Granick MS, Posnett J, Jacoby M, Noruthun S, Ganchi PA, Datiashvili RO. Efficacy and cost-effectiveness of a high-powered parallel waterjet for wound debridement. Wound Repair Regen. 2006;14(4):394–7.
36. Clemens MW, Attinger CE. Angiosomes and wound care in the diabetic foot. Foot Ankle Clin. 2010;15(3):439–64.
37. Attinger C, Cooper P, Blume P, Bulan E. The safest surgical incisions and amputations applying the angiosome principles and using the Doppler to assess the arterial-arterial connections of the foot and ankle. Foot Ankle Clin. 2001;6(4):745–99.
38. Christensen KS, Klarke M. Transcutaneous oxygen measurement in peripheral occlusive disease. An indicator of wound healing in leg amputation. J Bone Joint Surg Br. 1986;68(3):423–6.
39. Got I. [Transcutaneous oxygen pressure (TcPO2): advantages and limitations]. Diabetes Metab 1998;24(4):379–84.
40. Du Clos TW. Function of C-reactive protein. Ann Med. 2000;32(4):274–8.
41. Goss DE, de Trafford J, Roberts VC, Flynn MD, Edmonds ME, Watkins PJ. Raised ankle/brachial pressure index in insulin-treated diabetic patients. Diabet Med. 1989;6(7):576–8.
42. Cho MJ, Kwon JG, Pak CJ, Suh HP, Hong JP. The role of duplex ultrasound in microsurgical reconstruction: review and technical considerations. J Reconstr Microsurg. 2020;36(7):514–21.
43. Romiti M, Albers M, Brochado-Neto FC, Durazzo AE, Pereira CA, De Luccia N. Meta-analysis of infrapopliteal angioplasty for chronic critical limb ischemia. J Vasc Surg. 2008;47(5):975–81.
44. Saqib NU, Domenick N, Cho JS, Marone L, Leers S, Makaroun MS, et al. Predictors and outcomes of restenosis following tibial artery endovascular interventions for critical limb ischemia. J Vasc Surg. 2013;57(3):692–9.
45. Yue DK, McLennan S, Marsh M, Mai YW, Spaliviero J, Delbridge L, et al. Effects of experimental diabetes, uremia, and malnutrition on wound healing. Diabetes. 1987;36(3):295–9.
46. Berman SJ. Infections in patients with end-stage renal disease. An overview. Infect Dis Clin N Am. 2001;15(3):709–20, vii.
47. Hong JP. The use of supermicrosurgery in lower extremity reconstruction: the next step in evolution. Plast Reconstr Surg. 2009;123(1):230–5.
48. Randon C, Jacobs B, De Ryck F, Van Landuyt K, Vermassen F. A 15-year experience with combined vascular reconstruction and free flap transfer for limb-salvage. Eur J Vasc Endovasc Surg. 2009;38(3):338–45.
49. Bush HL Jr, Nabseth DC, Curl GR, O'Hara ET, Johnson WC, Vollman RW. In situ saphenous vein bypass grafts for limb salvage. A current fad or a viable alternative to reversed vein bypass grafts? Am J Surg. 1985;149(4):477–80.
50. Suh HP, Kim Y, Suh Y, Hong J. Multidetector computed tomography (CT) analysis of 168 cases in diabetic patients with Total superficial femoral artery occlusion: is it safe to use an anterolateral thigh flap without CT angiography in diabetic patients? J Reconstr Microsurg. 2018;34(1):65–70.
51. Shestak KC, Hendricks DL, Webster MW. Indirect revascularization of the lower extremity by means of microvascular free-muscle flap—a preliminary report. J Vasc Surg. 1990;12(5):581–5.
52. Chang N, Mathes SJ. Comparison of the effect of bacterial inoculation in musculocutaneous and random-pattern flaps. Plast Reconstr Surg. 1982;70(1):1–10.
53. Ecker ML, Jacobs BS. Lower extremity amputation in diabetic patients. Diabetes. 1970;19(3):189–95.
54. Goldner MG. The fate of the second leg in the diabetic amputee. Diabetes. 1960;9:100–3.
55. Kucan JO, Robson MC. Diabetic foot infections: fate of the contralateral foot. Plast Reconstr Surg. 1986;77(3):439–41.
56. Abdelfattah U, Power HA, Song S, Min K, Suh HP, Hong JP. Algorithm for free perforator flap selection in lower extremity reconstruction based on 563 cases. Plast Reconstr Surg. 2019;144(5):1202–13.
57. Adedeji R, Oragui E, Khan W, Maruthainar N. The importance of correct patient positioning in theatres

and implications of mal-positioning. J Perioper Pract. 2010;20(4):143–7.
58. Winfree CJ, Kline DG. Intraoperative positioning nerve injuries. Surg Neurol. 2005;63(1):5–18. discussion
59. Jeong HH, Hong JP, Suh HS. Thin elevation: a technique for achieving thin perforator flaps. Arch Plast Surg. 2018;45(4):304–13.
60. Goh TL, Park SW, Cho JY, Choi JW, Hong JP. The search for the ideal thin skin flap: superficial circumflex iliac artery perforator flap—a review of 210 cases. Plast Reconstr Surg. 2015;135(2):592–601.
61. Altiparmak M, Cha HG, Hong JP, Suh HP. Superficial circumflex iliac artery perforator flap as a workhorse flap: systematic review and meta-analysis. J Reconstr Microsurg. 2020;36(8):600–5.
62. Kim HB, Altiparmak M, Pak CJ, Suh HP, Hong JP. Reconstruction using free flaps for diabetic heel defects: outcomes and risk factor analysis. J Reconstr Microsurg. 2020;36(7):494–500.
63. McGregor IA, Jackson IT. The groin flap. Br J Plast Surg. 1972;25(1):3–16.
64. Daniel RK, Taylor GI. Distant transfer of an island flap by microvascular anastomoses. A clinical technique. Plast Reconstr Surg. 1973;52(2):111–7.
65. Koshima I, Nanba Y, Tsutsui T, Takahashi Y, Urushibara K, Inagawa K, et al. Superficial circumflex iliac artery perforator flap for reconstruction of limb defects. Plast Reconstr Surg. 2004;113(1):233–40.
66. Hsu WM, Chao WN, Yang C, Fang CL, Huang KF, Lin YS, et al. Evolution of the free groin flap: the superficial circumflex iliac artery perforator flap. Plast Reconstr Surg. 2007;119(5):1491–8.
67. Wei FC, Mardini S. Free-style free flaps. Plast Reconstr Surg. 2004;114(4):910–6.
68. Hong JP, Koshima I. Using perforators as recipient vessels (supermicrosurgery) for free flap reconstruction of the knee region. Ann Plast Surg. 2010;64(3):291–3.
69. Choi DH, Goh T, Cho JY, Hong JP. Thin superficial circumflex iliac artery perforator flap and supermicrosurgery technique for face reconstruction. J Craniofac Surg. 2014;25(6):2130–3.
70. Hong JP, Sun SH, Ben-Nakhi M. Modified superficial circumflex iliac artery perforator flap and supermicrosurgery technique for lower extremity reconstruction: a new approach for moderate-sized defects. Ann Plast Surg. 2013;71(4):380–3.
71. Suh YC, Hong JP, Suh HP. Elevation technique for medial branch based superficial circumflex iliac artery perforator flap. Handchir Mikrochir Plast Chir. 2018;50(4):256–8.
72. Hong JPJ, Goh TLH, Choi DH, Kim JJ, Suh HS. The efficacy of perforator flaps in the treatment of chronic osteomyelitis. Plast Reconstr Surg. 2017;140(1):179–88.
73. Suh HS, Jeong HH, Choi DH, Hong JP. Study of the medial superficial perforator of the superficial circumflex iliac artery perforator flap using computed tomographic angiography and surgical anatomy in 142 patients. Plast Reconstr Surg. 2017;139(3):738–48.
74. Fuse Y, Yoshimatsu H, Yamamoto T. Lateral approach to the deep branch of the superficial circumflex iliac artery for harvesting a SCIP flap. Microsurgery. 2018;38(5):589–90.
75. Yoshimatsu H, Iida T, Yamamoto T, Hayashi A. Superficial circumflex iliac artery-based iliac bone flap transfer for reconstruction of bony defects. J Reconstr Microsurg. 2018;34(9):719–28.
76. Yoshimatsu H, Steinbacher J, Meng S, Hamscha UM, Weninger WJ, Tinhofer IE, et al. Superficial circumflex iliac artery perforator flap: an anatomical study of the correlation of the superficial and the deep branches of the artery and evaluation of perfusion from the deep branch to the Sartorius muscle and the iliac bone. Plast Reconstr Surg. 2019;143(2):589–602.
77. Baek SM. Two new cutaneous free flaps: the medial and lateral thigh flaps. Plast Reconstr Surg. 1983;71(3):354–65.
78. Song YG, Chen GZ, Song YL. The free thigh flap: a new free flap concept based on the septocutaneous artery. Br J Plast Surg. 1984;37(2):149–59.
79. Wei FC, Jain V, Celik N, Chen HC, Chuang DC, Lin CH. Have we found an ideal soft-tissue flap? An experience with 672 anterolateral thigh flaps. Plast Reconstr Surg. 2002;109(7):2219–26. discussion 27-30
80. Hong JP, Chung IW. The superficial fascia as a new plane of elevation for anterolateral thigh flaps. Ann Plast Surg. 2013;70(2):192–5.
81. Kehrer A, Sachanadani NS, da Silva NPB, Lonic D, Heidekrueger P, Taeger CD, et al. Step-by-step guide to ultrasound-based design of alt flaps by the microsurgeon—basic and advanced applications and device settings. J Plast Reconstr Aesthet Surg. 2020;73(6):1081–90.
82. Kim EK, Kang BS, Hong JP. The distribution of the perforators in the anterolateral thigh and the utility of multidetector row computed tomography angiography in preoperative planning. Ann Plast Surg. 2010;65(2):155–60.
83. Chen KT, Mardini S, Chuang DC, Lin CH, Cheng MH, Lin YT, et al. Timing of presentation of the first signs of vascular compromise dictates the salvage outcome of free flap transfers. Plast Reconstr Surg. 2007;120(1):187–95.
84. Ashjian P, Chen CM, Pusic A, Disa JJ, Cordeiro PG, Mehrara BJ. The effect of postoperative anticoagulation on microvascular thrombosis. Ann Plast Surg. 2007;59(1):36–9. discussion 9–40
85. Glicksman A, Ferder M, Casale P, Posner J, Kim R, Strauch B. 1457 years of microsurgical experience. Plast Reconstr Surg. 1997;100(2):355–63.
86. Hanasono MM, Butler CE. Prevention and treatment of thrombosis in microvascular surgery. J Reconstr Microsurg. 2008;24(5):305–14.
87. Suh HP, Jeong HH, Hong JPJ. Is early compression therapy after perforator flap safe and reliable? J Reconstr Microsurg. 2019;35(5):354–61.
88. Wraight PR, Lawrence SM, Campbell DA, Colman PG. Creation of a multidisciplinary, evidence based, clinical guideline for the assessment, investigation and management of acute diabetes related foot complications. Diabet Med. 2005;22(2):127–36.

10 BKA with TMR Are Changing the Options in Limb Salvage

Christopher Attinger and Grant Kleiber

10.1 Introduction

When considering salvaging a limb, it is critical to assess the type of function the reconstructed limb is capable of providing. One has to accurately assess the realistic activities that the patient is physically capable of. This then determines which options best meet those goals: the planned reconstructed limb versus an amputation. The function achieved with below knee amputations have improved dramatically with the application of myodesis, vascularized fibular graft, targeted muscle reinnervation (TMR) and the use of ever more sophisticated prosthesis. Because of this, salvaging a limb just to salvage the limb is no longer an acceptable goal. The surgeon's goal is to give patients a *functional* limb that meets their realistic physical goals, whether it be a reconstructed or amputated limb. The younger and/or more athletic patients, the more they will demand of their reconstructed leg. As such, the reconstructed limb may not be able to meet their desired goal and the decision to undergo an amputation may more appropriate. However, the older the patient, the less he/she may demand of the reconstructed leg. As a result, a less than perfectly functional leg may be sufficient to carry on acts of daily living and avoids the necessity of relying on a prosthesis.

We will initially cover the decision-making for amputation versus salvage. We will then cover the basics of doing a below knee amputation focusing on myodesis, ERTL, and TMR.

10.2 Preoperative Preparation

The decision to potentially perform an amputation occurs because of inadequate available soft tissue or bone for the reconstruction of a functional limb, inability to restore appropriate arterial blood flow or overwhelming infection. To assess the leg for possible reconstruction, one has to accomplish three things: ensure sufficient blood flow to heal, eradicate any residual infection, and have a functional result in mind that fits the patient's needs.

When facing a diabetic or radiated patient, it is often hard to assess blood flow. One had to keep the angiosome concept in mind at all times to be sure that the area in question is adequately perfused [1]. ABIs are unreliable in diabetics and renal failure patients because of calcified vessels. The most reliable is an angiogram with magnified views of the foot. This also allows the

C. Attinger (✉)
Department of Plastic and Orthopedic Surgery, Medstar Georgetown University Hospital, Washington, DC, USA
e-mail: Christopher.attinger@medstar.net

G. Kleiber
Department of Plastic Surgery, Medstar Georgetown University Hospital, Washington, DC, USA

J. P. Hong, H. Suh (eds.), *Diabetic Foot Reconstruction*,
https://doi.org/10.1007/978-981-16-9816-3_10

surgeon to visualize the rate of flow in each artery. This can be done with very little dye (<10 cc of dye), especially in patients with kidney function at risk. One has to be able to assess the contributions of each of the three arteries to the foot and the arterial-arterial connections between those arteries [2]

It is critical to have a good vascular team to rely on. One needs access to physician(s) who excel in angioplasty, bypass surgery, and venous surgery. Going over the angiogram with the respective vascular interventionist is critical so that he or she understands exactly what type of blood flow is needed for the reconstructive surgery to be successful. This is especially true if microsurgery is one of the possible reconstructive options [3]. Angioplasties tend to have a shorter half-life (30% occlusion rate at 3 months) when compared to that of a bypass and that has to be kept in mind during the reconstruction. The optimal flow to the downstream foot (as measured by TcO2) with bypass surgery occurs at 5–8 days post bypass versus as long as 30 days post angioplasty. The microsurgical anastomosis to a major artery should *always* be end to side so as not to sacrifice distal flow [4]. The exception is when plugging the flap pedicle into a small perforator where end to end is preferable. When doing microsurgery, the venous flow also has to be assessed to make sure that the venous return from the flap travels via the venous system (superficial or deep) that has the least amount of resistance [5].

Dealing with infection can be difficult because diagnosis is affected by the way the specimen is collected, by how the laboratory handles it, by the presence of biofilm and interpretation of the PCR data. In addition, one has to consider the host. The more medically compromised the host, the more vulnerable the host is to residual infection. We recommend removing all exposed tissue after painting the wound with blue dye to accurately demarcate the wound surface [6]. By excisionally debriding to normal red, yellow, and white tissue, one can be certain that one has removed all the surface bacteria. The more extensive the excisional debridement, the more likely one is to also remove any burrowing biofilm that can be as deep as 4 mm under the wound surface. The resection of any indurated tissue at the edges of the wound down to soft normal tissue removes all potentially infected tissue and is more likely to remove residual biofilm. The amount of indurated soft tissue that needs to be resected is always surprisingly thin and may only require 2–4 mm thick cuts. It is critical to obtain pre-debridement and post-debridement tissue cultures (versus culture swabs) to assess the quality of the debridement. Once the post-debridement results are available, the surgeon can then make the decision as to whether to close or not [7]. Working closely with infectious disease for the initial broad-spectrum antibiotics and subsequent narrowing of the antibiotic coverage is critical to minimizing the potential toxicity of the antibiotics on the patient. If bone infection has been resected and the post-debridement bone cultures are negative, one only needs antibiotics for 1 week as per both the IDSA [8] and ISID guidelines.

Finally, one has to decide on the type of reconstruction that will be used. Keep in mind that if an ulcer heals in a diabetic foot, the chances of ulcer recurrence at 2 years can be as high as 80% [9]. The result therefore has to be a functionally sound foot in order to minimize the risk of recidivism. If it is deemed by the surgeon that the function of the salvaged limb will not meet the physical capacity and expectations of the patient, then amputation has to be considered. It can either be a foot amputation or a below knee amputation. It is important to fully discuss those options with the family and the patient. Having a peer amputee and the prosthetist and orthotist talk to the patient about the consequences of shorter foot amputations versus below knee amputation is very productive The patient and the family can then make an intelligent decision as to which to choose.

10.3 Below the Knee Amputation

10.3.1 Preoperative Preparation

The amputations with the longest 5 year survival at our center include toe amputation, trans-metatarsal amputations and below knee amputations [10]. All other amputations (ray, Lisfranc, Chopart or Syme amputation) lead to higher recidivism and lower 5-year survival due to decreased function. There is no significant difference 5 year survival difference between the below knee amputation and the TMA. Since we recently added TMR to the BKA, the ambulatory rate has risen to 91% at 3 month and the 1 year survival rate was 95% (average non-traumatic BKA had a 35% mortality at 1 year) [11]. These results add to the ever-growing data that regular physical activity is the key determinant to increasing survival [12].

The level of the amputation is dependent on the available, viable soft tissue and bone after debridement of the foot and ankle or drainage amputation. If the leg is ischemic, review of the angiogram is helpful to better assess what angiosomes are well perfused. Even if the popliteal or superficial femoral artery is occluded, the collateral flow can be adequate to heal a below knee operation. The demarcation line between cold and warm tissue usually coincides with the level of ischemic pain. Only using tissue above the lines demarcating pain and temperature has proved to be remarkably accurate in determining amputation levels with only a 2% BKA to AKA conversion rate [13]. It also important that the patient meet with a prosthetist preoperatively so that the patient fully understands what is about to occur. The prosthetist also provides invaluable feedback to the surgeon so that the ideal residual limb can be designed. If possible, it is also very helpful for them to meet with another amputee who has gone through what the patient is about to experience. This pre-amputation consultation is invaluable not only in allaying the fears of the patient but to have a positive outlook and thus ensure the most functional outcome.

Preoperative and perioperative medical management is as important as surgical technique. Diabetes, end-stage renal disease, coronary artery disease, coagulopathy, and chronic anemia are associated with increased surgical complications and should be managed aggressively. Patients with ESRD should dialyzed the day before the amputation. Beta-blockers should be taken the morning of surgery, and perioperative antibiotics should cover the initial infection and re-dosed as needed. Glucose should be kept under 200 during the perioperative period [14].

The level of anesthesia may vary based on the planned procedure. Regional blocks, with sedation, are preferred so that the block can be continued during the first 4–5 days postoperatively. In our recent experience, regional nerve blocks and selected targeted motor nerve reinnervation have been very successful in controlling postoperative pain and minimizing phantom pain.

Amputations performed in the setting of infection should be done in two stages. Two-stage below knee amputation for ischemic and infectious causes have been shown to have significant decreased reoperation rates [15]. It give 24–48 h for the lymphatic system to clear residual bacteria and it limits possible cross-contamination that can occur when done in a single stage. It also gives time to obtain definite culture and sensitivities. When there is lymphedema in the leg, removing the infection will decrease the swelling. In addition, a lymphedema wrap applied by physical therapy to the residual limb post drainage amputation works remarkably well to get rid of the edema and make the residual tissue more pliable for the definitive amputation. If only the foot is involved, the initial drainage amputation should be an ankle disarticulation to minimize bone bleeding. If the ankle is involved, a guillotine amputation is planned above the level of infection. The completion amputation is then performed at least 2–3 days afterward.

10.4 Below Knee Amputation

10.4.1 Technique

Bickel popularized the use of the posterior myocutaneous flap (PMF) in 1943. Burgess later modified it by recommending that the deep posterior compartment be removed to limit unnecessary bulk in the posterior flap and limit the amount of tissue dependent on presumably diseased posterior tibial and peroneal arteries [16]. Interestingly, in popliteal or trifurcation disease, the sural arteries that feed the gastrocnemius muscles are usually spared and provide the necessary blood flow to the superficial posterior flap. This is reflected in our series of 294 flaps where the ratio of BKA to AKA was 4–1 with a 2% eventual conversion rate from BKA to AKA. Our institution uses a posterior myocutaneous flap (PMF) in which the superficial posterior compartment provides vascularized and durable coverage of the tibial/fibular osteotomies. Tenodesis and myodesis of the superficial posterior compartment serve several functions. Gastrocnemius muscles continue to function as a knee flexor and thus maintain soft tissue bulk and prevent muscle atrophy. A second benefit of the PMF is preventing a suture line and future scar over the distal mid-stump. A final benefit is that the musculature with their insertion restored by the myodesis still functions as a venous pump to help prevent lower leg edema.

The componentry below the socket in the average below knee prosthesis requires at least 8 inches of clearance from the ground. This leaves plenty of amputation length to allow increased leverage of a longer moment arm, increased surface area to disseminate pressure from the interaction of soft tissue with the socket, and it provides additional tissue for an adequate revision BKA should it ever be required. After consulting with the prosthetist, each BKA is planned with a tibial osteotomy at 12–18 cm from tibial tubercle if there is adequate distal soft tissue (Fig. 10.1a). Add 4 cm to the measurement (16–22 cm) if one picks the knee joint line to measure from. Waterproof stockinet and Coban is used to

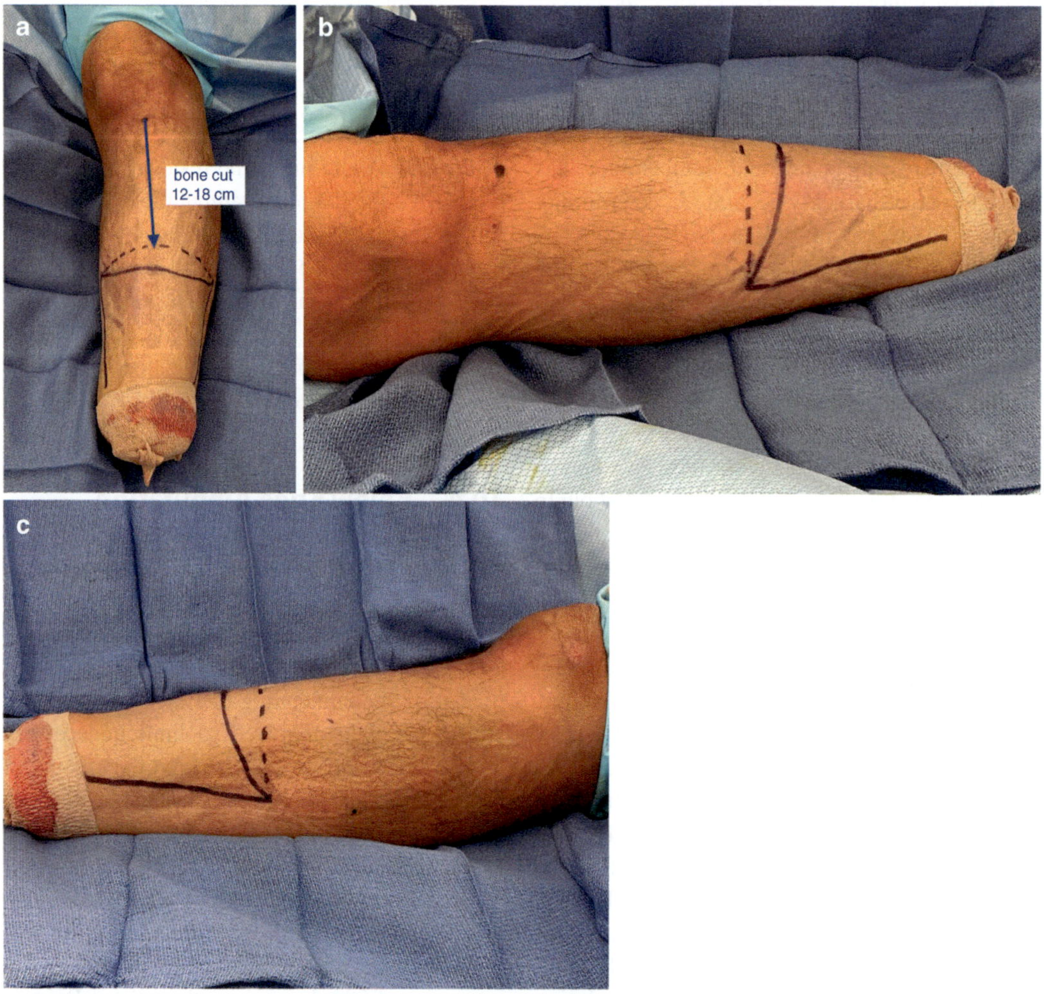

Fig. 10.1 (**a**) The length of the amputation is measured from the tibial tubercle to the planned bone cut. It should be anywhere between 12 and 18 cm in length. If measuring from the knee joint line, add 4 cm. The actual skin incision line is drawn 2–4 cm. distal to the bone cut line so that the incision does not lie on the bone cut. (**b**, **c**) The medial margin (**b**) stops just below the posterior aspect of the tibia. The lateral margin (**c**) goes just above the fascia separating the posterior from the lateral compartment. Both lines slope up distally to maintain width of distal flap

isolate the distal drainage wound or foot and prevent contamination of the field and proximal clean tissue. A proximal tourniquet is placed on the thigh for the nerve portion of the surgery.

An anterior skin line is drawn at the planned tibial osteotomy site encompassing approximately 2/3 the circumference of the leg (Fig. 10.1a). The medial limit is just below the posterior tibia, and the lateral limit is above the fascia separating the lateral from the posterior compartment. This gives a slightly skewed posterior flap with the medial side being more anterior than the lateral side. The anterior skin incision line is then drawn so that it starts at the same point medially and laterally but extends 2–4 cm distal to the planned tibial bone cut line (Fig. 10.1a). This ensures that the suture line does not fall at the level of the osteotomy site.

Medially and laterally, the skin incision is carried distally with a slight anterior slant toward the ankle to maintain the same flap width as the leg narrows (Fig. 10.1b, c). The skin cuts are through fascia taking great care to ligate or clip the saphenous vein and small arteries and veins (Fig. 10.2a). The saphenous nerve is identified and preserved. The superficial peroneal nerve lies just deep to the superficial fascia and just lateral to the fascia separating the anterior from the lateral compart-

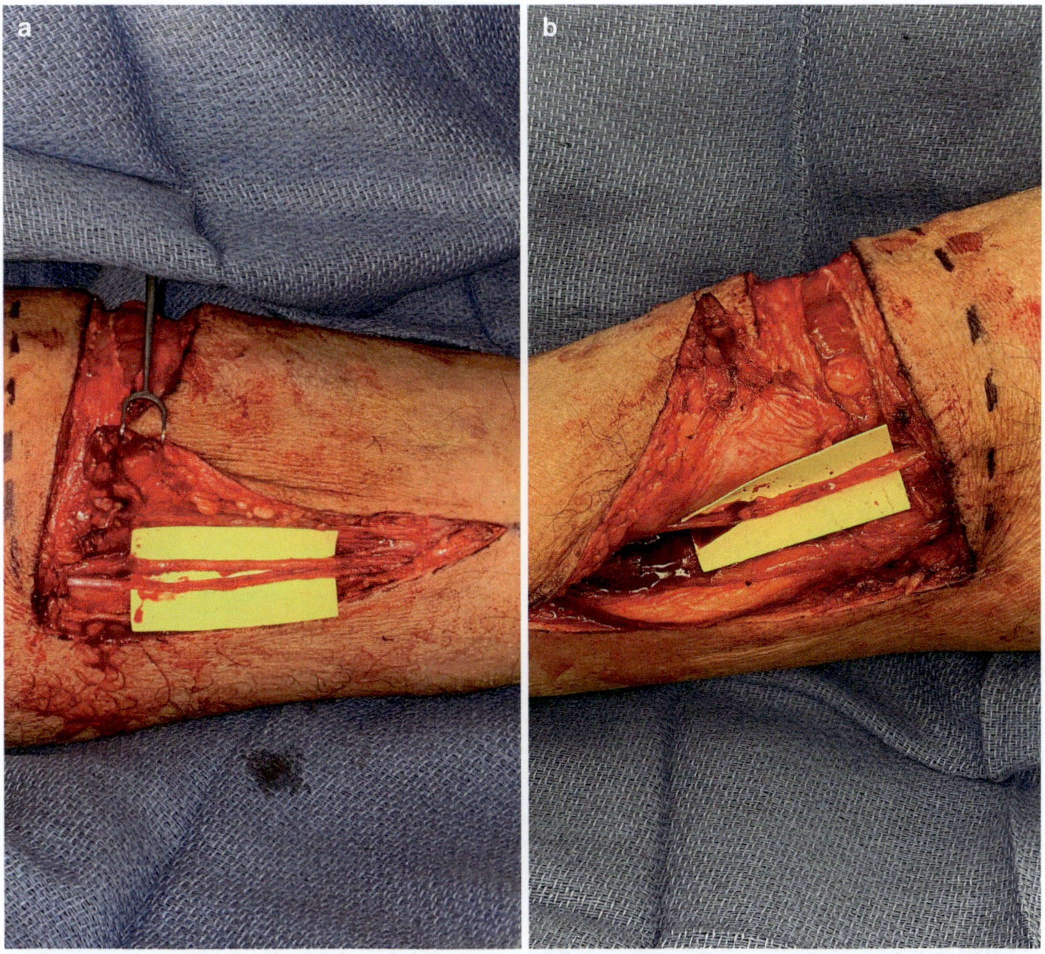

Fig. 10.2 (**a**) The medial incision is made above the saphenous vein, and the saphenous nerve are preserved. In this picture, 2 branches of the saphenous nerve lie just below the saphenous vein. (**b**) The superficial peroneal nerve is just lateral to the septum dividing the anterior from the lateral compartment. It is dissected out to its full length to the planned distal cut of the posterior flap

ment (Fig. 10.2b). It should be dissected out carefully along its distal length when the incision is made along the lateral compartment and should be identified and preserved. Special attention is paid to preserve the distal lateral compartment peroneus longus and brevis muscles that will be used for myodesis later. The anterior muscle compartment is then cut using electric cautery at just distal to the planned tibial bone cut (Fig. 10.3a). The anterior tibial artery and vein are identified and suture ligated. The deep peroneal nerve is isolated and cut as long as possible (Fig. 10.3b).

The tibia is exposed and the planned osteotomy is verified at pre-planned bone cut distance. An army-navy retractor is passed posterior to the tibia and the osteotomy is made perpendicular to the longitudinal axis of the tibia. The fibular osteotomy is approximately 1.5 cm shorter with a bevel slightly oriented from lateral to medial (Fig. 10.4a–c).

After both osteotomies, a bone hook into the open end of distal tibia provides anterior retraction to expose the deep posterior compartment. A 10 blade is used to sharply dissect the lateral and deep posterior compartment muscles off the distal tibia and fibula (Fig. 10.5a, b). The distal leg is then amputated at a distance that guarantees sufficient posterior flap length to fold anteriorly to close the amputation

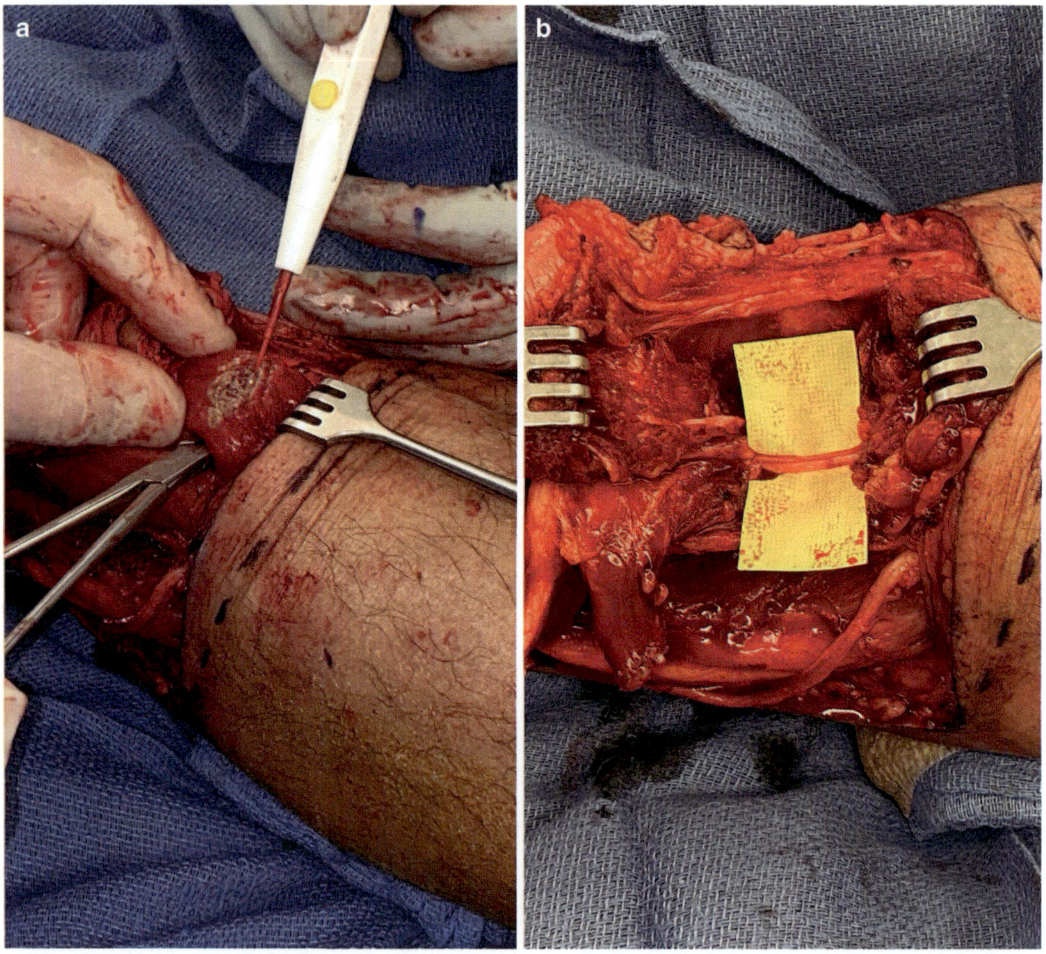

Fig. 10.3 (**a**) The anterior tibial muscles are cut at the level of the planned tibial bone cut. (**b**) the anterior tibial artery and vein are cut, and the deep peroneal nerve is preserved

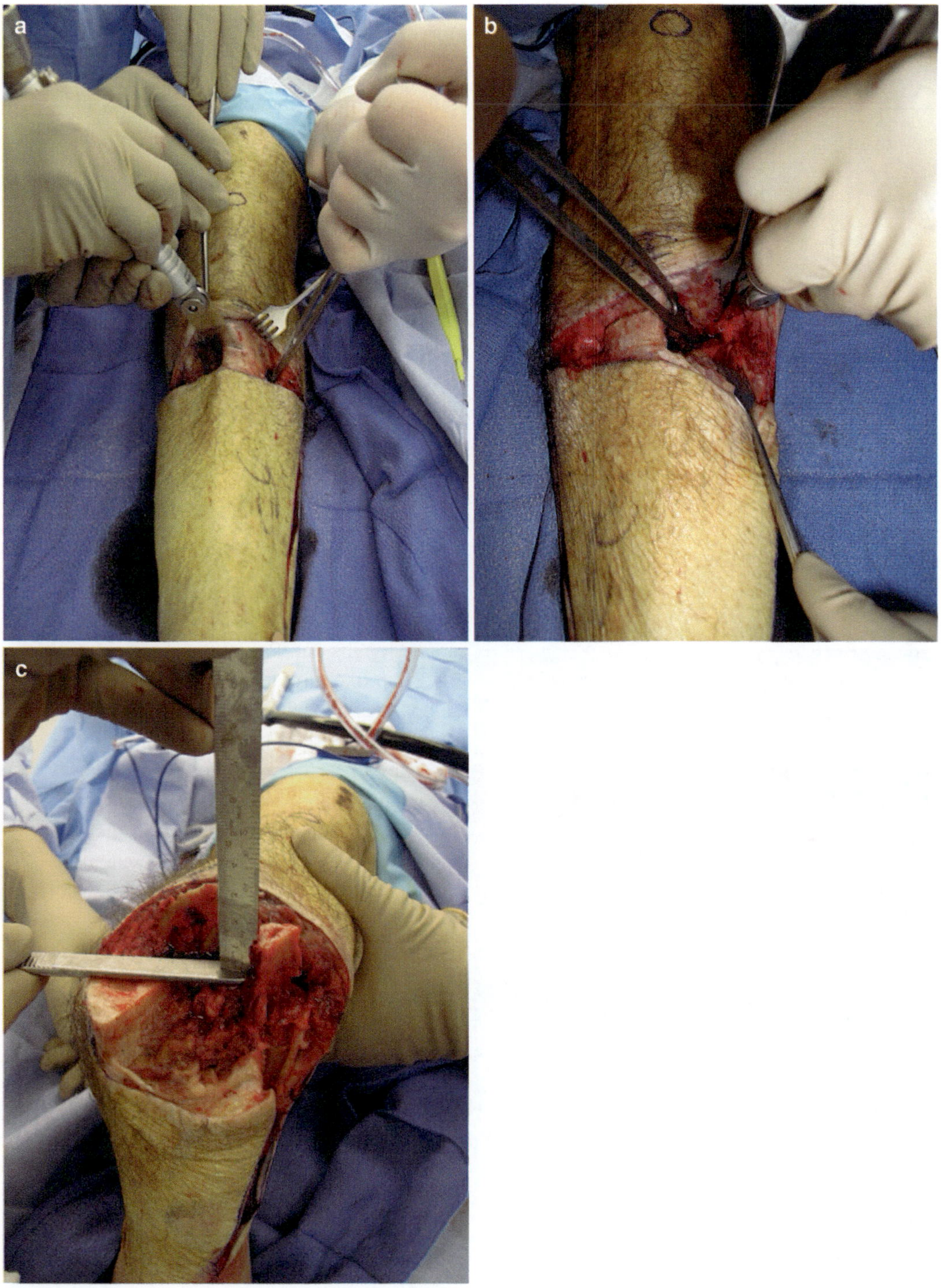

Fig. 10.4 (**a**) Osteotomy of tibia. (**b**, **c**) The fibular cut is 1–1.5 cm shorter than the tibia and is done carefully not to damage the peroneal artery and nerves

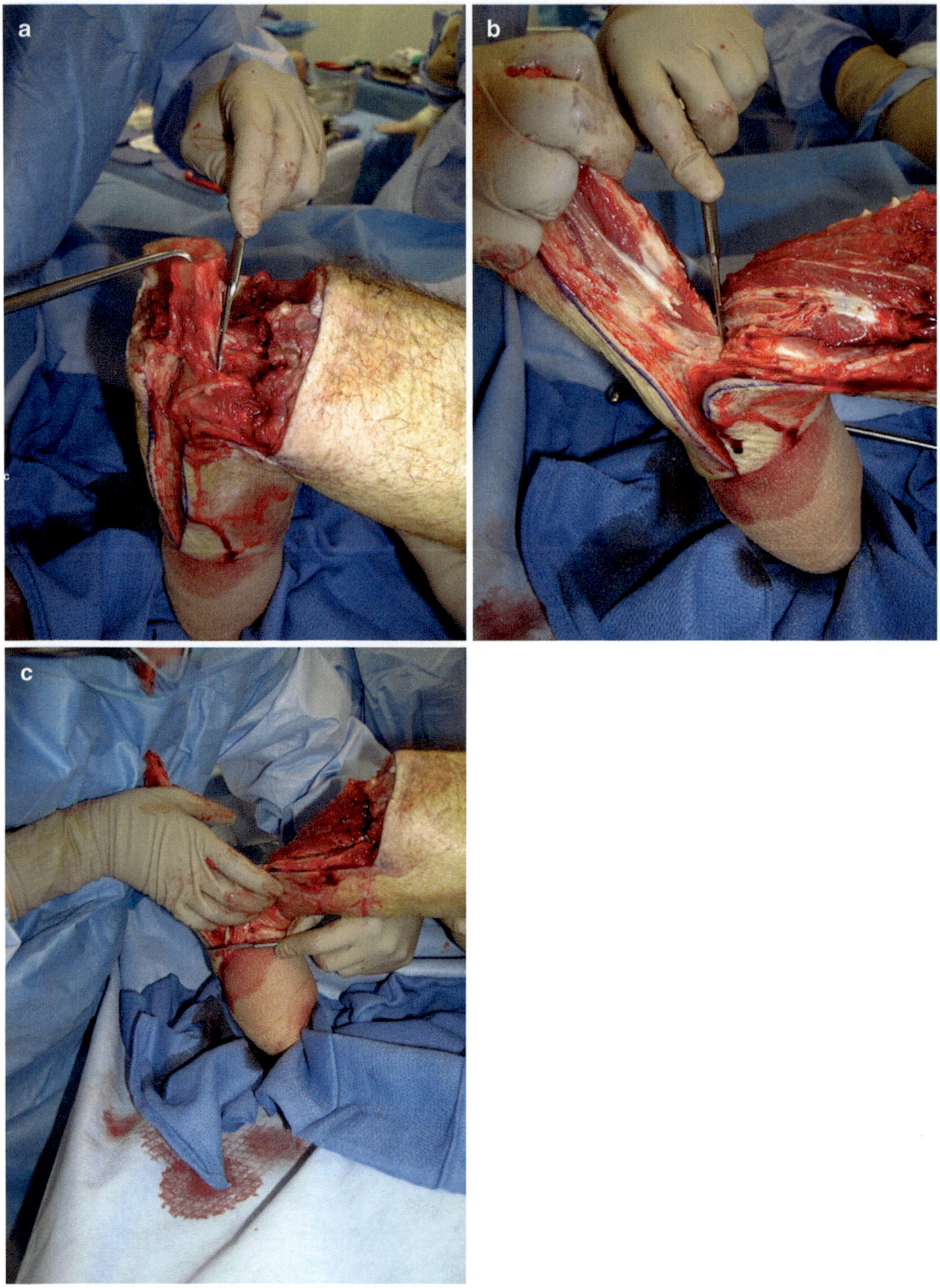

Fig. 10.5 (**a**, **b**) The posterior flap tissue is dissected off of the tibia and fibula taking great care to preserve the peroneal muscles. (**c**) The leg is cut off at a level where the flap is long enough to easily reach the anterior portion of the tibia for closure

(Fig. 10.5c). After discarding the distal leg, the deep posterior compartment is dissected off of the superficial compartment (Fig. 10.6a, b) and removed with careful ligation of the peroneal and posterior tibial perforators to the superficial posterior department. Then post tibial nerve is dissected out and preserved (Fig. 10.6c). The deep posterior compartment muscles are left a centimeter longer than the tibia for future myodesis to the tibia. The posterior tibial and peroneal arteries are tied off and the posterior tibial nerve is preserved. All four nerves (saphenous nerve, deep peroneal nerve, posterior tibial nerve, and superficial tibial nerve) are carefully preserved for future TMR or traction neurectomy (Fig. 10.7).

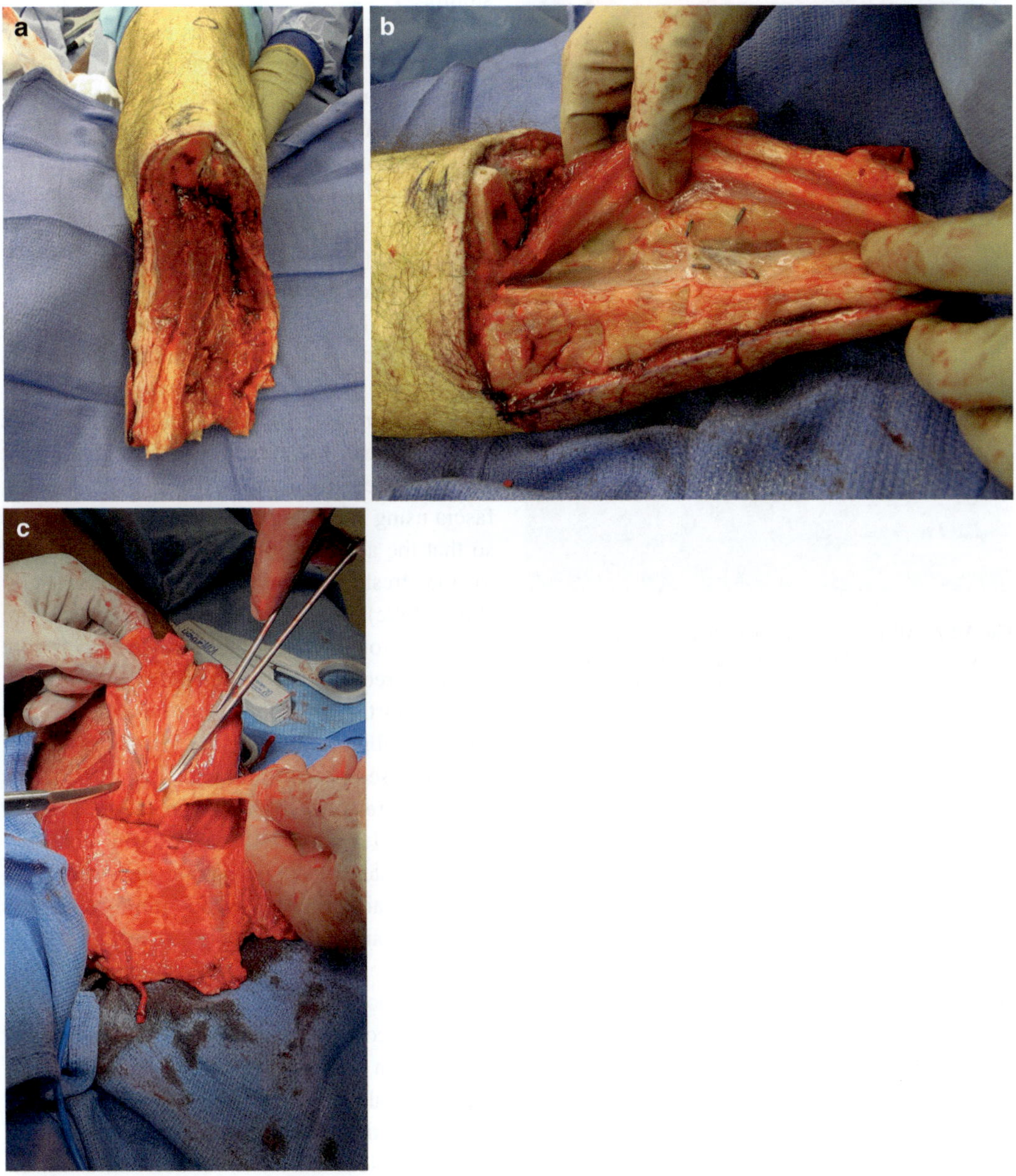

Fig. 10.6 (**a–c**) The deep posterior compartment is then removed off of the posterior compartment fascia taking care to ligate all perforators

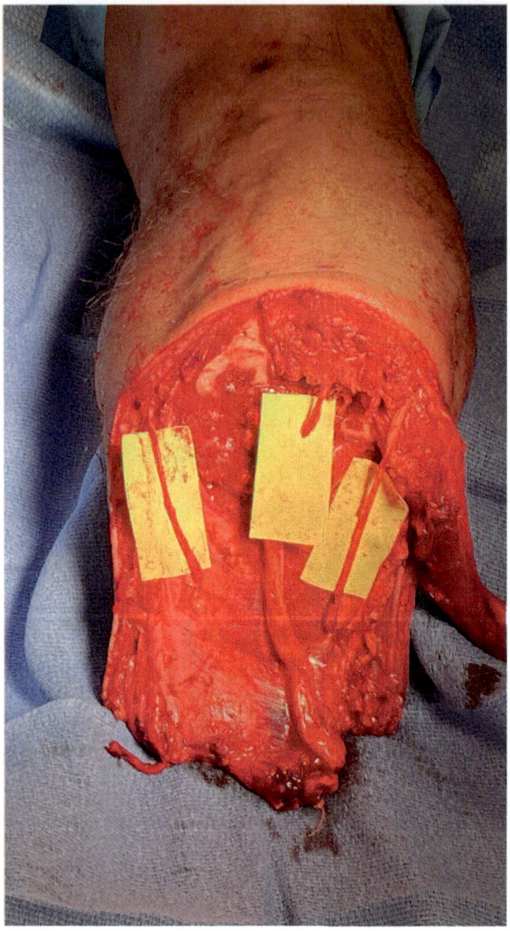

Fig. 10.7 All four nerves (saphenous n., deep peroneal nerve, posterior tibial nerve and superficial peroneal nerve) are carefully preserved for future TMR or traction neurectomy

The peroneal muscles are then freed up from the attachments to superficial posterior compartment muscle fascia all the way up to the cut fibula. Minor pedicles from the peroneal muscles are tied off.

The anterior half of the tibial cortex is then beveled for about 1 cm using a sagittal saw (Fig. 10.8a, b) taking great care to keep the thickness of the remaining cortex at least equal to that of the rest of the tibia. The bevel is then sanded down by brushing the sagittal saw over that area. Three holes are drilled into the medial anterior tibia (left 10, 11 and 12 o'clock and right 2, 1, 12 o'clock) through the anterior cortex toward the center of the medullary canal and will be used for future tenodesis of the soleus and gastrocnemius muscles (Fig. 10.8c). A hole is drilled in the lateral tibial (right 9 o'clock, left 3 o'clock and both at 6 o'clock) to tenodese the peroneal and deep posterior muscles, respectively. Irrigation is performed to get rid of bone dust. New gloves and sterile drapes are placed while a clean table and set of instrumentation are used to avoid any possible contamination with the removed distal stump.

At this point, all the nerves can be addressed with either TMR or traction neurectomy. See nerve section in the final section of this chapter for the technique of TMR.

The peroneus muscles (Fig. 10.9a) are then rotated medially and cut at the level of the lateral tibial border and sewn into the lateral tibial predrilled hole (Fig. 10.9b) using a 0 monofilament. If the muscles are too bulky, the brevis is cut at the level to the fibula and only the longus is used for the myodesis. In that case, a tacking stitch is used to keep the peroneus brevis myodesed to the peroneus longus. The 0 monofilament stitch is then continued back and forth through anterior tibial muscle without incorporating the overlying fascia using a running horizontal mattress suture so that the anterior tibial muscles are myodesed to the freshly myodesed peroneal muscle(s) (Fig. 10.9c). The deep posterior muscles are tenodesed to the 6 o'clock tibial hole making sure that all three muscles are included. In addition, one can further myodese them by attaching the posterior tibial muscles to the inferior border of the tenodesed peroneal muscle (Fig. 10.9d) This maneuver restores the insertion to the anterior tibial muscles and the deep posterior compartment muscles so they maintain their ability to contract against resistance and minimize the loss of muscle bulk over time (Fig. 10.9e).

The posterior flap is then swung up to the level of the anterior portion of the tibia making sure that the soleus covers the entire tibia and a semilunar line is drawn on the soleus muscle at the level of the anterior tibial fascia to mark that level (Fig. 10.10a). One or two drains are placed along the base of the flap. The soleus muscle is then incised along the drawn line with a bovie or ten blade down to Achilles tendon with a slant proximal to distal angle

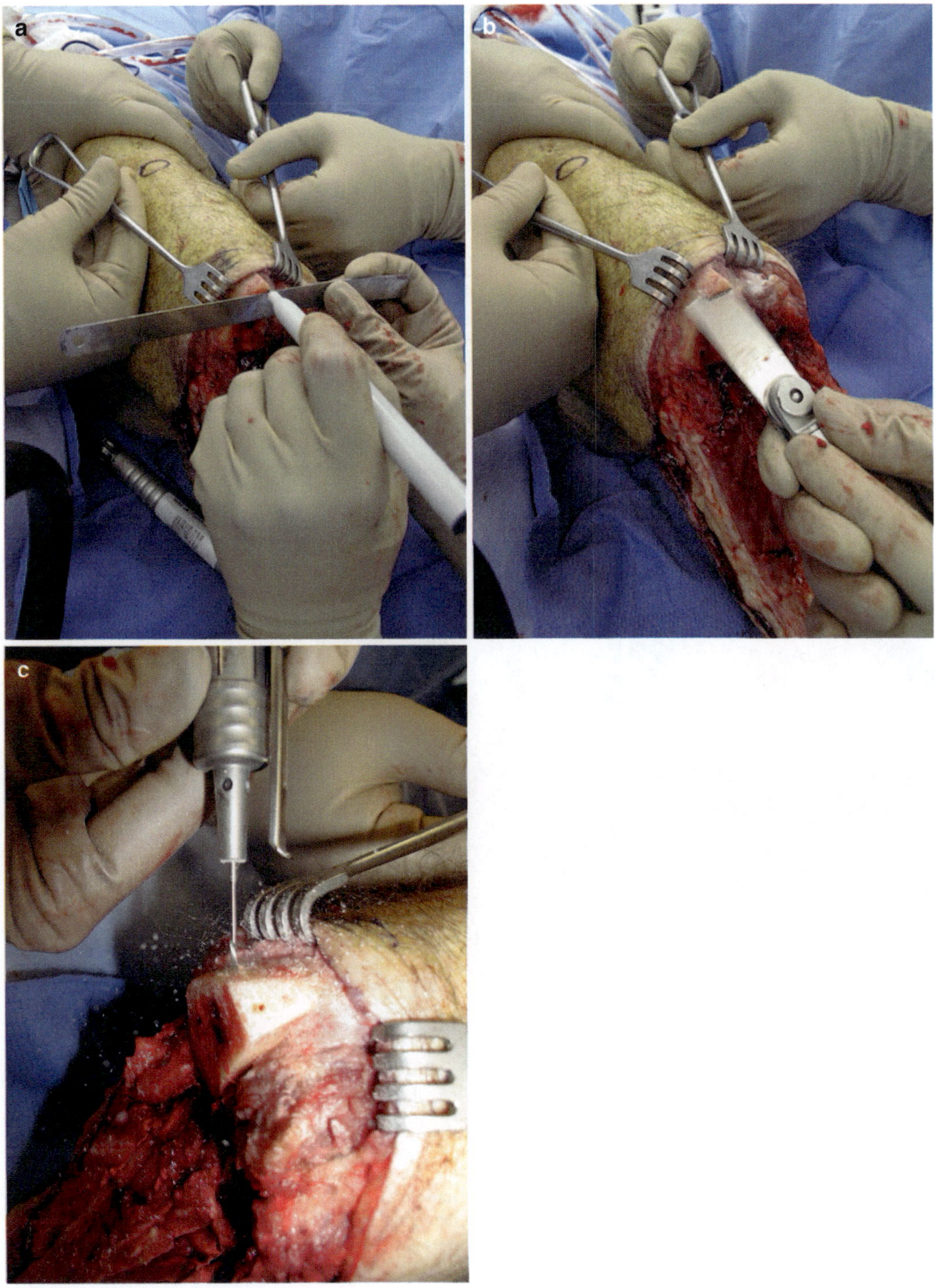

Fig. 10.8 (**a**, **b**) The anterior portion of the distal tibia is beveled and sanded down. Great care is taken to make the cut high enough to ensure that the circumferential thickness of the tibial cortex remains the same over the entire circumference. (**c**) Three holes are drilled into the medial anterior tibia (left 10, 11 and 12 o'clock and right 2, 1, 12 o'clock) through the anterior cortex toward the center of the medullary canal and will be used for future tenodesis of the soleus and gastrocnemius muscles. A hole is drilled in the lateral tibial (right 9 o'clock, left 3 o'clock and both 6 o'clock) to tenodese the peroneal and deep posterior muscles, respectively

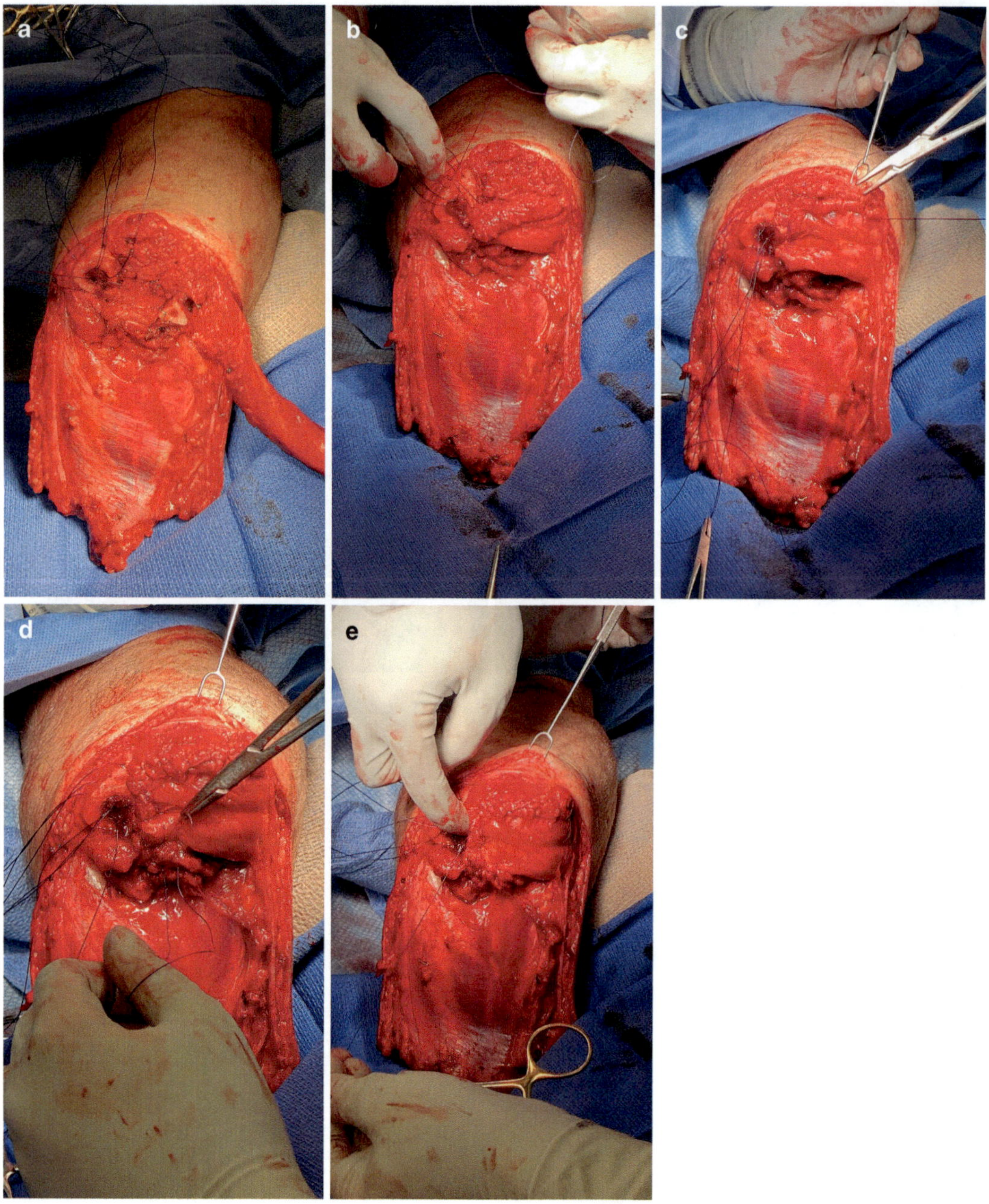

Fig. 10.9 (**a**, **b**) The peroneal muscle(s) (**a**) are rotated toward the tibia, cut along its lateral border and are then fixed to the lateral tibial cortex hole (**b**) using a 0 monofilament. (**c**) The stitch is then continued through anterior tibial muscle without incorporating the overlying fascia using a running horizontal mattress suture so that the latter are myodesed to the freshly myodesed peroneal muscle(s). (**d**, **e**) The deep posterior muscles are tenodesed to the 6 o'clock tibial hole making sure that all three muscles are included. In addition, one can attach the posterior tibial muscles to the inferior border of the tenodesed peroneal muscle

(Fig. 10.10b) so that when the posterior flap is rotated forward, the distal soleus muscle can be sewn into the anterior tibial cortex. The distal soleus muscle with the fascia-tendinous layer is then sewn into the three previously drilled holes in the tibia with 0 monofilament suture (Fig. 10.10c, d).

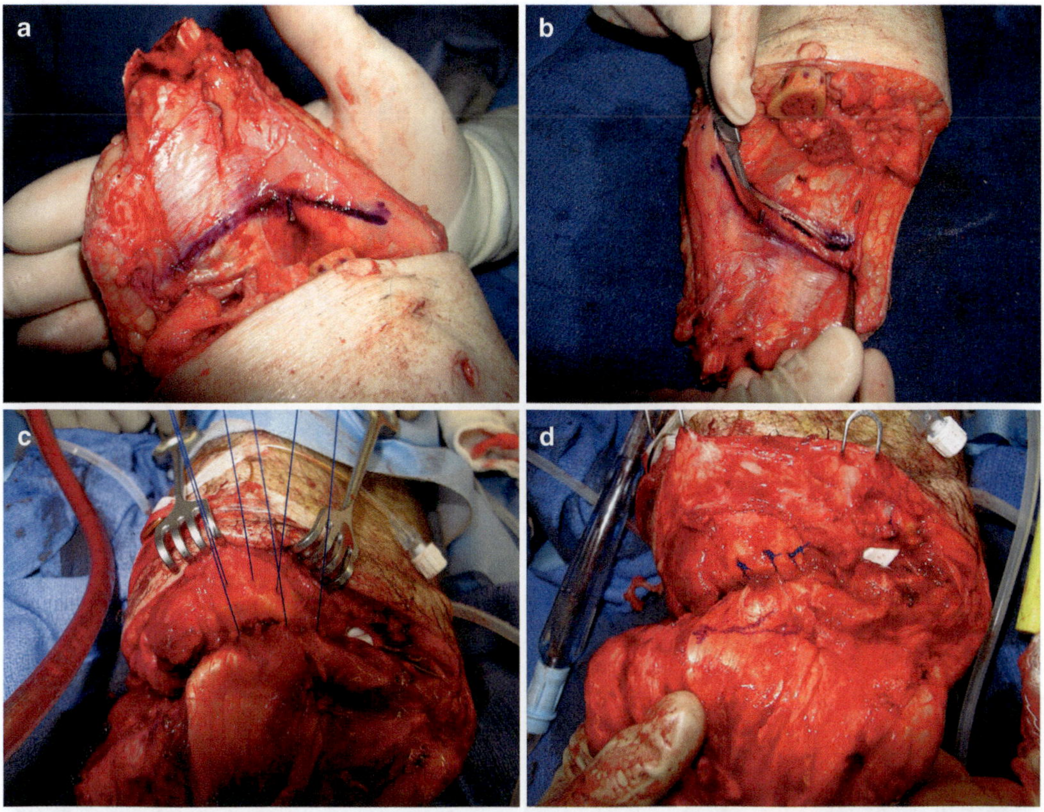

Fig. 10.10 (**a**) The posterior flap is folded up and a line is drawn at the level of the anterior fascia of the proximal leg. (**b**) The soleus distal to the line is removed either with a bovie or knife. Great care is taken to preserve the underlying Achilles tendon and fascia. (**c**, **d**) Three 0-monofilament dissolvable stitches are placed through the anterior tibial holes. They are sutured into the soleus muscle and underlying fascia. Great care is taken to make sure that the medial part of the soleus muscle covers the entire distal tibia bone with intact muscle

The skin and subcutaneous tissue are then dissected off the distal anterior tibial fascia for a width of about 2 cm (Fig. 10.11a). The Achilles tendon and posterior gastrocnemius tendinous fascia is then cut 2–3 cm distal to the distal end of the soleus tenodesis (Fig. 10.11b) and then sewn to the anterior tibial fascia with a running back and forth with 0 monofilament (Fig. 10.11c, d). The sural nerve and lesser saphenous vein are located at the distal central end of the posterior flap. The nerve is crushed 5 cm from the distal end, buried deep in its tunnel. The lesser saphenous vein is clipped. Skin is cut at a level where the wound can be closed without tension (Fig. 10.12a). Dog ears, if present at the medial and lateral edge of the closure, are removed (Fig. 10.12b) and the suture line re-contoured to create a smooth tapered end so that the leg is ready for a prosthesis as soon as the stitches are removed. The incision is closed with vertical mattress 2–0 monofilament and skin staples are used between each stitch to ensure good skin edge eversion (Fig. 10.12c). The incision line can be covered with an incisional negative pressure device to immobilize the suture line for 7–14 days (Fig. 10.12d). The wound is then dressed and the leg is placed in a knee immobilizer to protect it from falls and prevent possible knee flexion that may result in knee contracture. The skin clips are removed at 1 week and the stitches at 4 weeks (6 weeks for renal failure patients).

Evidence comparing PMF versus Skew or Sagittal flaps show no significant differences, although the level of evidence is poor. In our

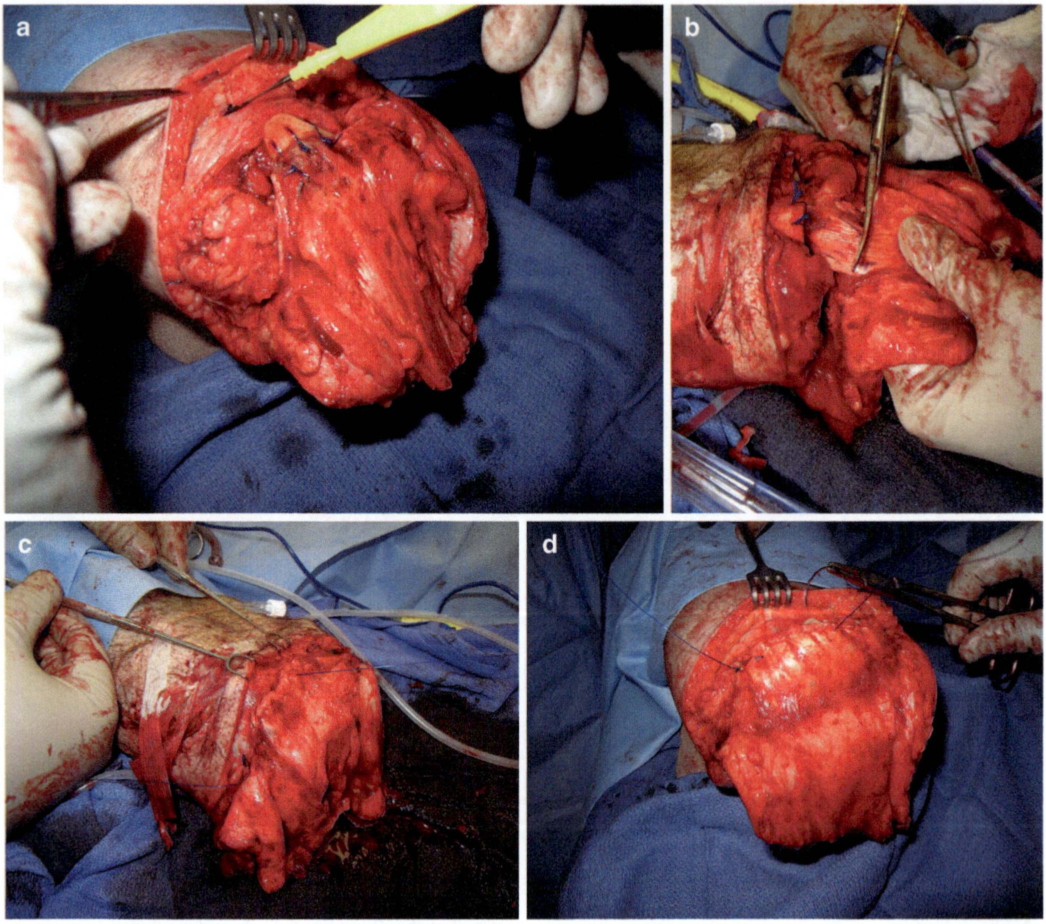

Fig. 10.11 (**a**) The distal skin and subcutaneous tissue is freed up from the underlying anterior compartment fascia for width of about 2 cm. (**b**) The Achilles tendon and posterior fascia are cut 2–3 cm distal to the tenodesed soleus muscle so they can be sewn into the anterior tibial fascia without tension. (**c, d**) The tenodesis of the Achilles tendon to the anterior tibial fascia is performed using a running zero monofilaments horizontal mattress suture in one direction and returned in the other with a running stitch

hands, however, the PMF provides sufficient vascularized soft tissue coverage over the tibial osteotomy to allow us to successfully perform below knee amputations in 80% of all patients who presented with an ischemic or a non-viable or non-functional foot. Without TMR up to 78% of those BKA's resulted ambulatory patients. With TMR, 92% are ambulatory at 3 months. In addition, only 2% of the below knee amputations had to undergo a higher level amputation [9]. This is the highest rate of BKA versus AKA in the literature, suggesting that the vascular supply to the PMF may be superior to that of other flap designs.

10.4.2 BKA Using the ERTL Technique

Alternatively, an ERTL modification to the BKA can be performed in patients who have the capacity of being physically active. The ERTL modification for below knee amputation involves placing a vascularized fibular bone graft between the distal tibia and fibula to promote distal bony fusion between the distal tibia and fibula. The distal bones with the interposed fibular graft fuse to form a solid "U" which allows better transfer of leg rotational torque to the artificial prosthetic ankle/foot [17]. It also

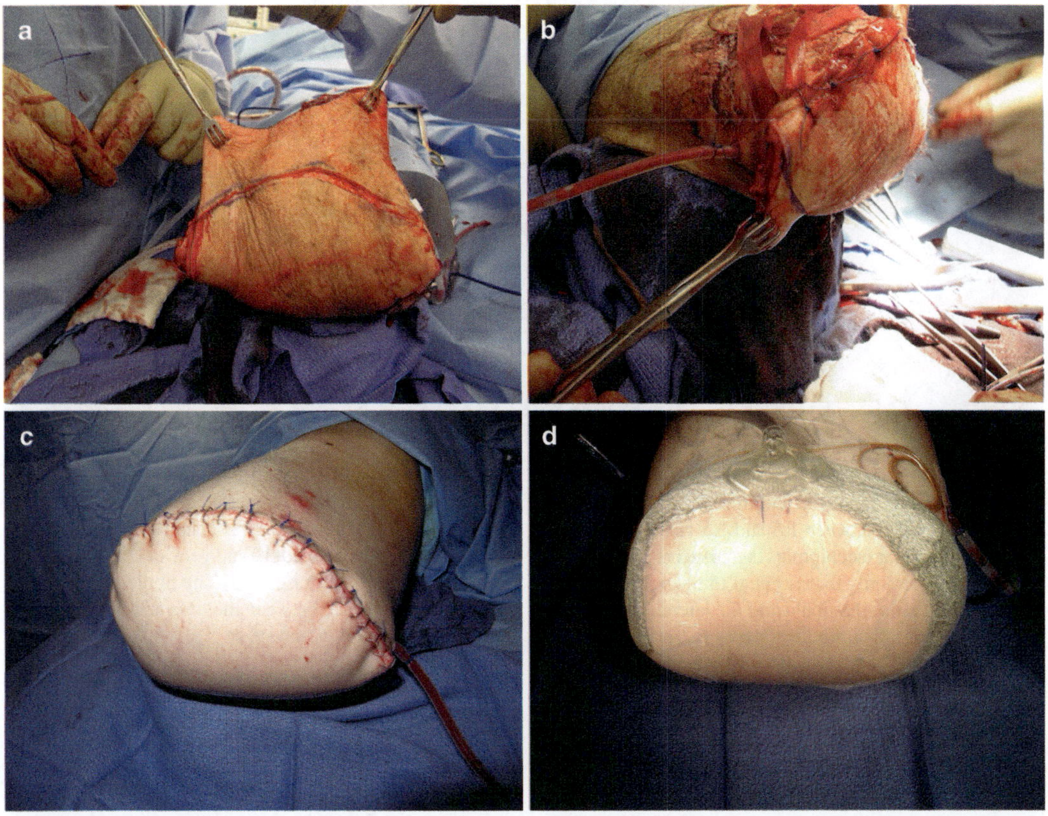

Fig. 10.12 (**a**) The skin is cut at a level where the wound can be closed without tension. (**b**) Dog ears, if present at the medial and lateral edge of the closure, are removed. (**c**) The incision is closed with vertical mattress 2–0 monofilament and skin staples are used between each stitch to ensure good skin edge eversion. (**d**) The incision line can be covered with an incisional negative pressure device to immobilize the suture line for 7–14 days

allows the distal stump to be end bearing when not wearing a prosthesis.

The initial surgical technique and markings are identical up to the planning of the fibular osteotomy. The distance between the lateral tibia and medial fibula at the planned tibial cut is measured (usually 1.5–2.5 cm) (Fig. 10.13a). The first of two fibular osteotomies is marked at a point distal to the tibial osteotomy that is equal to the width between the medial cortex of the fibula and the lateral cortex of the tibia (Fig. 10.13b). The distal fibula is then cut at that level, and the distal peroneal artery and vein are tied off at the same level. After the distal fibular osteotomy, the distal leg is removed (Fig. 10.5a–c) in the fashion described above.

The proximal fibulectomy is performed after re-confirming the fibular bone graft length is equal to the inter-osseous distance. We recommend a lateral approach to the fibular osteotomy with care when approaching the medial fibular cortex so as not to damage the peroneal artery and the thin medial and posterior cuff of muscle (Fig. 10.13c). The fibular bone graft is rotated into the space between the tibia and fibula to make sure that it fits well in that space (Fig. 10.13d).

The lateral cortex of the tibia and medial cortex of the distal fibula (Fig. 10.14a) are then burred down to aid in bony fusion and stable contact. The vascularized fibular bone graft is then interposed between the distal fibula and tibia and fixated with #20 wires after holes are drilled into both sides of the anterior part of the fibular strut graft, the medial distal fibula and lateral distal tibia (Fig. 10.14b, c). We used to use a cannulated

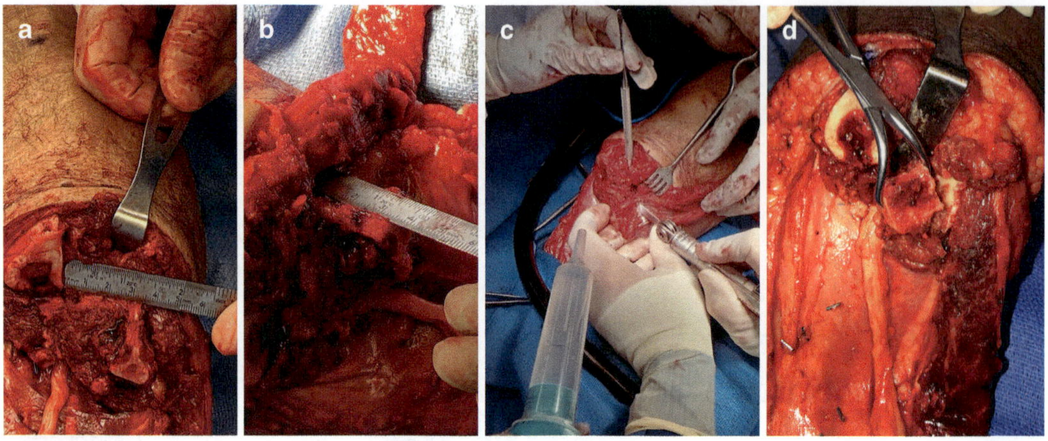

Fig. 10.13 (**a**) The distance between the lateral tibia and medial fibula determines the length of the distal cut of the fibula. It is usually between 1.5 and 2.5 cm. (**b**) The more distal of two fibular osteotomies is marked at a point distal to the tibial osteotomy that is equal to the width between the medial cortex of the fibula and the lateral cortex of the tibia. (**c**) The proximal fibulectomy is performed after reconfirming the fibular bone graft length is equal to the inter-osseous distance via a lateral approach to the fibula. The medial fibular cortex is approached carefully so as not to damage the peroneal artery and vein and the thin medial and posterior cuff of muscle. (**d**) The fibular bone graft is rotated into the space between the tibia and fibula to make sure that it fits well in that space

screw that had to be later removed in over 50% of the patients because it worked its way out over the following 5 years. We have not had such problems using wire fixation. The result (Fig. 10.14d) should lead to an excellent fusion at 2–3 months of the fibular strut with the distal fibula and tibia (Fig. 10.14e). We therefore no longer recommend using a screw. The myodesis and closure are same as described above for the normal BKA.

10.4.3 Postoperative Care

Postoperative care is a critical component in major lower extremity amputations. Pain control immediately the following surgery typically involves patient-controlled analgesia (PCA) via 5 day epidural or regional blocks. While the regional block is the best option, it often cannot used if there is anticoagulation on board. Alternatively, intra-operative use of long-lasting local anesthesia (Exparel) is strongly recommended along the five identifiable nerves.

After lower extremity amputation, there is a significant disturbance in the patient's sense of balance as their center of gravity has been altered significantly. Nursing care and physical therapy play an important role in protecting the patient as they learn to transfer. Falls after amputation can be devastating and frequently lead to reoperation. Nearly one in five amputees will require amputation revisions due to postoperative falls. Thus, it is important to protect the residual limb. A knee immobilizer is placed immediately after each below knee amputation to both protect the distal stump and to prevent knee contracture until the patient is ready for a prosthesis,

Gentle compression in the immediate postoperative period aids with the swelling but should be balanced when there is a question of possible ischemia. Compression should be avoided in patients with severe peripheral vascular disease. One can apply an incisional negative pressure device to the incision to protect it for 5–7 days postoperatively. Alternatively, the dressing is removed on day two to evaluate for signs of hematoma and ischemia. Drains should be observed and output recorded. Once the amount is less than 30 ml daily, the drain may safely be removed. Surgical staples are removed the day of discharge (5 days), and the sutures are typically removed at 4 weeks in clinic (6 weeks with renal failure patients).

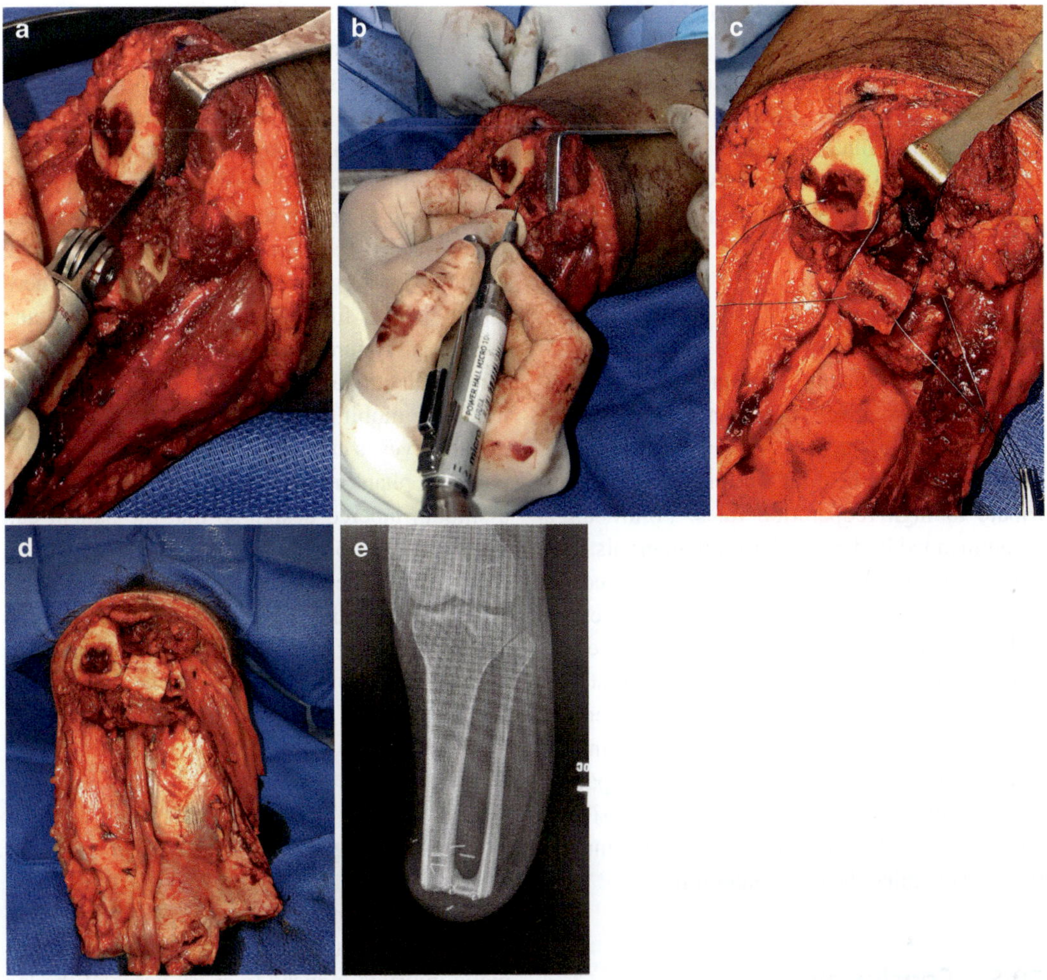

Fig. 10.14 (**a**) The lateral side of the tibia and the medial side of the fibula are sanded down using the saw to ensure a better fusion of the pedicled fibular graft. (**b**, **c**) Holes are drilled into the lateral tibia and medial fibula and the lateral and medial anterior aspect of the pedicled fibular graft for passage of the wires that will fixate the fibular graft between the tibia and fibula. (**d**) The wires are twisted until the fibular graft is solidly fixated to the tibia and fibula. (**e**) An x-ray of the fixation that occurs at 2–4 months after surgery. The wire is then cut and buried

10.4.4 Rehabilitation

The rehabilitation process begins immediately in the hospital. We typically keep each patient 4–5 days for inpatient pain control and evaluation by physical therapy. Physical therapy assesses each patient's strength and ability to transfer safely. Physical therapy determines the amount of assistance needed and recommends acute, sub-acute, or home-based rehabilitation. Our strong preference is an acute rehabilitation facility and it is important to have a center that is familiar with and trained in caring for amputees. The medical complexity and need for frequent follow up underscore the importance of open communication and a multidisciplinary approach.

The prosthetist now becomes the most important component in caring for amputees after the incision has healed. Once the sutures have been removed, the fitting of the prosthesis may begin. Patients should be educated on the care of the residual limb, compression devices, and the progression from initial prosthetic fitting to final prosthesis. After removal of the stitches, we advocate for fitting and ambulation as soon as it is safe for the patient. This prevents further deconditioning and promotes their return to normal functional status. Rehabilitation is recommended immediately after receiving the prosthesis to aid in teaching how to best use the prosthesis and how preventing injuries from falls.

10.4.5 Follow-Up

Reoperation following amputation is unfortunate, but it is relatively common occurring in up to 30% of amputations. Trauma, dehiscence, infection, wound healing, and ischemia all contribute to high reoperation rates. Follow-up is recommended in the 2 and 4 week intervals. At 2 weeks, the residual limb can be examined for signs of infection, dehiscence, or progressive ischemia. The 4-week visit typically involves the removal of sutures and arrangement of prosthetic fitting. If the postoperative course is uneventful, we aim to have each patient ambulating at 6–12 weeks. We then follow up with the patient 3 weeks after he has started using his prosthesis and then every 6 months to reassess the amputation and examine the contralateral foot.

10.5 Conclusion

The important lesson is to keep function in mind when making the decision to salvage or amputate a limb. Assuming biomechanical principles are followed, forefoot amputation, including toes, can yield good function. With trans-metatarsal amputation, it is critical to address possible equino-varus deformities. Shorter foot amputations (Lisfranc, Chopart amputations) all require significant AFO (assistant foot orthotic) devices in order to ambulate. These amputations also have to be performed functionally to keep recidivism low. For the less active patients, these shorter foot amputations provide an excellent solution and allow the patients to perform daily acts of living and stay independent. For the active patients, reliance on AFO devices may be too restrictive to allow them to do everything that they may want to do.

If the resulting function of the salvaged foot does not or will not meet the patient's physical needs, then a major amputation should be performed. It has to be done with the same amount of care and attention to detail and function that would have been carried out for limb salvage because the surgeon is actually creating a new, albeit shorter, limb. Focusing on myodesis and tenodesis ensures that the residual muscles remain functional and that the residual limb does not loose mobility and strength. Attention to the distal nerves is critical to minimize postoperative pain and phantom pain. The closure should have a smooth tapered design so that the patient can start wearing prosthesis as soon as the stitches are removed and the prosthesis is ready. Our duty as reconstructive surgeons is to give the patient the best possible leg (reconstructed or amputated) to return to as active a lifestyle as he or she may desire.

10.6 Nerve Stabilization in Amputation Surgery

With respect to peripheral nerves, an amputation is a massive neural injury. A complete neurotmetic injury is induced to every nerve of the leg at the amputation level. Often times, these nerves are ignored and left to form neuromas at the level of the weight-bearing amputation stump. An amputation stump neuroma can be severely disabling even in a relatively small sensory nerve such as the saphenous or superficial peroneal nerves, leading to phantom pain and severe residual limb pain. Patients with amputation stump neuromas often complain of pain when wearing their prosthesis, and this can substantially degrade their functional ambulation. The importance of functional ambulation in amputees cannot be overstressed, since non-ambulatory amputees can quickly become deconditioned, and non-ambulatory status is associated with a significantly greater mortality risk [18, 19]. In many ways, the philosophical view of amputation as failed limb salvage perpetuates this failure further downstream, leading to failure to provide a functionally ambulatory stump. Amputation must instead be seen as a form of limb salvage, the goal of which is to provide the patient with a well-padded and pain-free stump-prosthetic interface to allow for functional ambulation.

10.7 Pathogenesis of Neuroma Formation

After a nerve transection injury, there is axonal sprouting from the proximal stump. This is initially a disorganized proliferation of axons until continuity is established across the neural gap. This axonal continuity induces a pruning process through which the extraneous axons are removed, and the continuous axons continue distal growth into the downstream neural architecture. If the proliferating axons cannot establish continuity across the neural gap, or if there is no downstream nerve, the disorganized axonal proliferation continues until it is encased in fibrotic tissue and forms a terminal neuroma [20]. This is the case in amputation neuromas, as there is no downstream neural target for axonal growth. When stimulated, neuromas lead to neuropathic pain in the affected neural distribution. In amputees, this is often described as burning, electrical, or shooting pain to specific territories of the phantom leg or foot. When these terminal neuromas form at the weight-bearing stump, they are stimulated by stump-prosthetic interactions from walking or standing.

10.8 Incidence and Distribution of Amputation Stump Neuromas

Five nerves are cut in a below knee amputation: the tibial, superficial peroneal, deep peroneal, saphenous, and sural nerves. In more proximal below knee amputations the medial and lateral sural communicating nerves may be running individually. Any of these nerves has the potential to form a terminal neuroma at the amputation stump. In our experience with secondary neuroma management, the superficial peroneal nerve accounts for symptomatic neuroma formation in 76% of patients presenting with secondary amputation stump neuromas, with the saphenous affected in 64% of patients. The tibial nerve, while infrequently involved in neuroma formation, was frequently implicated as a source of plantar phantom pain [21, 22]. Upon review of the original amputation of patients presenting with secondary stump neuromas, the offending nerve was not identified in the operative report in 74% of cases, and failure to recognize a nerve at the time of amputation was associated with a significantly higher risk of stump neuroma formation in that specific nerve [23]. Whichever neuroma prevention technique a surgeon chooses to apply, recognizing the nerves at the time of amputation is the most important step in preventing stump neuroma formation.

10.9 Methods for Management and Prevention of Neuromas

Multiple methods exist for management of existing neuromas, but the gold standard after diagnosis of a terminal neuroma is excision of the neuroma. However, after the neuroma is excised back to healthy nerve, the process of axonal sprouting, which initially caused the neuroma begins again. For this reason, neuroma excision is almost always combined with some form of neuroma prevention technique. The most commonly practiced of these techniques is implanting the nerve end into muscle. This was initially thought to lead to reinnervation of the motor endplates by the implanted nerve axons. However, it is now well understood that innervated muscle will not accept new innervation. The success of this technique is likely due to relocating the nerve into a well-cushioned space with an ideal microenvironment, where the resulting terminal neuroma is less likely to be symptomatic. While this technique often results in improvement in symptomatic neuroma pain, the results are rather modest with incomplete resolution of pain [24, 25]. Other methods for neuroma prevention include an implanted device to cap the nerve end, centro-central coaptation, a dead-end nerve allograft, end-to-side nerve transfer, regenerative peripheral nerve interface, and targeted muscle reinnervation [26]. In centrocentral coaptation, the nerve is longitudinally neurolysed into two fascicular groups, which are then coapted end-to-end distally. Often a conduit or nerve graft is interposed between the coaptation. The goal of this procedure is to establish a nerve gap with axons on both sides, providing neurotrophic factors to guide axonal growth and induce [27]. This technique has been useful for pre-emptive management of the sciatic nerve at the time of amputation [28].

10.10 Regenerative Peripheral Nerve Interface

Regenerative peripheral nerve interface (RPNI) was initially described as a method for enhanced myoelectric prosthetic control. The technique involves wrapping a free muscle graft around the terminal end of the nerve, which heals as a graft [29]. The muscle is completely separated from its neurovascular supply to ensure total denervation and wrapped over the terminal nerve as a thin graft. This allows for signal amplification and superficialization, which can be transduced by an implanted or surface electrode for prosthetic control [30–33]. This technique has since been expanded to secondary management of terminal neuromas of the upper and lower extremity [34, 35], and for treatment of post-amputation pain [36, 37]. Recently RPNI has been advocated for prophylactic prevention of amputation stump neuromas at the time of primary amputation [38]. As a technique for nerve stabilization at the time of amputation, RPNI has several advantages. There is an abundance of muscle graft to be harvested from the discarded portion of the amputated limb, leaving no donor site morbidity to the patient. The technique is technically simple and does not require specialized equipment or magnification, and can be performed quickly and efficiently by any surgeon who can identify the terminal nerve ends. Additionally, RPNI provides superior fascicular coverage of the distal nerve end relative to any other technique, and is particularly helpful for management of large nerves, which would have an unacceptable size match for nerve transfer. There are disadvantages to this technique that must also be discussed. The muscle grafts used for RPNI are usually completely separated from their vascular supply, and must survive by imbibition until neovascularization occurs, either from the nerve end or the surrounding tissue. The method by which free muscle grafts survive and heal is not well understood, since muscle has a very low tolerance for ischemia due to its high metabolic activity. There are no other accepted indications for free muscle grafts.

10.11 Targeted Muscle Reinnervation

Targeted muscle reinnervation (TMR) is a nerve transfer of a proximal nerve into a distal motor target nerve. Similar to RPNI, this directs the regenerating proximal axons into denervated muscle, in this case through a nerve transfer rather than a muscle graft. TMR was initially described by Dumanian and Kuiken et al. for prosthetic control in proximal upper extremity amputees, redirecting the terminal branches of the brachial plexus into proximal muscle targets around the shoulder girdle. Once these muscles were reinnervated, they were mapped to a surface electrode array to allow for enhanced myoelectric control [39]. Serendipitously, these patients were found to have a substantial reduction in their phantom pain and residual limb pain. TMR has since been applied for management of post-amputation pain [20, 40]. After TMR was proven successful for management of secondary pain after amputation, Valerio and colleagues began to perform TMR nerve transfers at the time of primary amputation, showing superior outcomes in pain prevention [41].

10.11.1 Principles

Targeted muscle reinnervation is a nerve transfer, requiring a proximal nerve and a distal (target) nerve. Certain principles should be applied to targeted muscle reinnervation in amputees to optimize outcomes and minimize loss of function. These are similar to the standard principles of nerve and tendon transfers.

1. Expendable Motor Target.

   When selecting a motor target nerve for transfer, it is important that the nerve transfer not lead to loss of function. In a lower extremity amputee, there are many muscles to target since the foot and ankle have been removed. However, considering that the gastrocnemius and soleus muscles have now been repurposed for stump padding, surgeons should consider other motor targets whenever possible to minimize stump atrophy. When a muscle is innervated by more than one motor nerve, one of the redundant nerves may be selected as a target for transfer since native innervation is still preserved.
2. Anatomic Feasibility of Transfer.

   For the nerve transfer to be acceptable, the nerve ends much reach each other to allow for a tension-free coaptation. When possible, the motor target should be within the same muscle compartment as the proximal nerve. This not only allows for a tension-free transfer, but avoids crossing fascial planes, which may lead to entrapment. There are multiple expendable target nerves in each compartment to select.
3. Size Match.

   When possible, target nerves should be selected that are a similar caliber to the proximal nerve. However, this is often not possible, particularly for large nerves such as the tibial nerve. When such a size mismatch exists, the proximal nerve may be split into multiple fascicular groups which can each be independently transferred to different targets. Alternatively, the transfer can be performed to a single smaller nerve, centering the target as best as possible onto the proximal nerve stump, and anchoring the entire coaptation into the denervated muscle surrounding the neuromuscular junction of the target nerve. This creates a combined TMR/RPNI effect.
4. Nerve Transposition with Proximal Transfers.

   When possible, the ends of the proximal nerves should be transposed away from the weight-bearing stump. Target nerves can be identified more proximally, and the transfer can be performed at that level. This prevents the coaptation site from being stimulated during prosthetic ambulation.

10.11.2 Author's Technique

During the amputation, the nerve ends are identified and length is preserved (Fig. 10.15). We typically transfer the superficial peroneal (SPN) and tibial nerves, and occasionally the saphenous

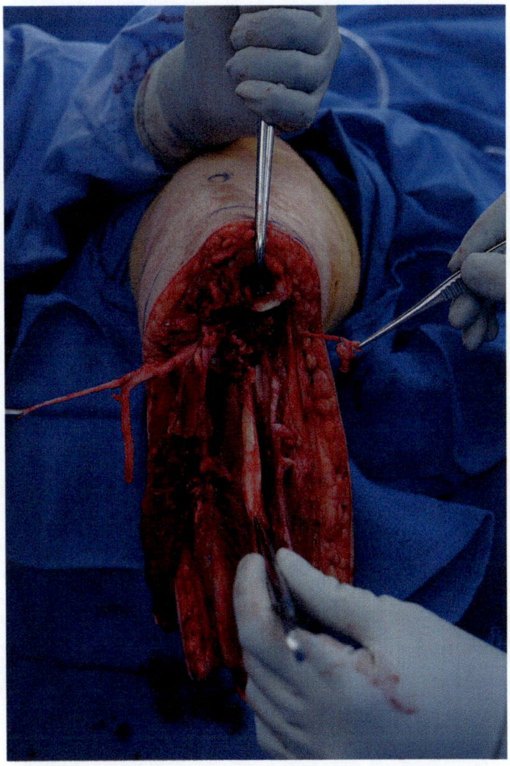

Fig. 10.15 The tibial, saphenous, and superficial peroneal nerves preserved with length at the time of below knee amputation

nerve. The superficial peroneal nerve is identified most commonly in the anterior corner of the lateral compartment just posterior to the anterolateral septum. Occasionally the nerve may run in the lateral corner of the anterior compartment, and infrequently it is located within the anterolateral septum itself. There may be two branches of the superficial peroneal nerve, in which case each should be identified and preserved.

The knee is positioned flexed and the fibular head is palpated. A two-centimeter incision is made at an oblique angle, one centimeter inferior to the fibular head. The common peroneal nerve (CPN) is identified at this level beneath the crural fascia, as it courses beneath the posterior crural intermuscular septum (PCIS) that separates the lateral compartment from the superficial posterior compartment. The fascia over the lateral compartment is incised at its posterior aspect, and the peroneus longus muscle is retracted superficially away from the PCIS. This allows the surgeon to sharply release the PCIS over the CPN and under the peroneus longus. The nerve may be decompressed further distally, releasing the anterior crural intermuscular septum as well. At this point, an internal neurolysis is performed to separate the common peroneal nerve into its fascicular groups. A nerve stimulator is used to map the fascicular groups to the muscles in the anterior and lateral compartments. We advocate preservation of the tibialis anterior innervation, since this is the largest muscle in the anterolateral leg and is important for padding of the tibial bone stump. Our preferred target is the extensor digitorum longus or peroneus longus (Fig. 10.16). The SPN is then translocated from the distal wound into the proximal CPN incision by passing a clamp retrograde along the SPN, and pulling the nerve out proximally (Fig. 10.17). The SPN and the target nerve will usually match closely in caliber, and the coaptation is performed through the small proximal incision [42].

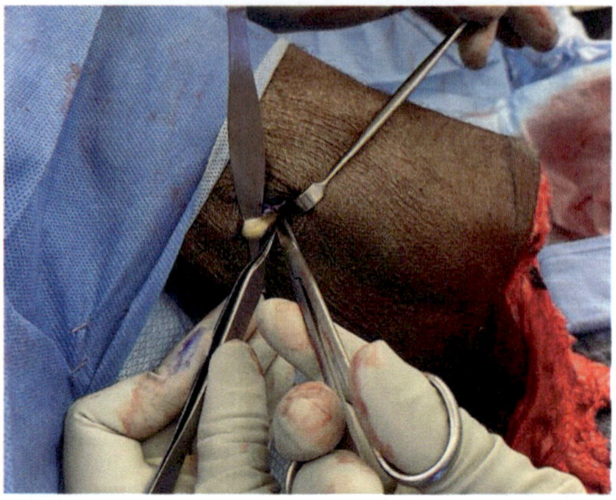

Fig. 10.16 The common peroneal nerve is exposed and decompressed through a small oblique incision just below the fibular head

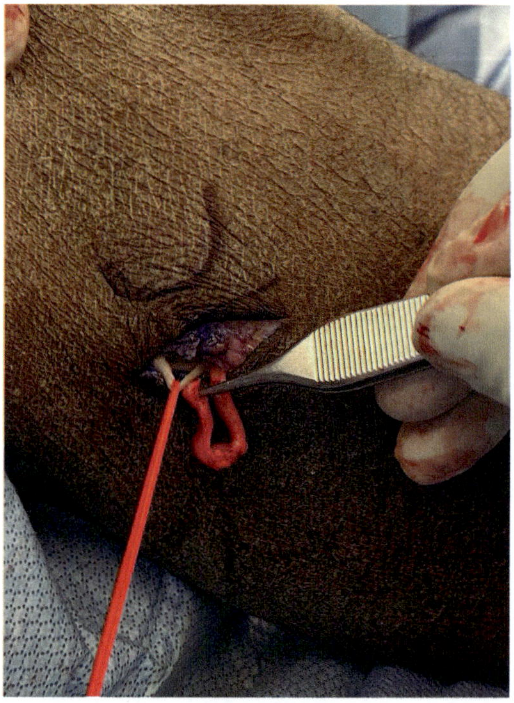

Fig. 10.17 The superficial peroneal nerve is translocated into the proximal wound in preparation for transfer to the extensor digitorum longus motor nerve (looped)

The tibial nerve is dissected retrograde from the distal amputation wound until a motor branch is identified from the nerve. At this level, any branch from the tibial nerve is a motor branch. We preferentially select target nerves for the deep posterior compartment, since these muscles are cut flush at the amputation level and are not used for stump padding. The tibialis posterior is the most commonly identified target at the amputation level. The motor target nerve is carefully neurolysed from the tibial nerve as far proximally as can be reached, then transected proxi-

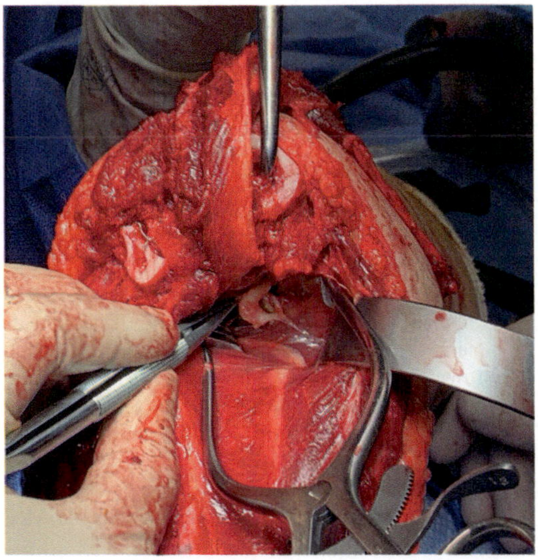

Fig. 10.18 The tibial nerve is transferred to a deep flexor motor nerve (in this case FHL) through the distal wound, in the interval between the superficial and deep posterior compartments

mally and brought distally into the wound. The tibial nerve is then transected, and an antegrade end-to-end coaptation is performed, usually with significant size mismatch (Fig. 10.18). The coaptation is then anchored to the denervated muscle at the neuromuscular junction with suture or fibrin glue.

If a transfer is performed for the saphenous nerve, it is brought through the fascia to the medial gastrocnemius muscle. Intramuscular dissection is performed until a distal motor nerve branch is identified, usually within a small fat stripe. The target nerve is transected, and coaptation is performed at this level. More often, the saphenous nerve is managed with a crush-and-bury neurectomy, and a more proximal TMR transfer is performed if the patient develops saphenous nerve symptoms, which is rare in our experience. This transfer is performed at the level of the adductor canal to the sartorius or vastus medialis motor nerves.

10.11.3 Outcomes

The initial studies mentioned above were mostly conducted on healthy patients having amputations for traumatic or oncologic processes. However, the majority of patients who require amputations have progressive peripheral vascular disease or diabetic foot infections. After performing successful TMR procedures for secondary post-amputation neuroma pain, we designed and applied a TMR protocol for major amputees at our institution, and TMR transfers are now performed concurrently for every major amputation at our center. Compared to patients undergoing standard BKA, significantly fewer patients undergoing TMR reported phantom pain (17 vs. 52%) or residual limb pain (13 vs. 51%). Significantly fewer TMR patients required narcotics for pain control at 3-month follow-up (9 vs. 27%). Significantly more TMR patients were ambulatory with a prosthesis (92 vs. 71%) [43].

10.12 Conclusions

Post-amputation pain is often attributable to a failure to recognize and properly managed the nerves transected at the amputation level. Multiple options exist for the stabilization of these distal nerve ends. At our institution, we favor targeted muscle reinnervation nerve transfers at the time of the amputation, which allows for axonal redirection into denervated motor endplates, without leaving non-vascularized tissue in the amputation stumps of patients with peripheral vascular disease or diabetic foot infections. This technique is efficient and reproducible, and can be applied to patients with severe medical comorbidities. When performed at the time of amputation, TMR nerve transfer is effective at preventing phantom limb pain or stump neuroma formation in most patients.

References

1. Attinger C, Cooper P, Blume P, Bulan E. The safest surgical incisions and amputations applying the angiosome principles and using the Doppler to assess the arterial-arterial connections of the foot and ankle. Foot Ankle Clin. 2001;6(4):745–99.
2. Bekeny JC, Alfawaz A, Day J, Naz I, Attinger CE, Fan KL, Evans KK, Akbari CM. Indirect endovascular

revascularization via collaterals: a new classification to predict wound healing and limb salvage. Ann Vasc Surg. 2020;S0890–5096(20):31074–8.
3. Janhofer DE, Lakhiani C, Kim PJ, Akbari C, Naz I, Tefera EA, Attinger CE, Evans KK. The utility of preoperative arteriography for free flap planning in patients with chronic lower extremity wounds. Plast Reconstr Surg. 2019;143(2):604–13. https://doi.org/10.1097/PRS.0000000000005265.
4. Black C, Fan KL, Defazio MV, Luvisa K, Reynolds K, Kotha VS, Attinger CE, Evans KK. Limb salvage rates and functional outcomes using a longitudinal slit arteriotomy end-to-side anastomosis for limb-threatening defects in a high-risk patient population. Plast Reconstr Surg. 2020;145(5):1302–12. https://doi.org/10.1097/PRS.0000000000006791.
5. Janhofer DE, Lakhiani C, Kim PJ, Naz I, Black CK, Tefera EA, Akbari C, Hashmi A, Attinger CE, Evans KK. Plast the utility of preoperative venous testing for lower extremity flap planning in patients with lower extremity wounds. Plast Reconstr Surg. 2020;145(1):164e–71e. https://doi.org/10.1097/PRS.0000000000006384.
6. Endara M, Attinger C. Using color to guide debridement. Adv Skin Wound Care. 2012;25(12):549–55.
7. Elmarsafi T, Garwood CS, Steinberg JS, Evans KK, Attinger CE, Kim PJ. Effect of semiquantitative culture results from complex host surgical wounds on dehiscence rates. Wound Repair Regen. 2017;25(2):210–6. https://doi.org/10.1111/wrr.12509.
8. Lipsky BA, Berendt AR, Cornia PB, Pile JC, Peters JG. 2012 Infectious Disease Society of America clinical practice guidelines for diagnosis and treatment of diabetic foot infections. Clin Infect Dis. 2012;54(12):e132–73.
9. Mueller MJ, Sinacore DR, Hastings MK, Strube MJ, Johnson JE. Effect of Achilles tendon lengthening on neuropathic plantar ulcers. A randomized clinical trial. Jn Bone Joint Surgery AM. 2003;85-A(8):1436–45.
10. Zolper EG, Fan KL, Meshkin D, Bekeny JC, Hill C, Mishu MD, Connolly P, Evans KK, Attinger C, A call for a new limb salvage paradigm for patients with diabetes. ADA Abstract.
11. Meshkin DH, Zolper EG, Chang K, Bryant M, Bekeny JC, Evans KK, Attinger CE, Fan KL. Long-term mortality after nontraumatic major lower extremity amputation: a systematic review and meta-analysis. J Foot Ankle Surg. 2020;60(3):567–76. https://doi.org/10.1053/j.jfas.2020.06.027.
12. Chudasama YV, Khunti KK, Zaccardi F, Rowlands AV, Yates T, Gillies CL, Davies MJ, Dhalwani NN. Physical activity, multimorbidity, and life expectancy: a UK Biobank longitudinal study. BMCmed. 2019;17(1):108.
13. Brown BJ, Iorio ML, Klement M, Conti Mica MR, El-Amraoui A, O'Halloran P, Attinger CE. Outcomes after 294 transtibial amputations with the posterior myocutaneous flap. Int J Low Extrem Wounds. 2014;13(1):33–40.
14. Endara M, Masden D, Goldstein J, Gondek S, Steinberg J, Attinger C. The role of chronic and perioperative glucose management in high-risk surgical closures: a case for tighter glycemic control. Plast Reconstr Surg. 2013;132(4):996–1004. https://doi.org/10.1097/PRS.0b013e31829fe119.
15. Fisher DF Jr, Clagett GP, Fry RE, Humble TH, Fry WJ. One-stage versus two-stage amputation for wet gangrene of the lower extremity: a randomized study. J Vasc Surg. 1988;8(4):428–33.
16. Burgess EM, Romano RL, Zettl JH, Schrock RD Jr. Amputations of the leg for peripheral vascular insufficiency. J Bone Joint Surg Am. 1971;53(5):874–90.
17. Brown BJ, Iorio ML, Hill L, Carlisle B, Attinger CE. Below-knee amputation with a vascularized fibular graft and headless compression screw. Plast Reconstr Surg. 2013;131(2):323–7.
18. Sen N, Gigi R, Haim A, et al. Mortality and reoperations following lower limb amputations. Isr Med Assoc J. 2014;16:83–7.
19. Stern JR, Wong CK, Yerovinkina M, et al. A meta-analysis of long-term mortality and associated risk factors following lower extremity amputation. Ann Vasc Surg. 2017;42:322–7.
20. Souza JM, Cheesborough JE, Ko JH, Cho MS, Kuiken TA, Dumanian GA. Targeted muscle reinnervation: a novel approach to postamputation neuroma pain. Clin Orthop Relat Res. 2014;472:2984–90.
21. Nigam M, Webb A, Harbour P, Devulapalli C, Kleiber G. Lower extremity amputation stump neuromas: Implications for pre-emptive targeted muscle reinnervation. American Society of Plastic Surgeons annual meeting. San Diego CA, 9/19.
22. Nigam M, Harbour P, Kleiber G. Lower extremity amputation stump neuromas: Patterns of occurrence, treatment, and outcomes. American Society for Peripheral Nerve annual meeting, Ft Lauderdale FL, 1/20.
23. Fleury C, Chang BL, Harbour P, Kleiber GM. Symptomatic neuroma formation after below-knee amputation preferentially occurs in nerves unrecognized at initial amputation. American Society for Peripheral Nerve annual meeting, Ft Lauderdale FL, 1/20.
24. Decrouy-Duruz V, Christen T, Raffoul W. Evaluation of surgical treatment for neuropathic pain from neuroma in patients with injured peripheral nerves. J Neurosurg. 2018;128(4):1235–40.
25. Domeshek LF, Krauss EM, Snyder-Warwick AK, et al. Surgical treatment of neuromas improves patient-reported pain, depression, and quality of life. Plast Reconstr Surg. 2017;139(2):407–18.
26. Eberlin KR, Ducic I. Surgical algorithm for neuroma management: a changing treatment paradigm. Plast Reconstr Surg Glob Open. 2018;6(10):e1952.
27. Barberá J, Gonzalez J, Gil JL, Sanjuán MA, García F, Lopez A. The quality and extension of nerve fibre regeneration in the centrocentral anastomosis of the peripheral nerve. Acta Neurochir Suppl (Wien). 1988;43:205–9.

28. Economides JM, DeFazio MV, Attinger CE, Barbour JR. Prevention of painful neuroma and phantom limb pain after transfemoral amputations through concomitant nerve coaptation and collagen nerve wrapping. Neurosurgery. 2016;79(3):508–13.
29. Frost CM, Wei B, Baghmanli Z, Cederna PS, Urbanchek MG. PEDOT electrochemical polymerization improves electrode fidelity and sensitivity. Plast Reconstr Surg. 2012;129(4):933–42.
30. Kung TA, Langhals NB, Martin DC, Johnson PJ, Cederna PS, Urbanchek MG. Regenerative peripheral nerve interface viability and signal transduction with an implanted electrode. Plast Reconstr Surg. 2014;133(6):1380–94.
31. Vu PP, Vaskov AK, Irwin ZT, et al. A regenerative peripheral nerve interface allows real-time control of an artificial hand in upper limb amputees. Sci Transl Med. 2020;12(533):eaay2857.
32. Ursu DC, Urbanchek MG, Nedic A, Cederna PS, Gillespie RB. In vivo characterization of regenerative peripheral nerve interface function. J Neural Eng. 2016;13(2):026012.
33. Urbanchek MG, Kung TA, Frost CM, et al. Development of a regenerative peripheral nerve interface for control of a neuroprosthetic limb. Biomed Res Int. 2016;2016:5726730.
34. Ives GC, Kung TA, Nghiem BT, et al. Current state of the surgical treatment of terminal neuromas. Neurosurgery. 2018;83(3):354–64.
35. Hooper RC, Cederna PS, Brown DL, et al. Regenerative peripheral nerve interfaces for the management of symptomatic hand and digital neuromas. Plast Reconstr Surg Glob Open. 2020;8(6):e2792.
36. Woo SL, Kung TA, Brown DL, Leonard JA, Kelly BM, Cederna PS. Regenerative peripheral nerve interfaces for the treatment of postamputation neuroma pain: a pilot study. Plast Reconstr Surg Glob Open. 2016;4(12):e1038.
37. Kubiak CA, Kemp SWP, Cederna PS. Regenerative peripheral nerve interface for management of postamputation neuroma. JAMA Surg. 2018;153(7):681–2.
38. Kubiak CA, Kemp SWP, Cederna PS, Kung TA. Prophylactic regenerative peripheral nerve interfaces to prevent postamputation pain. Plast Reconstr Surg. 2019;144(3):421e–30e.
39. Kuiken TA, Dumanian GA, Lipschutz RD, Miller LA, Stubblefield KA. The use of targeted muscle reinnervation for improved myoelectric prosthesis control in a bilateral shoulder disarticulation amputee. Prosthet Orthot Int. 2004;28:245–53.
40. Dumanian GA, Potter BK, Mioton LM, et al. Targeted muscle reinnervation treats neuroma and phantom pain in major limb amputees: a randomized clinical trial. Ann Surg. 2019;270(2):238–46.
41. Valerio IL, Dumanian GA, Jordan SW, et al. Preemptive treatment of phantom and residual limb pain with targeted muscle reinnervation at the time of major limb amputation. J Am Coll Surg. 2019;228(3):217–26.
42. Devulapalli C, Kotha V, Harbour P, Attinger CE, Kleiber G. Targeted muscle fascicular reinnervation in the lower extremity: prevention of neuroma and phantom limb pain at the time of below-knee amputation, American Society for Peripheral Nerve annual meeting, Palm Desert CA, 2/19.
43. Chang BL, Fleury C, Harbour P, Attinger CE, Kleiber GM. Targeted muscle reinnervation effectively reduces pain and improves ambulation rates in a highly comorbid patient population undergoing lower limb amputation. American Society for Peripheral Nerve annual meeting, Ft Lauderdale FL, 1/20.

11 Understanding Autologous Stem Cell as Future Minimal Invasive Modalities for Treatment

Rica Tanaka

Key Points

- Ischemic diabetic foot ulcers are difficult to cure with conventional treatment modalities.
- Autologous stem cell therapy is one of therapeutic options for nonhealing ischemic diabetic ulcers as an adjunctive therapy with reconstructive surgery for limb salvage.
- None of stem cell products are yet approved for conventional use for ischemic diabetic foot, but previous studies have shown safety and efficacy of autologous stem cell therapies. Further studies with higher evidence are needed.

R. Tanaka (✉)
Division of Regenerative Therapy, Juntendo University Graduate School of Medicine, Tokyo, Japan

Department of Plastic and Reconstructive Surgery, Juntendo University School of Medicine, Tokyo, Japan

Juntendo Hospital, Podiatry Center, Tokyo, Japan

Juntendo University Graduate School of Medicine, Intractable Diseases, Intractable Disease Research Center, Tokyo, Japan
e-mail: rtanaka@juntendo.ac.jp

11.1 Introduction

Peripheral arterial disease (PAD) causing ischemia of lower limb is one of the most severe complications of diabetes and increasing the risk of lower limb loss. Patients with severe lower limb ischemia have high risk of major amputation within 1 year after diagnosis, and the average 5-year mortality rate range from 39 to 68% [1]. And this mortality rate is higher for PAD patients with unhealed ulcers [2]. Considering that more than 50% of diabetic foot patients have PAD as coexisting disease [3], evaluating the vascular perfusion level of these patients prior to surgical approach is one of the important factors for successful wound closure.

Diabetes has many factors that lead to decreased angiogenesis, endothelial dysfunction that can cause lower limb ischemia. In diabetes, there are macrovascular disorders and microcirculatory disorders in vascular lesions. As a treatment for a low blood circulation due to a large blood vessel disorder, vascular bypass surgery or an endovascular treatment is an option. However, there is no effective treatment for microvascular disorder. Therefore, if macrovascular treatments are ineffective and tissue ischemia is still present due to microvascular insufficiency, the wound will not heal and tissue necrosis expands. Failure of all treatment modalities leads to limb amputation as the only solution [4]. A novel therapy to

J. P. Hong, H. Suh (eds.), *Diabetic Foot Reconstruction*,
https://doi.org/10.1007/978-981-16-9816-3_11

reconstruct or to regenerate microvascular circulation is essentially needed in order to salvage diabetic foot patients with ischemia.

Autologous stem cells therapy is one of the therapeutic options for microvascular reconstruction for ischemic diabetic foot. Currently, bone marrow and peripheral blood is considered to be the most accessible and enriched source of stem cells for widespread medical treatments. In 1997, vascular stem cell named endothelial progenitor cells (EPCs) was first established as part of bone marrow and peripheral blood mononuclear cell components (CD34-positive fraction) [5]. Since EPCs reside in the bone marrow and the peripheral blood possessing the function to regenerate vessels by differentiating in the mature endothelial cells, intense research has done to establish vascular regenerative therapy using bone marrow and peripheral blood EPCs to treat ischemic diseases.

Presently, the following two methods are widely used for revascularization treatment using EPC for ischemic limbs. One is bone marrow or peripheral blood-derived mononuclear cell transplantation method in which a mononuclear cell component containing EPC is fractionated and transplanted from bone marrow or peripheral blood, which was previously reported by Tateishi-Yuyama et al. [6]. The other is a method of isolating and purifying cells that are positive for the EPC marker CD34 or CD133 from bone marrow or peripheral blood and transplanting highly pure EPCs. Because of the scarcity of CD133 or CD34positive cells in the bone marrow and peripheral blood, MNCs are collected after administration of G-CSF, which stimulates the production of CD133 or CD34positive cells in the bone marrow. These cells are amplified internally within the bone marrow and then mobilized to the peripheral blood. The first phase I/II clinical trial using autologous G-CSF mobilized peripheral blood CD34-positive cell therapy for nonhealing diabetic ulcers was performed by our group [7]. In this study, nonhealing diabetic ulcers were treated with G-CSF-mobilized peripheral blood CD34-positive cells as an EPC-enriched population in five patients. No serious adverse effects were observed in any of the cases, there were no cases of major amputation of the lower limbs, and complete wound closure was observed in all patients at an average of 18 weeks. Interestingly, patients who were treated with cells having higher numbers of vasculogenic colonies and higher percentages of CD34/KDR double-positive cells showed better clinical outcomes, as demonstrated by faster wound healing and positive prognosis without recurrence or heterotopic ulcers. These results suggested that the vasculogenic potential of EPCs and the numbers of EPCs transplanted directly affect the efficacy of cell transplantation therapy using EPCs. Since diabetic patients demonstrate decreased number of EPCs, with dysfunction in proliferation, migration, endothelial cell differentiation and angiogenic potential [8, 9], the efficacy of autologous EPC therapy for diabetic patients may be limited for patients with low EPC function.

Another limitation is the physical burden of cell isolation. Since EPC resides only 0.01% of the peripheral blood cells and 0.1% of the bone marrow cells, a large amount of bone marrow aspiration or peripheral blood apheresis and injection of G-CSF are needed for cell therapy applications. Based on these experiences, we believe that in order to solve the problem, we need to establish a cell therapy that can collect cells by a more non-invasive method and transplant more functional cells [9].

In order to overcome these limitations and to establish minimal invasive and highly effective vascular regenerative therapy ischemic diabetic ulcer patients, we have established a new method called Quality and Quantity culture for generating EPCs with enhanced vasculogenic and angiogenic potential [10–13]. Mononuclear cells (MNCs) harvested from peripheral blood are cultured in vitro with our quality and quantity controlled culture (QQ culture) system in the presence of five different kinds of cytokines [14]. MNCs harvested after QQ culture (MNC-QQ) showed enrichment of EPCs (CD34+, CD133+) and M2 macrophages (CD206+ cell) populations with increased vasculogenic functions. Preclinical animal studies have shown the potential of QQ culture-treated PBMNCs as a promising therapeutic option for ischemic diseases [15]. We have recently conducted a PhaseI/IIa clinical trial to treat nonhealing ischemic ulcers with MNC-QQ therapy and obtained a promising data showing safety and efficacy (unpublished data). This chapter will introduce the possibility of limb salvage by autologous stem cell therapy for ischemic diabetic foot introducing my experience.

11.2 Indications and Contraindications of Your Preferred Reconstruction

Stem cell therapy has shown efficacy in various types and disease entity of diabetic foot. Ischemic diabetic foot is the most difficult to cure, and sufficient blood flow is the major factor necessary to obtain complete closure. Any surgical interventions such as direct closure of the wound, skin graft, flap reconstruction cannot not be done successfully without sufficient blood flow. Diabetic foot with ischemia will first be treated by vascular surgeon or interventionist by EVT or bypass to obtain enough flow to the wound. However, there are times when the wound does not heal after large vessel vascular intervention and needs further vascular perfusion through microvascular reconstruction. Stem cell therapy, especially vascular stem cell therapy, becomes effective in these cases when large vessel intervention and other treatment modalities are exhausted and further therapy to enhance microvascular perfusion is needed.

Transplanted stem/progenitor cells may or may not directly differentiate into endothelial lineage cells for vasculogenesis but also secrete cytokines/growth factors inducing angiogenesis, vasodilatation, or anti-inflammation. EPCs (BM or PB-derived CD34 positive cells) and MNC-QQ cells are preclinically shown to indirectly and directly differentiate to endothelial cells and promote vessel formation. Newly formed blood vessels after stem cell therapy are mainly capillaries or arterioles, but not arteries. Therefore, blood flow recovery might be slower after cell therapy compared with conventional revascularization. In addition, the mechanism of action of cell therapy is more complicated than conventional interventions. Multiple biological actions of stem cells may result in the improvement of clinical and functional parameters in a unique time course. The blood flow parameters would start as early as week 2–4. Therefore, surgical intervention such as debridement with direct wound closure, flap reconstruction, skin graft, etc., should be at least 2–4 weeks after the cell therapy confirming the blood perfusion is enough for the wound to be operated.

Since most cell therapy for ischemic diabetic foot is under clinical investigation, the indications for treating ischemic diabetic foot with cell therapy are not yet well established. The heterogeneity among the studies leads to variety of indications and different end points. Therefore, the future clinical trials should have comparable protocols to establish the true indication for ischemic diabetic foot ulcers. Presently, most of the studies using stem cell therapy targetting non-option ischemic wound patient uses the following indication.

1. Nonhealing wound for more than 1 month after standard of care and surgical intervention necessary for improving the blood flow and wound closure.
2. Wound size

   Clinical trials using stem cells for diabetic foot target wound grade of Wagner 1–4. For critical limb ischemia (CLI), many of the target is Fontaine III–IV [16], Rutherford 5 [17–19]. Due to the heterogeneity of the trials, there is no answer to what wound size is suitable for stem cell therapy. In general, the larger the wound, the more vascularity is required for the wound to heal. Therefore, high stem cell efficacy will be expected to promote enough vascular perfusion to a larger wound for it to heal.
3. Level of Ischemia

   Many of the studies do not indicate exact grade of ischemia that is suitable for stem cell therapy for ischemic diabetic foot. Our group, Kawamoto et al. and others, performed G-CSF mobilized CD34 cell therapy for ischemic ulcers targeting patients with >70% luminal stenosis in the leg arteries [17, 20]. The metanalysis data of stem cell therapy for diabetic foot reported by Xuan Shu et al. showed the baseline TcPO2 of the patients indicated range from 16.3 ± 11 to 44.5 ± 10.5 mmHg [21]. Since stem cells are efficacious at promoting capillaries and not regenerating large arterioles, patients with total occlusion of all three lower limb arteries will be difficult to cure. It is ideal to have some perfusion left in the wound bed for the cells to survive to function their potency. There are four previously reported studies treating ischemic diabetic foot with stem cells in adjunction with percutaneous transluminal angioplasty. The results demonstrated the superiority of combination therapy of angioplasty and cell therapy with higher wound healing [22, 23].

4. Level of Infection

   Most of the clinical trials exclude patients with severe infection of the wound. Active infection should be controlled with antibiotics and proper wound care prior to cell therapy.

11.3 Relevance to Surgical Outcome

Stem cell therapy is expected to increase the vascular flow of the peripheral capillaries in the foot and the wound bed. Therefore, stem cells therapy should be performed prior to surgical procedure after stem cell showing its effect of increasing vascular flow at the surgical site. Previous studies have shown that vascular flow of TcPO2 over 25–40 mmHg or over and skin perfusion pressure 40 mmHg or over is necessary predicting wound healing after surgical approach [24, 25]. Therefore, it will be ideal if the stem cell therapy can be performed prior to the surgery to make the surgical site vascularized. If possible, stem cell injection at the time of surgery may provide more secure blood flow. Combination of stem cell therapy with surgery may have high possibility of increasing the success rate of surgical outcome.

11.4 Preoperative Evaluation and Special Considerations (Surgical Chapters)

The previous clinical trials had set an exclusion criteria for patients receiving stem cell therapy. Since the function of vascular regenerative therapy is angiogenesis, tumor growth and the malignancy become a worrying factor for recipients. Therefore, history of malignancy within past 5 years and diabetic retinopathy are excluded from receiving the therapy.

11.5 Procedures for Cell Therapy

Isolation of patient's cell or tissue is necessary for autologous stem cell therapy. Since most of stem cell therapy origins are bone marrow, peripheral blood-derived EPCs or adipose-derived stem cells, the cells are isolated by bone marrow aspiration, apheresis, or liposuction. Since EPC resides only 0.01% of the peripheral blood cells and 0.1% of the bone marrow cells, a large amount of bone marrow aspiration or peripheral blood apheresis and injection of granulocyte-colony stimulating factor (G-CSF) are needed for cell therapy applications. Therefore, achieving clinically sufficient number functional EPCs from diabetic patients remains a limiting factor [7]. In order to overcome this issue, we have established a cell culture system called Quality and Quantity cell culture of peripheral blood mononuclear cells (MNC-QQ cell therapy), where tissue and vascular regenerative cells can be generated by just a blood draw of 100–200 ml. In our study with MNC-QQ cells, 100–200 ml of blood is collected in outpatients setting, and patients wait for a week for the cells to be cultured. The blood is delivered to GMP controlled cell processing facility for QQ culture. Briefly, mononuclear cells are separated from whole PB and suspended in serum-free media composed of Stemline II (Sigma-Aldrich) containing thrombopoietin (TPO) 20 ng/ml, stem cell factor (SCF) 100 ng/ml, interleukin-6 (IL-6) 20 ng/ml, vascular endothelial growth factor

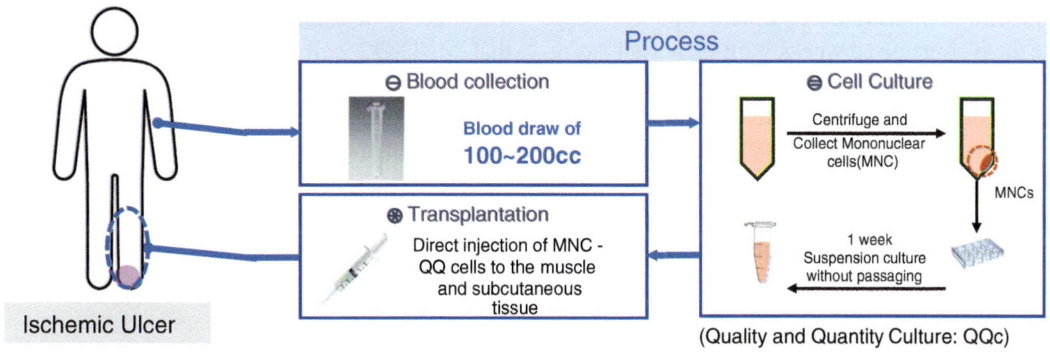

Fig. 11.1 Process of MNC-QQ therapy. Peripheral blood mononuclear cells (PbMNCs) are isolated from100 to 200 ml of blood. PbMNCs is cultured in a serum free suspension culture for one week and injected in the lower limb, the foot and the wound

(VEGF) 50 ng/ml, Fms-like tyrosine kinase-3 ligand (FLT-3 L) 100 ng/ml (all growth factors are human recombinant proteins purchase from PeproTech, Rocky Hill, NJ) and antibiotics (penicillin 100 unit/ml and streptomycin 100 ng/ml, Thermo Fisher). The cells were cultured in CO2 incubator at 37 °C for 7 days without passaging. After 7 days, the cells were ready as MNC-QQ cells for injection in patients [14, 15] (Fig. 11.1).

Promising results in the treatment of diabetic foot have been achieved by administering stem cells either via intramuscular or intra-arterial injection into the diseased lower limb or by direct application over the wound [26]. Although evidence has not shown which delivery method is the best way to cure diabetic ischemic wounds with stem cells, considering the delivery of stem cells to the wound bed and surrounding ischemic tissue, I believe that the method of direct injection is most reasonable. In our G-CSF mobilized CD34 cell therapy [7] and first MNC-QQ study by single-dose treatment, we had directly injected the cells in intramuscularly within 20 cm surrounding the wound in the plantar area of the wound. Each patient received a total of 2×10^7 cells by administration of injections at 20 cites (1.5–2.0 cm deep) with 27 gaze needle. Each injection containing 1×10^6 cells suspended in 0.25 ml saline. In the second stage of MNC-QQ clinical trial, we had performed three time injection of MNC-QQ cells at 1 month interval. At that time, we have changed our protocol to injecting the cells not just in the plantar area but also in the lower limb calf muscle at total of 50 sites. We had to change our protocol to further increase the vascular flow from the lower limb area to the foot near the wound.

11.6 Postoperative Care

In our study, saline gauze dressing was placed over the treated wound immediately after the treatment to avoid cell damage and standard of wound care was continued starting postoperative day 1. The patient was discharged from the hospital the following day, provided there were no side effects due to the cell therapy and standard care regime for diabetic foot was continued starting from the day of discharge.

11.7 Expected Outcome

Majority of previous studies demonstrate the efficacy of various stem cell therapy for ischemic diabetic foot. Until now, we have previously reported the safety and efficacy of G-CSF mobilized autologous peripheral blood CD34 positive cell therapy, single-dose MNC-QQ therapy (unpublished data), and multiple-dose MNC-QQ (unpublished data) for nonhealing ischemic diabetic ulcers. Our first trial with G-CSF mobilized peripheral blood CD34 cell therapy demonstrated complete wound closure at an average of 18 weeks with increased vascular perfusion in all patients [7]. The patient receiving this therapy was nonhealing for a more than 3 months after PTA along with other surgical intervention and was prepared for lower limb amputation, but with cell therapy, the wound started to heal without additional skin graft or flap surgery or NPWT. With debridement, the open wound healed with only standard of care and topical treatment. The study with MNC-QQ cell therapy demonstrated significantly higher SPP and $TcPO_2$ after cell therapy measuring over 40 mmHg starting 2 weeks after the cell therapy lasting until more than 3 months post-therapy. Complete wound closure occurred in seven of 10 cases at 12 weeks. The average wound closure rate was 73.2 ± 40.1% post 12 weeks after the therapy. Since patients had well vascular perfused wound after 2 weeks of cell therapy, the patients were able to receive minor amputation with complete healing within 2 weeks post-surgery [27]. We are presently performing three times dosage of MNC-QQ cell therapy with 1 month interval, and the results look promising, with higher efficacy than the previous method.

MNC-QQ cells include hematopoietic and EPCs with CD34 and/or CD133 markers and M2 macrophage cells with CD206 cells. Quantitative real-time polymerase chain reaction (qRT-PCR) assay reveals high expression of proangiogenic gene expressions in MNC-QQ cells. Using murine ischemic hindlimb models, MNC-QQ intramuscular transplantation had higher blood perfusion recovery in ischemic hindlimbs compared to non-cultured PB MNCs and G-CSF mobilized CD34 cells. Histological evaluations and qRT-PCR assays in ischemic hindlimbs demonstrated that MNC-QQ cells have high angio-vasculogenesis and myogenesis and inhibited inflammation and fibrosis vs. compared to PB MNCs [14]. In porcine wounds treated with MNC-QQ cells, the wounds healed significantly faster and developed granulated tissue with larger capillary networks. Also confirmed the direct vascular formation of MNC-QQ cells by the presence of differentiated human MNC-QQ cells in newly formed vessels in porcine wounds [15]. These preclinical and clinical results demonstrate that MNC-QQ cell therapy has the potency to provide microvascular perfusion to the wound bed for it to withstand surgical intervention such as skin graft and flap coverage, etc. In the future, stem cell therapy will be a great therapeutic option for patients that need combination therapy with surgical wound coverage.

11.8 Management of Complications

Presently, most of stem cell therapy studies including ours are performed autologously. Therefore, it is reported to be safe without any immune response, and most of the studies do not report major adverse effects related to stem cell therapy. Gao et al. reported that eight of the studies receiving autologous stem cell therapy for PAD with RCT had side effects associated with cell therapy. These include slight edema of limbs, transient increase of serum creatine phosphokinase, bleeding, pain, infection, and cellulitis after puncture or injection, hematocrit, proliferative retinopathy, moderate hypotension, and chest distress during mobilization and severe worsening of CLI in the target leg after injection. Most serious side effect was wound sepsis ending with amputation [16].

11.9 Revision or Subsequent Procedures

There are no revision or subsequent procedures after stem cell application. As another adjunctive therapy to increase peripheral vascular perfusion, hyperbaric oxygen therapy (HBO) is commonly used along with standard wound care in many types of wounds, including ischemic wounds. Although HBO therapy has gained popularity as an adjunctive treatment for diabetic foot wounds, there are surprisingly few published reports that support its efficacy and to determine if the wound would benefit from HBO therapy [28]. Previously there are three RCT studies performed to investigate the efficacy of HBO for ischemic diabetic foot ulcers [29–31]. By exploring the results of the individual studies, some evidence was found that HBOT improves wound healing in ischemic diabetic ulcers in the longer term, as opposed to non-ischemic diabetic ulcers [32]. However, HBOT should not be considered a substitute for optimal revascularization and it should be considered after angioplasty. Although there are no study performed to compare the efficacy of HBO and stem cell therapy until now, considering the power and potency of both therapies, stem cell therapy may be effective to be performed prior or adjunctive to HBO for severe ischemic diabetic patients in the future.

11.10 Case Demonstrations

Case 1: Case receiving autologous G-CSF mobilized peripheral blood CD34 positive cells. A 63-year-old male with non healing chronic wound for more than 6 months with past medical history of 20 years of diabetes and 4 years of CRF on hemodialysis. Figure 11.2a: Pretherapy: The ulcer located on the left third, fourth, and fifth toes to metatarsus did not heal for 26 weeks. SPP was 10 mmHg at this point. Figure 11.2b: The ulcer at time of debridement prior to cell therapy. Figure 11.2c: The wound significantly

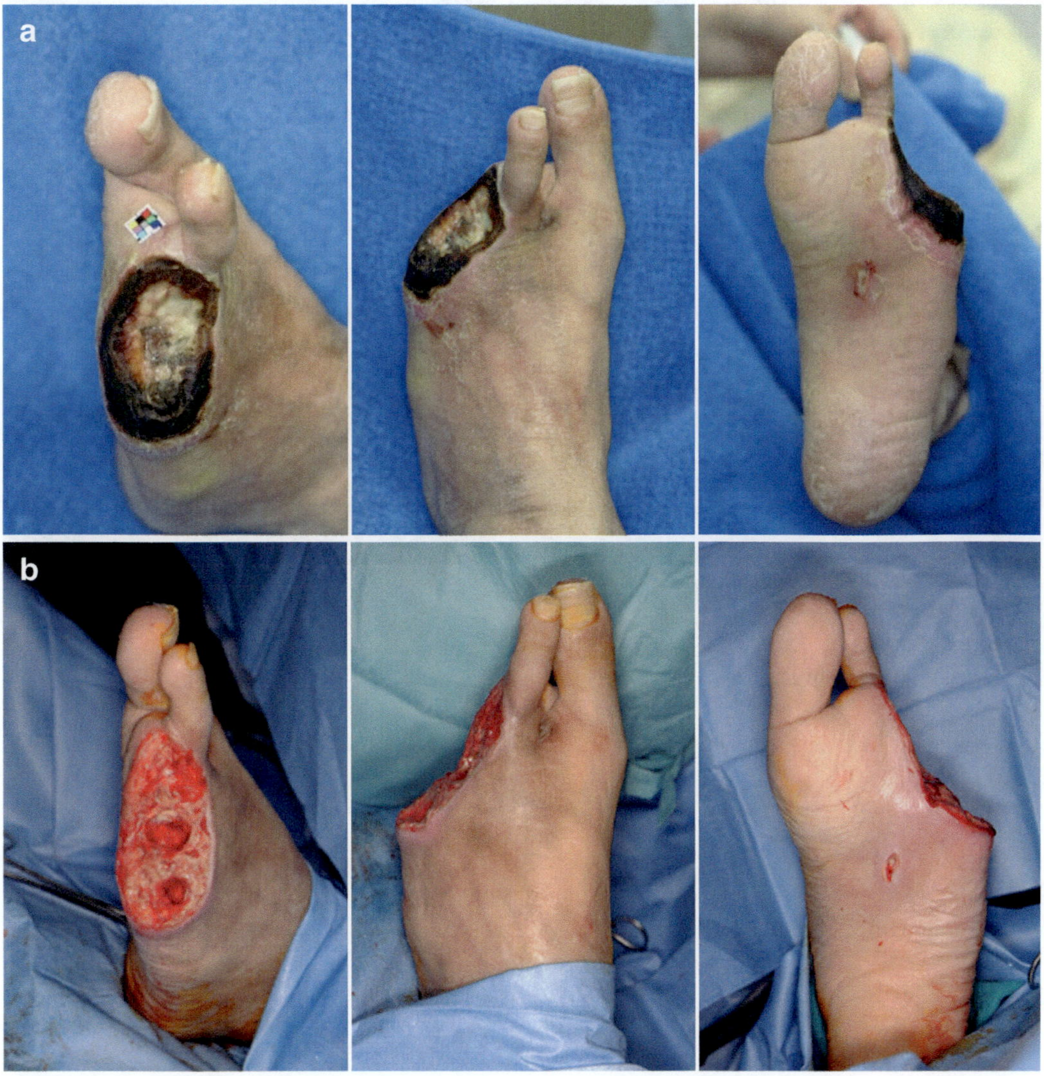

Fig. 11.2 Case receiving autologous G-CSF mobilized peripheral blood CD34 positive. (**a**) pretherapy. (**b**) The ulcer at time of debridement prior to cell therapy. (**c**) 16 weeks post therapy. (**d**) 11 years after posttherapy

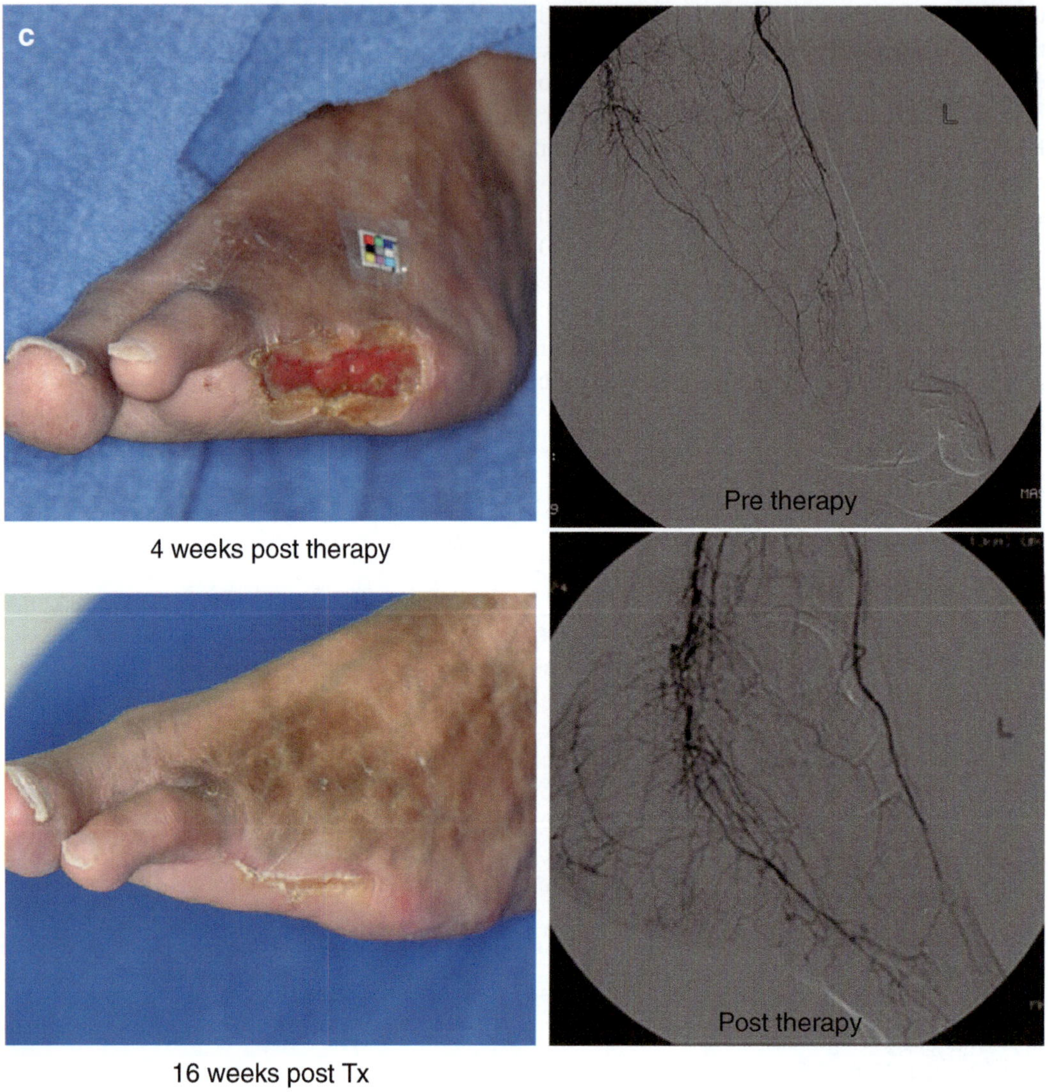

Fig. 11.2 (continued)

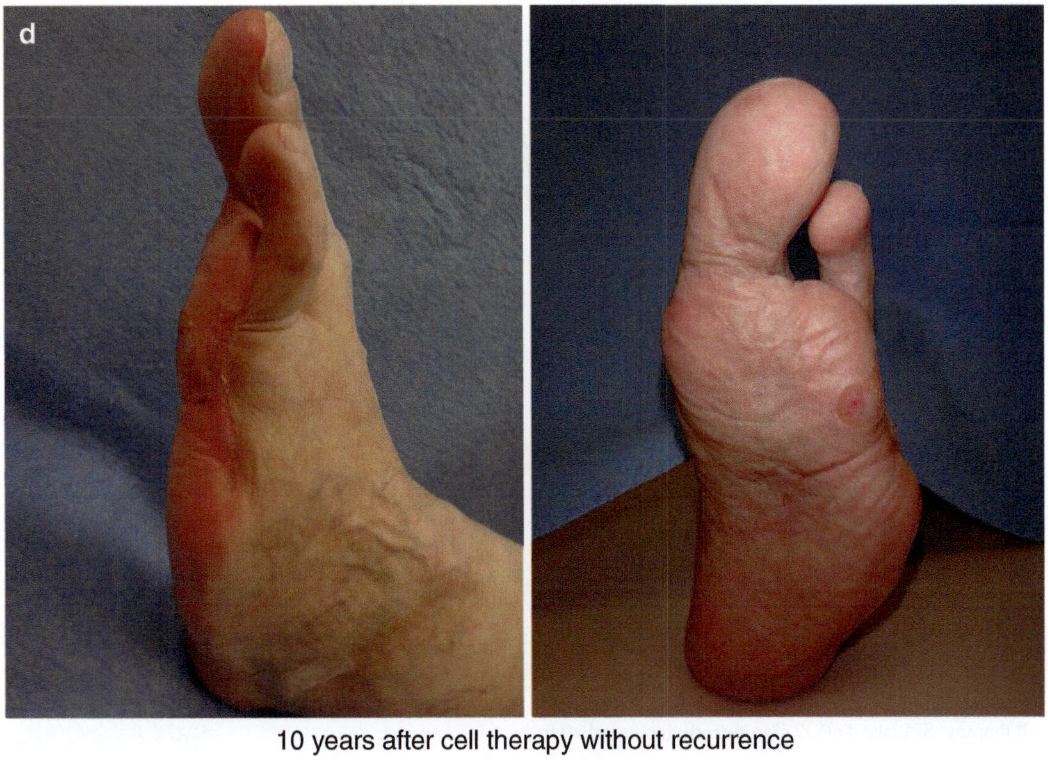

Fig. 11.2 (continued)

closed after the cell therapy and completely healed after 16 weeks post-therapy. SPP was 67 mmHg 12 weeks post-therapy. Angiography pretherapy shows avascular area, however after cell therapy, angiography post 12 weeks showed enhanced vascular perfusion. Figure 11.2d: At 11 years after post-therapy. Currently, patient is ambulant throughout the period after therapy without any recurrence and heterotopic ulcer in the same foot for 11 year with stable SPP of 66 ± 23 mmHg without any PTA intervention of the full 12 years.

Case 2: Effects of MNC-QQ therapy on wound healing is shown in Fig. 11.3. Single-dose cell therapy of MNC-QQ cell injection was performed for 61-year-old man with nonhealing wound of metatarsals due to CLI. Medical History included hypertension, chronic renal failure on hemodialysis, CLI, hypothyroidism, post-myocardial infarction, post cerebral infarction. The patient was admitted with necrosis of third, fourth, and fifth toe and underwent debridement and minor amputation surgery for wound closure. However, the wound opened after suture removal and the wound was not healing for 197 days and underwent MNC-QQ cell therapy. After cell therapy, the wound completely healed after 179 days. SPP and TcPO2 significantly increased after the cell therapy. Red dotted line denotes the level of SPP and TcPO2 needed for wound healing as previously reported. The patient was wound free for at least 1 year after the therapy.

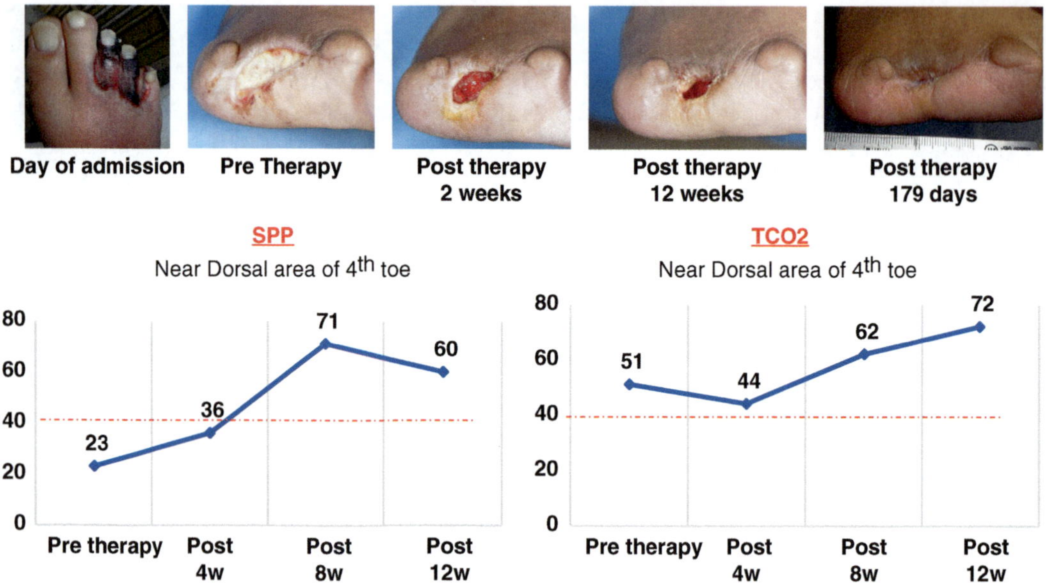

Fig. 11.3 Effects of MNC-QQ therapy on wound healing, SPP and TcPO2 in Case 10. 61-year-old man with non-healing wound of metatarsals for 197 days due to CLI. The wound completely healed after 179 days post cell therapy. SPP and TcPO2 significantly increased after the cell therapy. Red dotted line denotes the level of SPP and TcPO2 needed for wound healing as previously reported. Red dotted line is the amount of SPP needed for wound healing previously reported

11.11 Discussion

Diabetic wounds with severe ischemia do not have many options for its treatment to enhance vascular perfusion. Angioplasty is currently an acceptable first-line treatment for selected patients with lower limb ischemia, and once other treatment modalities such as HBO are exhausted, major amputation will be the only option. Investigation of the efficacy of bone marrow cells in peripheral vascular disease started in the early 2000s [6] and we are starting to realize that stem cell therapy may be the new option to limb salvage for patients with no-option other than major amputation due to ischemia [33].

Currently, endothelial progenitor cells (EPCs) and mesenchymal stem cells (MSCs) are the major source of stem cell therapy for vascular regeneration therapy. Table 11.1 demonstrates the characteristics of different types of cell therapy. Stem cell therapy using EPCs has been introduced in the introduction of this chapter. Since EPC resides within the MNC population of bone marrow and the peripheral blood as CD34+ cells, bone marrow aspiration and apheresis are performed to collect these cells. EPCs are known to have a high vasculogenic and angiogenic potential to promote vascular regeneration. MSCs are multipotent stromal cells that have high tendency to differentiate into osteoblasts, chondrocytes, and adipocytes. It is also reported that MSC can also promote angiogenesis [34]. Since adipose tissue and bone marrow are the source to collect mesenchymal stem cell, liposuction and bone marrow aspiration is performed to collect MSCs. Recently, our group introduced a next generation cell therapy with MNC-QQ cells. MNC-QQc are an ex vivo cultured peripheral blood MNCs with highly vascular regenerative potential with a very small amount of blood. Compared to other therapies, MNC-QQ cell therapy can be performed with just a blood draw without patient's physical burden. Therefore, if it is approved for practical use, it will be the first minimally invasive, highly effective vascular regenerative therapy in the future.

Table 11.1 Comparative characteristics of therapeutic approach for vascular regeneration

	Mesenchymal stem cell therapy	MNC cell therapy	CD34+ cell (EPC) therapy	MNC-QQc therapy
Cell isolation technique	Bone marrow aspiration, liposuction	Bone marrow aspiration, apheresis	Apheresis with G-CSF mobilization	100–120 ml Blood draw
Risk/patient physical burden	High to middle	High to middle	Middle	Low
Culture (duration)	Several weeks	None	None	One week
Angiogenic potential	+	+	++	++++

EPC endothelial progenitor cells, *MNC* mononuclear cells, *MNC-QQ* quality and quantity ex vivo cultured mononuclear cells, *G-CSF* granulocyte colony stimulating factor

However, none of the stem cell therapies are yet approved by FDA as conventional therapy for diabetic ischemic foot. Presently, many clinical trials are under investigation for approval [21, 35]. And it is difficult to conclude which cell therapy will be most suitable for ischemic DFU patients due to the heterogeneity among the studies. All of the studies conducted with heterogeneity of the protocol, including different inclusion and exclusion criteria, different end points, and different procedures. Therefore, it is not yet clear what is 'the best' stem cell type and best indication of ischemic DFU for cell therapy. Although, safety of autologous adult stem cells is justified by simpler isolation protocol, free of immune response due to rejection and ethical issues.

Most recent meta-analysis of randomized controlled trials of autologous stem cell therapy for peripheral arterial disease reported that stem cell therapy for ischemic diabetic wounds can reduce the amputation rate of cell therapy up to 2.8% when the control is 20%: (3/109 vs. 32/155; OR 0.17, 95% CI 0.06–0.45, $I^2 = 0\%$) and improve wound healing rate to 54% when it is 29% for the controls (167/305 vs. 89/304; OR 4.34, 95% CI 2.96–6.38, $I^2 = 23\%$) [16]. These results demonstrate that many ischemic diabetic foot patients have high possibility to benefit from stem cell therapy. However, when considering autologous cell therapy, diabetic patients are reported to have reduced autologous stem cell function, thereby decreasing the stem cell therapy effectiveness [9]. We have previously reported that efficacy of autologous EPC therapy relies on the function of cells transplanted, suggesting that key to successful cell therapy is to enhance the function of diabetic stem cell prior to deliver. As a result, we have established MNC-QQ therapy for more and effective cell therapy. Six of the 10 cases with nonhealing wound with CLI including diabetes and collagen diseases showed complete wound closure with average wound closure rate was 73.2 ± 40.1% at 12 weeks receiving MNC-QQ therapy [27]. The study is still ongoing as an open-label single-center non-blinded clinical trial by conducting three times injection of MNC-QQ cells with 1 month interval. Presently, we have improved and stabilized our culture method from MNC-QQ and now established a newly type peripheral blood regenerative cells (Repri cells; product code:RE-01) for clinical trials in 2022 FY. Our goal is to establish stem cell therapy as a conventional therapy for nonhealing ischemic wounds including diabetic foot by getting global approval of our minimal invasive highly regenerative cell therapy in the near future.

11.12 Conclusion

Non-option nonhealing ischemic diabetic foot patients have a high possibility to benefit from stem cell therapy. However, there is not product approved for conventional use until now. Further studies with larger randomized, double-blinded, placebo-controlled, multi-center trials with long-term follow-up is necessary to efficacy of stem cell therapy for these patients. In addition, it should be understood that these wounds can never be treated only by cell therapy and that effective treatment is achieved by controlling the underlying disease and performing appropriate wound management.

Disclosure Statement The author is a Chief Scientific Officer of ReEir Co. ReEir is a company conducting Phase II Clinical trial of ex vivo cultured peripheral blood MNCs.

References

1. Izumi Y, Satterfield K, Lee S, Harkless LB, Lavery LA. Mortality of first-time amputees in diabetics: a 10-year observation. Diabetes Res Clin Pract. 2009;83(1):126–31.
2. Yoshikawa H, Kujime S, Iwasaki M, Yoshikawa M. Poor survival of dialysis patients with unhealed wounds because of critical limb ischemia: limb salvage and survival requires wound healing. Int Wound J. 2019;16(5):1112–8.
3. Dubsky M, Jirkovska A, Bem R, Nemcova A, Fejfarova V, Jude EB. Cell therapy of critical limb ischemia in diabetic patients—state of art. Diabetes Res Clin Pract. 2017;126:263–71.
4. Butt T, Lilja E, Orneholm H, Apelqvist J, Gottsater A, Eneroth M, et al. Amputation-free survival in patients with diabetes mellitus and peripheral arterial disease with heel ulcer: open versus endovascular surgery. Vasc Endovasc Surg. 2019;53(2):118–25.
5. Asahara T, Murohara T, Sullivan A, Silver M, van der Zee R, Li T, et al. Isolation of putative progenitor endothelial cells for angiogenesis. Science. 1997;275(5302):964–7.
6. Tateishi-Yuyama E, Matsubara H, Murohara T, Ikeda U, Shintani S, Masaki H, et al. Therapeutic angiogenesis for patients with limb ischaemia by autologous transplantation of bone-marrow cells: a pilot study and a randomised controlled trial. Lancet. 2002;360(9331):427–35.
7. Tanaka R, Masuda H, Kato S, Imagawa K, Kanabuchi K, Nakashioya C, et al. Autologous G-CSF-mobilized peripheral blood CD34+ cell therapy for diabetic patients with chronic nonhealing ulcer. Cell Transplant. 2014;23(2):167–79.
8. Tanaka R, Wada M, Kwon SM, Masuda H, Carr J, Ito R, et al. The effects of flap ischemia on normal and diabetic progenitor cell function. Plast Reconstr Surg. 2008;121(6):1929–42.
9. Sukmawati D, Tanaka R. Introduction to next generation of endothelial progenitor cell therapy: a promise in vascular medicine. Am J Transl Res. 2015;7(3):411–21.
10. Tanaka R, Masuda H, Fujimura S, Ito-Hirano R, Arita K, Kakinuma Y, et al. Quality-quantity control culture enhances vasculogenesis and wound healing efficacy of human diabetic peripheral blood CD34+ cells. Stem Cells Transl Med. 2018;7(5):428–38.
11. Tanaka R, Vaynrub M, Masuda H, Ito R, Kobori M, Miyasaka M, et al. Quality-control culture system restores diabetic endothelial progenitor cell vasculogenesis and accelerates wound closure. Diabetes. 2013;62(9):3207–17.
12. Geeroms M, Hamdi M, Hirano R, Hagiwara H, Fujimura S, Mizuno H, et al. Quality and quantity-cultured murine endothelial progenitor cells increase vascularization and decrease fibrosis in the fat graft. Plast Reconstr Surg. 2019;143(4):744e–55e.
13. Hagiwara H, Higashibata A, Ogawa S, Kanazawa S, Mizuno H, Tanaka R. Effectiveness of endothelial progenitor cell culture under microgravity for improved angiogenic potential. Sci Rep. 2018;8(1):14239.
14. Masuda H, Tanaka R, Fujimura S, Ishikawa M, Akimaru H, Shizuno T, et al. Vasculogenic conditioning of peripheral blood mononuclear cells promotes endothelial progenitor cell expansion and phenotype transition of anti-inflammatory macrophage and T lymphocyte to cells with regenerative potential. J Am Heart Assoc. 2014;3(3):e000743.
15. Kado M, Tanaka R, Arita K, Okada K, Ito-Hirano R, Fujimura S, et al. Human peripheral blood mononuclear cells enriched in endothelial progenitor cells via quality and quantity controlled culture accelerate vascularization and wound healing in a porcine wound model. Cell Transplant. 2018;27(7):1068–79.
16. Gao W, Chen D, Liu G, Ran X. Autologous stem cell therapy for peripheral arterial disease: a systematic review and meta-analysis of randomized controlled trials. Stem Cell Res Ther. 2019;10(1):140.
17. Fujita Y, Kinoshita M, Furukawa Y, Nagano T, Hashimoto H, Hirami Y, et al. Phase II clinical trial of CD34+ cell therapy to explore endpoint selection and timing in patients with critical limb ischemia. Circ J. 2014;78(2):490–501.
18. Ohtake T, Kobayashi S, Slavin S, Mochida Y, Ishioka K, Moriya H, et al. Human peripheral blood mononuclear cells incubated in vasculogenic conditioning medium dramatically improve ischemia/reperfusion acute kidney injury in mice. Cell Transplant. 2018;27(3):520–30.
19. Norgren L, Weiss N, Nikol S, Hinchliffe RJ, Lantis JC, Patel MR, et al. PLX-PAD cell treatment of critical limb Ischaemia: rationale and design of the PACE trial. Eur J Vasc Endovasc Surg. 2019;57(4):538–45.
20. Ohtake T, Mochida Y, Ishioka K, Oka M, Maesato K, Moriya H, et al. Autologous granulocyte colony-stimulating factor-mobilized peripheral blood CD34 positive cell transplantation for hemodialysis patients with critical limb ischemia: a prospective phase II clinical trial. Stem Cells Transl Med. 2018;7(11):774–82.
21. Shu X, Shu S, Tang S, Yang L, Liu D, Li K, et al. Efficiency of stem cell based therapy in the treatment of diabetic foot ulcer: a meta-analysis. Endocr J. 2018;65(4):403–13.
22. Dubsky M, Jirkovska A, Bem R, Fejfarova V, Pagacova L, Nemcova A, et al. Comparison of the effect of stem

cell therapy and percutaneous transluminal angioplasty on diabetic foot disease in patients with critical limb ischemia. Cytotherapy. 2014;16(12):1733–8.
23. Qin HL, Zhu XH, Zhang B, Zhou L, Wang WY. Clinical evaluation of human umbilical cord mesenchymal stem cell transplantation after angioplasty for diabetic foot. Exp Clin Endocrinol Diabetes. 2016;124(8):497–503.
24. Forsythe RO, Apelqvist J, Boyko EJ, Fitridge R, Hong JP, Katsanos K, et al. Performance of prognostic markers in the prediction of wound healing or amputation among patients with foot ulcers in diabetes: a systematic review. Diabetes Metab Res Rev. 2020;36(Suppl 1):e3278.
25. Berli MC, Wanivenhaus F, Kabelitz M, Gotschi T, Boni T, Rancic Z, et al. Predictors for reoperation after lower limb amputation in patients with peripheral arterial disease. Vasa. 2019;48(5):419–24.
26. Badiavas EV, Falanga V. Treatment of chronic wounds with bone marrow-derived cells. Arch Dermatol. 2003;139(4):510–6.
27. Tanaka R, Fujimura S, Kado M, Fukuta T, Arita K, Hirano-Ito R, Mita T, Watada H, Kato Y, Miayuchi K, Mizuno H. MNC-QQ therapy for non-healing wounds. Stem Cells Transl Med. 2022;10(6):895–909.
28. Wunderlich RP, Peters EJ, Lavery LA. Systemic hyperbaric oxygen therapy: lower-extremity wound healing and the diabetic foot. Diabetes Care. 2000;23(10):1551–5.
29. Faglia E, Favales F, Aldeghi A, Calia P, Quarantiello A, Oriani G, et al. Adjunctive systemic hyperbaric oxygen therapy in treatment of severe prevalently ischemic diabetic foot ulcer. A randomized study. Diabetes Care. 1996;19(12):1338–43.
30. Abidia A, Laden G, Kuhan G, Johnson BF, Wilkinson AR, Renwick PM, et al. The role of hyperbaric oxygen therapy in ischaemic diabetic lower extremity ulcers: a double-blind randomised-controlled trial. Eur J Vasc Endovasc Surg. 2003;25(6):513–8.
31. Londahl M, Katzman P, Nilsson A, Hammarlund C. Hyperbaric oxygen therapy facilitates healing of chronic foot ulcers in patients with diabetes. Diabetes Care. 2010;33(5):998–1003.
32. Stoekenbroek RM, Santema TB, Legemate DA, Ubbink DT, van den Brink A, Koelemay MJ. Hyperbaric oxygen for the treatment of diabetic foot ulcers: a systematic review. Eur J Vasc Endovasc Surg. 2014;47(6):647–55.
33. Rigato M, Monami M, Fadini GP. Autologous cell therapy for peripheral arterial disease: systematic review and meta-analysis of randomized, nonrandomized, and noncontrolled studies. Circ Res. 2017;120(8):1326–40.
34. Hutchings G, Janowicz K, Moncrieff L, Dompe C, Strauss E, Kocherova I, et al. The proliferation and differentiation of adipose-derived stem cells in neovascularization and angiogenesis. Int J Mol Sci. 2020;21(11):3790.
35. Lopes L, Setia O, Aurshina A, Liu S, Hu H, Isaji T, et al. Stem cell therapy for diabetic foot ulcers: a review of preclinical and clinical research. Stem Cell Res Ther. 2018;9(1):188.

GPSR Compliance

The European Union's (EU) General Product Safety Regulation (GPSR) is a set of rules that requires consumer products to be safe and our obligations to ensure this.

If you have any concerns about our products, you can contact us on ProductSafety@springernature.com

In case Publisher is established outside the EU, the EU authorized representative is:

Springer Nature Customer Service Center GmbH
Europaplatz 3
69115 Heidelberg, Germany

Batch number: 10731385

Printed by Printforce, the Netherlands